# HEALTH PSYCHOLOGY

## A PSYCHOBIOLOGICAL
## PERSPECTIVE

# HEALTH PSYCHOLOGY

## A PSYCHOBIOLOGICAL
## PERSPECTIVE

### MICHAEL FEUERSTEIN

*University of Rochester School of Medicine and Dentistry*
*Rochester, New York*

### ELISE E. LABBÉ

*University of Miami School of Medicine*
*Miami, Florida*

*and*

### ANDRZEJ R. KUCZMIERCZYK

*University of Rochester School of Medicine and Dentistry*
*Rochester, New York*

PLENUM PRESS • NEW YORK AND LONDON

Library of Congress Cataloging in Publication Data

Feuerstein, Michael.
  Health psychology.

  Includes bibliographies and index.
  1. Medicine and psychology. 2. Health behavior. 3. Psychology, Physiological. I. Labbé,
Elise E. II. Kuczmierczyk, Andrzej R. III. Title. [DNLM: 1. Behavioral Medicine. 2. Disease
—psychology. 3. Health. 4. Psychophysiologic Disorders. WM 90 F423h]
R726.5.F48    1985                          616′.0019                          85-25884
ISBN 0-306-42037-6

© 1986 Plenum Press, New York
A Division of Plenum Publishing Corporation
233 Spring Street, New York, N.Y. 10013

Printed in the United States of America

To my wife Michele, daughter Sara Elizabeth, and son Andrew Scott
Michael Feuerstein

To Rebecca Marcon, Ph.D.—a constant source of inspiration
Elise E. Labbé

To my sister Hania
Andrzej R. Kuczmierczyk

Over 90 percent of us are born healthy and suffer premature death and disability only as a result of personal misbehavior and environmental conditions.

Knowles, J. H., *Science,* 1977, *198,* 1104 (Editorial)

# PREFACE

Although it has been assumed since early recorded history that psychological factors influence health and illness, it has only been within the past few years that a group of investigators and clinicians with a shared interest in the application of psychological principles and techniques to health and illness has existed. Over this same period of time, a number of multi-author books on the topic of health psychology and an associated field, behavioral medicine, have been published. Although these books are major resources for the investigator and the clinician in the field, it is often difficult for students, both undergraduate and graduate, to learn the basics of health psychology from such books. Thus, *Health Psychology: A Psychobiological Perspective* was written to provide such basics. The need for such a textbook in health psychology became apparent to the first author when he was searching for reading material for an undergraduate course in health psychology at McGill University. This book grew out of the course in health psychology, and its structure represents the course content.

The purpose of the book is to present the theoretical, empirical, and clinical aspects of the rapidly developing field of health psychology. Data from a number of subdisciplines within psychology and the behavioral and health-related sciences are integrated throughout each chapter in an effort to provide a balanced perspective. *Health Psychology* explores the development of the field and its research methodologies, theoretical models, and intervention possibilities. The text uses three major problem areas—coronary heart disease, smoking, and pain—as models in which the principles and techniques presented earlier are applied. The contributions of a psychobiological approach to the understanding of these disorders and to prevention and/or treatment are also illustrated.

This book is intended for senior level undergraduates and first- or second-year predoctoral graduate students in psychology, although advanced undergraduates in the behavioral or biological sciences with some background in psychology will also be able to use the text. In addition, senior and graduate-level nursing students, students in the health-related professions, and first-year medical students will find the content and depth of analysis useful either in similar courses or in more general courses on the behavioral contributions to disease or psychosocial care of the medical patient.

This volume can also serve as a useful introduction to the field of health psychology for the practicing health care professional interested in the integration of psychological principles and techniques in the practice of medicine. The review of current concepts of stress, health and illness behaviors, and recent intervention strategies for such major problem areas as coronary heart disease, smoking, and pain, provides the physician and nurse clinician with perspectives on several critical issues related to the psychological aspects of health care. This book reviews much of the theory and research that forms the foundation for the modern application of a psychological approach to health and illness.

The book itself is divided into three major parts. Part One reviews the foundations of health psychology, including a definition and its general scope, in addition to historical perspective. Research strategies used in health psychology, with an emphasis on epidemiological research, are covered next. Chapter 4 reviews the principles of psychophysiology that underlie the various concepts and problem areas within health psychology.

Part Two covers current concepts in the field, which includes stress, stress and illness, stress management, health behavior, and illness behavior. These general concepts are presented to introduce the student to their theoretical complexities. Also, these topic areas illustrate how research approaches are used in studying these complex phenomena. The concepts reviewed in Part Two were chosen because they represent a cross section of the key issues in health psychology. Stress and the effects of stress on illness are assumed to play a major role in a variety of health problems. Stress management is a major clinical activity in health psychology. In Chapter 7, principles and techniques of clinical psychology as applied to health and illness are discussed using stress management as a model. The role life-style plays in health and illness also is of major interest in health psychology. Chapter 8 thus is a review of the theoretical and practical aspects of the health behavior concept. Chronic illness often involves a set of complex problems experienced by the patient, his or her family, and the health care system in general. The construct of illness behavior is invoked to help explain these problems. Chapter 9 provides an overview of the factors that contribute to the development, exacerbation, and maintenance of maladaptive illness behavior. It also addresses the management of such problematic behavior.

Case material is provided throughout Part Two to illustrate many of these concepts.

Part Three integrates basic principles and current concepts for specific problem areas in health psychology. Coronary heart disease (Chapter 10) is used to illustrate how an understanding of stress and stress and illness contributes to our understanding of the etiology of this major problem. Stress management as an intervention technique, is also discussed. Smoking behavior (Chapter 11) presents a model problem for the application of principles related to health behavior, whereas Chapter 12, on pain, gives the student an opportunity to consider several of the concepts presented in Part Two.

MICHAEL FEUERSTEIN
ELISE E. LABBÉ
ANDRZEJ R. KUCZMIERCZYK

# ACKNOWLEDGMENTS

The authors wish to acknowledge the support of the Department of Psychiatry, Division of Behavioral and Psychosocial Medicine, University of Rochester School of Medicine and Dentistry, and the Department of Psychology, Virginia Polytechnic Institute and State University. Michael Feuerstein would also like to express his gratitude to the Departments of Psychology and Psychiatry at McGill University for the encouragement and opportunity to develop this project.

The initial support of the senior editor and others at Plenum Publishing Company, at the onset of this project, was most appreciated. Leonard Pace's belief in the importance of this work continuously inspired the authors. Eliot Werner, who as new senior editor at Plenum directed this project during its latter stages, provided significant support and guidance for which we are indebted. We are also appreciative of the professional editorial effort of Daniel Spinella, production editor, to hasten the publication of this volume. Lastly we acknowledge the competent reviews of an earlier manuscript by Patricia Dobkin, M.S. and Lawrence J. Siegel, Ph.D.

The highly professional technical support of Cherie D. Rynerson, Cynthia C. O'Keefe, and Karen R. Nelson was most helpful. Their assistance facilitated the completion of this project, for which we are most thankful. We also wish to thank Cathy Drechsler for her assistance with the references.

# CONTENTS

# FOUNDATIONS

*Part One is designed to orient the reader to several basic issues and meth odologies found in the rapidly emerging field of health psychology. Early definitions of the field are reviewed, followed by an attempt to place the field in historical perspective. Chapter 3 presents important basic principles of research methods in the field that students are not usually exposed to unless they have taken courses in research methodology related to health and epidemiology. Because the book's goal is to integrate basic and clinical research, clinical research methods are also presented. Chapter 4 reviews the principles and techniques of human psychophysiology, which has played an important role in the development of knowledge on mechanisms and treatment of several health problems. In sum, a technical framework is provided for the interpretation of the material in the remainder of the book.*

# CHAPTER 1

# DEFINITION AND SCOPE

---

Definition of Health Psychology
Health Psychology versus Behavioral Medicine
Coronary-Prone Behavior: The Case for Health Psychology

---

## DEFINITION OF HEALTH PSYCHOLOGY

In this chapter, the field of health psychology and what differentiates it from behavioral medicine is discussed, and this discussion is followed by an illustration of how health psychology can contribute to the understanding and management of a major health problem.

Psychologists have a long history of interest in issues of health; however, only within the past few years has there been a movement within psychology that can be designated *health psychology*. Matarazzo's definition of health psychology has been widely accepted and was endorsed by the recently established Division of Health Psychology of the American Psychological Association (Matarazzo, 1982). The definition is as follows:

> Health Psychology is the aggregate of the specific educational, scientific and professional contributions of the discipline of psychology to the promotion and maintenance of health, the prevention and treatment of illness, the identification of etiologic and diagnostic correlates of health, illness and related dysfunction, and the analysis and improvement of the health care system and health policy formation. (p. 4)

The meaning of this definition is quite clear: any activity of psychology relating to any aspect of health, illness, the health care system, or health policy formation is considered to be within the field of health psychology. What is important to note is that the activities of diverse areas of psychology, such as developmental, physiological, cognitive, and industrial-organizational, should be considered in definitions of health psychology. Health psychology deals with such basic questions as, What are the physiological bases of emotion and how do they relate to health and illness? Can biobehavioral risk factors for illness be identified and what are their mechanisms of action? What is stress? What factors contribute to the development of both health and illness behaviors? How does psychological knowledge contribute to the basic understanding of the etiology and management of a number of major medical problems? What roles can the psychologist play within the health care system? Health psychology should be able to integrate data from several levels of psychology when addressing these basic questions. Figure 1-1 depicts the various psychologically based sources of input in the field of health psychology.

Although health psychology as defined by Matarazzo is a relatively recent subdiscipline, models for conceptualizing the field of health psychology have already been proposed. In one such model, Stone (1982) emphasizes the concept of the health system and problems of interaction within this system. The health system, as protrayed in Figure 1-2, involves complex transactions among several of its components, ranging from the individual whose health is at issue to a number of sociocultural support systems. Stone suggests that the health psychologist may intervene at any point within the health care system. A psychologist may focus on the exchanges among various aspects of the system. For example, these could involve such psychosocial investigations as studies of the verbal interaction between patient and physician, with the goal of determining the optimal way to increase communication and ensure compliance to medical regimens.

Some psychologists focus on the prevention of disease and the promotion of health through the modification of behaviors that contribute to health risk (Weiss, 1982). Weiss points out that three general themes appear in the recent literature in health psychology: (a) health care costs are out of control, (b) chronic illness is a major concern to those involved in health, and (c) consumerism is rampant. More and more citizens are concerned with health issues and are willing to take responsibility for

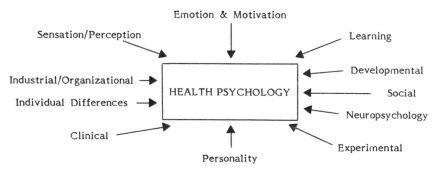

**FIGURE 1-1.** Disciplines in psychology that contribute to the field of health psychology.

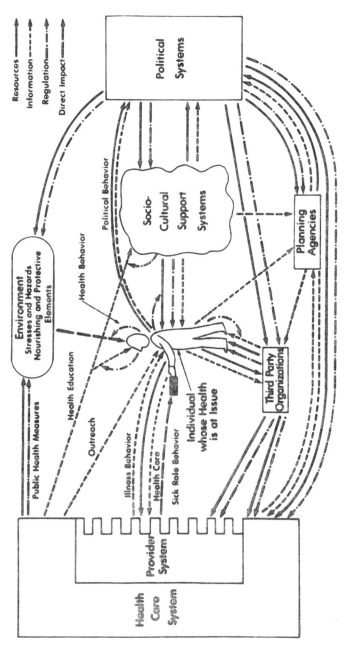

FIGURE 1-2. Schematic representation of the health system. From "Health Psychology: A New Journal for a New Field" by George C. Stone, 1982, *Health Psychology*, 1(1), p.2. Copyright 1982 by Lawrence Erlbaum Associates, Inc. Reprinted by permission.

them. Thus, the economic, social, and political need for psychologists to work in the prevention of disease and in the promotion of health is considerable. Although a challenge to the psychologist, it is also an avenue for psychologists to contribute socially, as well as to further the concepts of health psychology generally.

There is considerable excitement about health psychology and many have jumped on the bandwagon. If health psychology is to make important contributions to health care, the health psychologist must be well rounded and open to advances in the basic medical sciences, in addition to the field of psychology. A knowledge of research design and methodology, as well as general psychology, is essential. The ability to integrate several areas within psychology and the health sciences, coupled with an awareness of the parameters of the health system and patient care, are important skills for the health psychologist.

## HEALTH PSYCHOLOGY VERSUS BEHAVIORAL MEDICINE

Health psychology and behavioral medicine are often thought to be synonymous, yet there has been concern over distinguishing the fields (Agras, 1982). The definition of *behavioral medicine* that evolved from the Yale Conference on Behavioral Medicine (Schwartz & Weiss, 1978, addendum), is the first attempt to formally delineate this rapidly developing area:

> The *interdisciplinary* field concerned with development and integration of behavioral and biomedical science, knowledge and techniques relevant to the understanding of physical health and illness and the application of this knowledge and these techniques to prevention, diagnosis, treatment, and rehabilitation.

Health psychology represents the specific contribution of the discipline of psychology to this base of knowledge and techniques termed *behavioral medicine.* Perhaps the most important distinction between behavioral medicine and health psychology is the interdisciplinary versus the discipline-specific approach to health and illness. As Figure 1-3 illustrates, several health care and basic science fields contribute to behavioral medicine, with health psychology making one important contribution. This book does not focus on behavioral medicine, although it is agreed that the potential contributions psychology can make to the understanding of health and illness and the consequent intervention strategies that evolve from such an understanding depend, in part, on the interdisciplinary orientation of behavioral medicine. Indeed, the contributions of the basic biomedical sciences (e.g., physiology, biochemistry, neurobiology) and epidemiology, coupled with health psychology

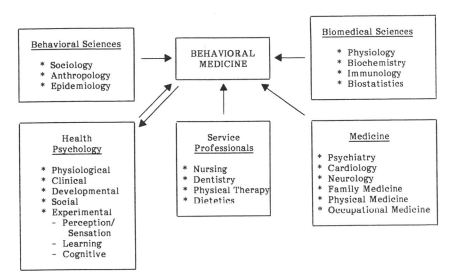

FIGURE 1-3. Sources of input to behavioral medicine.

(clinical, experimental, social, developmental, neuropsychology, and physiological psychology) hold the most promise for gaining an understanding of the complexities of health and illness. This book offers an introduction to such an approach from a health psychologist's vantage point. The next section illustrates how various areas within psychology can contribute to an integrative psychobiological understanding of a major worldwide health problem, that is, coronary heart disease.

## CORONARY-PRONE BEHAVIOR: THE CASE
## FOR HEALTH PSYCHOLOGY

Whereas health psychology has begun to contribute to the basic understanding and treatment of a variety of health problems, this is perhaps more the case with coronary heart disease. The terms *coronary heart disease* (CHD), *atherosclerotic heart disease*, and *ischemic heart disease* are used interchangeably to refer to cardiac disease resulting from *myocardial ischemia*, in which insufficient oxygen reaches the heart. Clinical problems associated with CHD often include angina pectoris (chest pain), sudden arrhythmic death (ventricular fibrillation), and myocardial infarction (blockage of a blood vessel in the heart, with subsequent death of heart tissue). Coronary heart disease is a major cause of death in our culture.

Several long-term prospective studies have identified a number of risk factors that contribute to CHD (Kannel, McGee, & Gordon, 1976). These factors include a family history of heart disease, elevated serum cholesterol, high blood pressure (hypertension), smoking, lack of exercise, obesity, age, sex, and the Type A personality or coronary-prone behavior pattern. It should be apparent that five of the nine involve some type of specific *behavior*, and six of the nine involve psychobiological factors. However, to illustrate how psychology contributes to the understanding of CHD, we will focus on the Type A behavior pattern.

Most of us know people, perhaps even ourselves, who frequently experience feelings of impatience when waiting in line at the bank or the grocery store or who find it extremely difficult to find time for a haircut or who gulp down their food. These people feel they simply do not have enough time in the day to complete all the tasks that "must" be accomplished, yet they find themselves taking on more and more responsibilities. These behaviors characterize the Type A individual. The Type A behavior pattern includes such characteristics as time urgency, impatience, hard drivenness, ambitiousness, competitiveness, hostility, and achievement-oriented behavior (Cooper, Detre, & Weiss, 1981). The importance of this behavior pattern rests in its ability to predict CHD (Rosenman *et al.*, 1975). Individuals who display the Type A pattern are at approximately twice the risk of developing CHD than are those individuals termed *Type B* (Rosenman *et al.*, 1975) not displaying the pattern. The specifics of the Type A pattern will be discussed in Chapter 10. The behavior pattern itself actually predicts the development of heart disease independently of other risk factors.

Type A is a construct, and psychological literature is replete with constructs. Anxiety, depression, stress, and ego are all constructs. Experimental, social, developmental, physiological, and clinical psychology have all contributed to a greater understanding of the Type A construct. Researchers in these fields have addressed such critical questions as, Does experimental manipulation of time pressure, achievement striving, or challenge actually facilitate Type A-like behavior in those who display a cluster of these characteristics during an interview or who endorse these behaviors on self-report forms? What environmental and cognitive factors contribute to the display of such behaviors? Are these behaviors somehow the result of early familial modeling; is there a genetic predisposition toward such behaviors, or is there some interaction among these behaviors? Because CHD is an illness complex, with documented pathophysiology, how does the Type A behavior pattern contribute to its etiology? If the behavior pattern predicts CHD, is it possible that a modification of some aspects of the behavior pattern will help prevent heart disease of this type?

Psychophysiological research has begun to contribute to an understanding of the possible mechanisms linking Type A behavior to CHD. Given that Type A is considered by some investigators to be a self-induced reaction pattern to challenge or a complex stress response, the role of the sympathetic nervous system, in general, and stress-related hormones (catecholamines), in particular, have been emphasized. Psychophysiologists have observed greater autonomic reactivity in Type A people, compared to Type Bs, in challenging situations (Cooper *et al.*, 1981). This greater physiological reactivity has been observed in those who are competitive, impatient, and hostile. Investigators have argued that this increased reactivity elevates serum cholesterol levels, increases blood clotting times, and imposes a greater workload on the heart. These factors, coupled with an impaired coronary blood flow, may set the stage for a myocardial infarction.

In addition to research on the psychophysiology of the Type A behavior pattern, clinical research has demonstrated that components of the behavior pattern can be modified (e.g., Suinn, 1982). Stress management programs with asymptomatic Type A managers have modified such CHD risk factors as blood pressure and serum cholesterol, as well as Type A behavior. Recently, a large-scale evaluation of intervention strategies for Type A patients with a history of myocardial infarction indicated that efforts at modifying Type A behavior are associated with a significant reduction in the recurrence rate of heart attacks (Friedman *et al.*, 1984).

Although Type A behavior is used here as an example of the input from two areas of psychology to the understanding and treatment of health problems, a number of other problem areas could have served equally well. The potential contribution of health psychology to behavioral medicine and, more broadly, to health and illness is considerable, as will be seen in the following chapters. After a historical review of the field and a study of current models in the area, major research methods will be presented in depth. Such general concepts as stress, health behavior, and illness behavior illustrate current trends in the field. These methods and concepts are integrated in Part Three, which deals with specific health problems. Each chapter integrates basic research and clinical research and practice to emphasize the contributions from several areas of psychology.

## REFERENCES

Agras, S. W. (1982). Behavioral medicine in the 1980's: Nonrandom connections. *Journal of Consulting and Clinical Psychology, 50,* 797–803.

Cooper, T., Detre, T., & Weiss, S. M. (1981). Coronary-prone behavior and coronary heart disease: A critical review. *Circulation, 63*(6), 1199–1215.

Friedman, M., Thoresen, C. E., Gill, J. J., Powell, L. H., Ulmer, D., Thompson, L., Price, V. A., Rabin, D. D., Breall, W. S., Dixon, T., Levy, R., & Bourg, E. (1984). Alteration of Type A behavior and reduction in cardiac recurrences in postmyocardial infarction patients. *American Heart Journal, 108*(2), 237–248.

Kannel, W., McGee, D., & Gordon, T. (1976). A general cardiovascular risk profile: The Framingham Study. *American Journal of Cardiology, 38*(1), 46–51.

Matarazzo, J. D. (1982). Behavioral health's challenge to academic, scientific and professional psychology. *American Psychologist, 37*(1), 1–14.

Rosenman, R. H., Brand, R. J., Jenkins, D., *et al.* (1975). Coronary heart disease in the Western Collaborative Group Study: Final follow-up experience of 8½ years. *Journal of the American Medical Association, 233*(8), 872–877.

Schwartz, G. E., & Weiss, S. M. (1978). *Proceedings of the Yale Conference on Behavioral Medicine* (U.S. Department of Health, Education, and Welfare No. [NIH] 78–1424). Washington, DC: U.S. Government Printing Office.

Stone, G. C. (1982). Health psychology: A new journal for a new field. *Health Psychology, 1*(1), 1–6.

Suinn, R. M. (1982). Intervention with Type A behaviors. *Journal of Consulting and Clinical Psychology, 50,* 933–949.

Weiss. S. M. (1982). Health psychology: The time is now. *Health Psychology, 1*(1), 81–91.

# CHAPTER 2

# HISTORICAL PERSPECTIVE

## ANTECEDENTS: FROM HIPPOCRATES TO THE FOUNDING OF THE DIVISION OF HEALTH PSYCHOLOGY

Holistic conceptions of health and disease can be traced to Oriental physicians around 2600 B.C. and Greek physicians, particularly of the Hippocratic school, around 500 B.C. Good habits and the avoidance of excesses were considered essential for good health. It was also realized that individuals have some control over their health, instead of emphasizing magical thinking or blaming the gods for illness. The physician was seen as a guide, helping the patient restore a natural balance, physical and emotional. For the ancient Greeks, health was thought of as a harmonious mixture of the humors (blood, phlegm, choler, melancholy [yellow or blackbile]) and disease was considered a disharmonious mixture. It is noteworthy that with our increasing communication with Oriental and Eastern Indian cultures over the past two decades, we have become interested in the health practices and theories of these cultures. Acupuncture, biofeedback, self-hypnosis, and autogenic training represent some of the practices that have arisen from the holistic approach to health care and are currently considered useful adjuncts to the treatment of certain health problems in our Western culture (e.g., stress-related medical disorders and pain).

11

### Early Psychosomatic Medicine

From the 1930s to the 1950s, much work was done on the role of anxiety and distress in the development and exacerbation of a variety of physical illnesses. The work of Franz Alexander and Harold G. Wolff best represents this era. Alexander proposed the symbolic mediation of physiological processes. He endorsed the idea that unconscious conflicts trigger psychological disorders and that these conflicts are directly related to the malfunction of various organs of the body. Wolff, at Cornell University Medical Center (New York), spent 30 years in innovative experimental work on the effects of psychosocial stressors on peripheral physiological measures (e.g., muscular activity) assumed to be related to specific medical disorders. He is especially known for his work on the mechanisms and treatment of headache.

Although the work of these clinical researchers broke ground and encouraged others to consider the possible association between "mind" and "body," the research strategies were mostly of a case study nature. These case studies involved careful analyses of individual patients, but it is difficult to generalize from such a limited methodology. They did, however, generate several hypotheses for further testing (Weiner, 1977).

### Development of Experimental Psychophysiology

*Psychophysiology,* or the study of the physiological basis of psychological processes, has been defined in terms of its methods and procedures. It is a discipline that attempts to explain a variety of behavioral processes by the interaction of their psychological and biological components. Improved instrumentation, new methodologies, and empirical findings relating to the psychophysiological bases of emotion, motivation, and consciousness have contributed to the growth of health psychology.

In the early 1900s, researchers focused on the effects of nonspecific stress on the organism. An example is the elucidation by physiologist Walter Cannon of the fight–flight reaction (Cannon, 1932). Cannon's research provided the basis for early psychosomatic investigations that suggested that adaptive, defensive psychophysiological response patterns might produce tissue damage and illness when repeated or prolonged. More recently, Schacter and Singer (1962) emphasized the role of biocognitive processes in emotion. Other researchers have directed their efforts at delineating neural mechanisms that underlie the experience of emotion. Their theories postulate that the interaction of neurophysiological systems, including those that process discrete patterns of postural and facial mechanisms, may interact (Plutchik, 1980; Strongman, 1978).

Another area of psychophysiological research contributing to the foundation of health psychology is the study of consciousness. There is evidence that patterning of peripheral and central nervous system activity in human consciousness occurs (Schwartz, 1978), a concept that furthers our understanding of this complex phenomenon. One line of research involves recording a subject's differential patterns of electrocortical and peripheral physiological responses while he or she is engaged in complex cognitive tasks. For example, Schwartz and colleagues (1977) observed that, in right-handed subjects, verbal versus spatial cognitive processes differentially invoke activity in the left and right hemispheres, respectively. Several psychophysiologists have attempted to map conscious processes physiologically in order to develop models of such activity.

Animal models have also been used in experimental psychophysiology. Theories involving behavioral and physiological interactions may be readily tested using such animal models. Selye's work on gastrointestinal lesions in rats is an example. Selye demonstrated that several forms of immobilization produced gastric lesions, depending on how much control the rat had over the conditions of the experiment. He also observed involution of the thymus and enlargement of the adrenal cortex following such immobilization and defined these physical changes as signs of the "stress syndrome." Animal models have also been used in the study of psychobiological mechanisms of heart disease, arthritis, gastrointestinal disorders, and pain. The use of animal models to investigate the role of psychosocial and learning factors in disorders of the immune system (e.g., cancer) represent a more recent application of behavioral science to the study of health and illness (Ader, 1981; Anisman & Sklar, 1984).

The increasing interest in studying such psychophysiological relationships, especially in humans, has stimulated advances in the technology used in psychophysiology. These allow a researcher to measure specific bodily reactions using electrodes or other sensors, which are usually placed on the surface of the body. Such physiological parameters as muscle tension, skin temperature, and electrical activity of the skin and brain can be detected, monitored, and recorded. Sophisticated computer systems have been developed to integrate these data and to present them graphically to facilitate analysis and interpretation.

For the past two decades, psychophysiologists have studied the basic processes of learning within the nervous system in a variety of species. Following the observation that yogis can regulate certain bodily processes, research with laboratory animals and humans was conducted, and it was found that such autonomic responses as heart rate and blood pressure could be reliably regulated, although the observed changes were small. This research thus challenged the concept of the "involuntary" nature of the autonomic nervous system and led to more research on the influence of psychological factors on this system, both theoretically and practically. Some investigators argue that by studying the phenomenon of biological self-regulation it is possible to determine the extent to which physiological responses, human behavior, and consciousness are interdependent. At the clinical level, biofeedback equipment was devised to aid patients in learning to regulate an overactive biological response or in modifying a physiological response assumed to heighten anxiety or tension. This clinical biofeedback uses such measures as heart rate, skin temperature, or skin resistance as target autonomic responses, and muscle tension as a target somatic response. Clinical biofeedback has played a significant role in stimulating the development of health psychology, particularly clinical health psychology.

In sum, psychophysiology has provided theory and applied technology that permit further exploration of the relationships among emotion, cognition, and physiology. As will be illustrated later, a knowledge of these interactions facilitates the understanding and management of a number of health problems.

## Development of Empirical Clinical Psychology

Clinical psychologists have become more interested in evaluating the outcome of therapy, especially in terms of cost efficiency. In particular, the social learning-based therapies emphasize empirically based, brief therapeutic approaches for behavioral problems. Before these techniques were developed, nonpsychiatric physicians often reported difficulty in determining the value of various psychological approaches to health problems, indicating that they were time-consuming, their goals were vague, and they were not applicable to the majority of their patients. Another problem with the use of these earlier approaches was that only minimal changes in symptoms were obtained (Kellner, 1975). Indeed, symptom reduction was often a secondary goal of these approaches. But with the development of behavioral and other brief therapies, observable and clinically relevant changes have been achieved within a reasonable period of time for a number of health problems (e.g., headache, chronic back pain, and arthritis).

The attitude of health professionals has always been pragmatic, and clinical psychologists, especially behaviorally oriented ones, have devised a language system and a technology health professionals can relate to. In general, health professionals have known for years that psychological factors affect both disease and health, at least in certain cases, but these factors were largely ignored, because they were not understood. Why is there a tendency toward greater acceptance by the larger core of health providers now? We think part of the answer is the availability of psychological technology that can be used to manage health problems. Although still in the developmental stage, such technology is being applied in many areas. Behavioral techniques are available for the treatment of acute and chronic pain; cognitive preparatory techniques are used to prepare patients for surgery or other medical treatments; and relaxation, biofeedback, and hypnotic therapies are used as adjuncts in the treatment of a variety of medical problems. Specific biobehavioral techniques have proved useful in the assessment, treatment, and management of headache.

## Government Support of Large-Scale Cardiovascular Risk Reduction Trials

Such large-scale, multicenter cardiovascular risk reduction trials as the MRFIT (Multiple Risk Factor Intervention Trial), sponsored by the National Heart, Lung and Blood Institute, the Stanford Heart Disease Prevention Program, and the North Karelia Project have also contributed to the development of health psychology. All three programs were aimed at reducing risk factors identified in the Framingham Heart Study. Three major factors were elevated serum cholesterol levels, hypertension (high blood pressure), and cigarette smoking. These prevention programs targeted several thousand individuals, including employed men (no employed women), children, and women working in the home. Behavioral interventions were a significant aspect of the program, as it was recognized that these risk factors involve such behavioral excesses as overeating or eating high-cholesterol foods and smoking and such behavioral deficits as infrequent exercise.

Although these innovative programs were comprehensive in focus, the behavioral interventions in the early stages of these programs were not as sophisticated as those implemented in later years. This may prove problematic in determining the effectiveness of the current behavioral techniques on long-term CHD risk reduction; however, the wide recognition of the need to modify risk behaviors, which was facilitated by these major risk reduction efforts, has stimulated much interest in this problem at both a research and a clinical level. The problems in initiating and maintaining such behavioral changes challenge health psychology; the behavioral changes have considerable potential to affect the long-term health of the individual and society.

## Reconceptualization of Pain

The *gate control theory* of Ronald Melzack and Patrick Wall (1965) has significantly changed the theory and treatment of pain. The theory proposes that pain is affected by both psychological *and* physiological factors and has provided, in part, a basis for research on psychological processes in pain. Melzack and Wall's theory represents a major shift away from conceptualizing pain as a purely sensory event. Neurosurgeons who had considered sectioning the so-called pain pathways as the treatment of choice for patients with several pain problems now consider the psychobiological nature of pain to a much greater extent. Referral of patients to interdisciplinary pain treatment facilities, which can offer alternatives to surgery, has increased over the past few years. Indeed, some neurosurgeons and anesthesiologists are now learning various psychological approaches to pain control and often treat their patients themselves.

Other psychologists involved in the study of pain include Fordyce (1976) and Sternbach (1978), who emphasized the behavioral nature of chronic pain. These investigators argue that pain is a subjective experience that cannot be objectively measured. Therefore, the only way pain can be communicated is through verbal responses or such bodily movements as crying, grimacing, or limping. This pain behavior can be reinforced, as can any behavior, in an operant manner, outside the patient's awareness. Attention, comfort, and the avoidance of negative consequences or any other potentially reinforcing event may follow the expression of pain thus increasing the chance of its reoccurrence. Inactivity, overeating, boredom, or an expectation of increased pain in certain situations may contribute to the problem. Because a variety of behavioral and cognitive factors appears to contribute to the experience of pain, behavioral interventions directed at modifying these components of pain have been developed for and applied to various pain problems with some success. This reconceptualization of pain and the clinical procedures for alleviating pain have also played major roles in the development of the field. Chapter 12 will focus on this area of health psychology.

## Holistic Philosophy of Health Care and Emphasis on Prevention

In the past, medical professionals tended to become specialists. Although this tendency continues, there has been a recent shift from a focus on specialized treatment to a desire to provide integrated medical care. Family medicine is again being seen as an important approach to caring for patients. The attitude that younger physicians have adopted is that the patient should be understood at a comprehensive level and that health and disease are multidimensional. Thus, the family physician may consult with various specialists, including neurologists, internists, cardiologists, or psychologists, but the ultimate responsibility for integrating the patient's care rests with him or her.

Although the physician with a holistic orientation to health care will have evaluated psychosocial factors in history-taking, what is different now is that he or she has a referral source, the clinical health psychologist, who can offer solutions to deal directly with several of these problems. For example, consider a patient presenting with angina. The physician weighs the physical findings, the results are significant, and medication is prescribed. The physician may note, during history-taking, a possible problem within the family or in the occupational area. He or she may then either attempt to deal with the problem or, more likely, refer the case for such psychological intervention as family or behavior therapy.

Physicians and patients have become increasingly concerned with the prevention of such illnesses as cancer and cardiovascular disease. Patients now are more educated and demanding, and some want to take greater responsibility for their own health care. Western nations are experiencing a movement toward self-care. People are increasingly monitoring their blood pressure, exercising systematically, stopping smoking, and watching their caloric intake. Although the patient can engage in these health behaviors without assistance, many preventive measures may require significant behavior change and necessitate the assistance of such behavior change professionals as health psychologists.

### Founding of the Division of Health Psychology

A number of disciplines within psychology (e.g., clinical, social, developmental, experimental, physiological), with a common interest in health-related issues, convened in 1978 to form the Division of Health Psychology of the American Psychological Association. The goals of the Division, as specified in its by-laws, are shown in Table 2-1 (Matarazzo, 1979). A survey found that a diversity of training opportunities are available within clinical psychology graduate training programs and other subspecialty areas in psychology (Belar, Wilson, & Hughes, 1982) for the

**TABLE 2-1**
Goals of the Division of Health Psychology

---

To advance contributions of psychology as a discipline to the understanding of health and illness through basic and clinical research and by encouraging the integration of biomedical information about health and illness with current psychological knowledge.

To promote education and services in the psychology of health and illness.

To inform the psychological and biomedical community, and the general public, on the results of current research and service activities in this area.

---

health psychology student. In addition, in 1983, a National Working Conference on Education and Training in Health Psychology was held to discuss the nature of future training in this rapidly developing field (Stone, 1983).

## THE NEED FOR ALTERNATIVE MODELS
## TO THE BIOMEDICAL MODEL

Three major interrelated factors appear to have stimulated interest in a more comprehensive theoretical and clinical approach to health and disease. These factors include (a) a shift from a prevalence of infectious, single causal agent diseases to multiply determined chronic illnesses, many the result of unhealthy life-styles; (b) the elevated cost of health care; and (c) a greater emphasis on the quality of life.

In the first half of this century, the average American's health and life span improved considerably through a reduction in infectious disease and epidemics and acute nutritional disease (Gori & Richter, 1978), but the incidence of *chronic* illness has increased. The major health problems today include cardiovascular and renal disease, malignant neoplasms, injuries, respiratory disease, and diabetes mellitus. These problems require a different approach to conceptualization and management, especially since many such illnesses are often considered the result of certain life-styles. Evidence for this has accumulated over the past three decades. The major diseases of modern life are multiply determined by such factors as poor diet, excessive drinking, smoking, drug abuse, lack of exercise, unsafe driving and working conditions and environmental pollution. This suggests that these major diseases could be prevented. One way in which this could occur is through a change in the life-style or in the behavior of individuals at risk for these disorders. Environmental pollution must also be cut down. The implication is that greater emphasis must be placed on the prevention of chronic disease. But once a chronic illness is diagnosed, effective management procedures must be undertaken that may involve intervention at biological, social, and psychological levels to contain the disease process, reduce pain and discomfort, and facilitate active coping behavior on the part of the patient and his or her family.

The second factor relates to the economic realities of health care and disease. Although it is difficult to place a dollar value on health, as might be expected, it has been done. Essentially, according to an economic analysis of disease prevention in the United States published in *Science* (Gori & Richter, 1978), the effects of such preventive measures had been established largely by 1950 (the result of a drop in infant and maternal mortality, better nutrition, and better hygiene). Economists have indicated that between 1940 and 1975, the average life span increased 15%, while per capita disease care expenditures increased 314% in constant 1967 U.S. dollars. Essentially, despite a large increase in financial support for health care, the health of the American people is not necessarily improving. Weiss (1982) has indicated that health care costs are essentially out of control. In the United States health care costs were over $200 billion in 1982, and the percentage increase in health care cost is growing twice as fast as inflation. These economic realities suggest the need for a change, and many institutions have been exploring alternative models of health care and have attempted to reduce delivery costs.

These economic data argue for a need to develop additional ways of enhancing longevity, as through primary disease prevention. This emphasis, of course, would not supplant present therapeutic efforts, but rather would be incorporated into them. It is questionable as to whether current preventive measures would significantly reduce the cost of disease in the near future. It should be emphasized that the economic models used to predict these gains are not without limitation. If, however, economic gains are not totally achieved, there are other reasons for eliminating chronic disease, such as the enhancement of the quality of life and the continuation of gainful employment by the patient.

The current discontent with health care delivery and the development of consumerism over the past several years have suggested the possibility of experimentation with innovative approaches. The general assumption that traditional health care is characterized by a certain insensitivity to patients, and less concern for the comfort of the patient than for specific procedure, is frequently being questioned by health care consumers. Patients want physicians who are communicative and willing to discuss the possible causes of their symptoms.

There has also been concern about the overuse and misuse of drugs and the sometimes adverse effects of medical treatment. The government has become more involved in the control of certain drugs, particularly the minor tranquilizers, that are frequently prescribed for relief of somatic symptoms. Some patients have become interested in nonpharmacological approaches to symptom control and often ask their physicians about them.

These three factors, along with the historical antecedents discussed, have created a need for health psychology as a specific subdiscipline of psychology and a subspecialty within behavioral medicine. It is the purpose of this book to illustrate in greater detail the methods health psychology uses to generate its knowledge base and how this information is used to enhance health and to manage disease.

## RECONCEPTUALIZATION OF HEALTH AND ILLNESS

Certain types of disorders, particularly chronic illness, often must be managed differently than acute disease states. These various clinical approaches can perhaps be best conceptualized by using alternative models to the basic biomedical model (Engel, 1977). For example, consider the treatment of a neck injury. Such an injury requires an immediate examination to determine if bones, and other structures in the neck, are damaged. After establishing that the injury is not severe, the attending physician may give the patient an analgesic and instruct him or her to take this medication as needed to control pain. After 2 to 3 weeks, if an examination reveals that the neck has returned to "normal," and if the pain has disappeared, medication is terminated. Often this represents the actual situation, and the classic biomedical model is quite appropriate for the conceptualization and treatment of the problem. However, what if the pain persists? A different sequence of events usually occurs. The patient may begin to search for other treatments, other drugs, or physical therapy; if the pain persists after these efforts, the patient often requests stronger pain relievers as the search for relief continues. Depression, anxiety, and anger often occur. Activity levels decrease and the patient's work and social life may also suffer. Addiction may also occur. The situation is now much different than before. The problem is now *chronic*, and it involves *psychological, environmental, social,* and *biological* components. The treatment must focus on (a) reducing drug intake rather than maintaining or increasing it, (b) treating the mood disturbance, (c) helping the patient develop the ability to manage pain, and (d) increasing activity levels, to name but a few areas of intervention. This type of clinical approach requires a different theoretical model for health and illness.

Engel (1977) has perhaps been one of the strongest medical proponents for the need of alternative models to the biomedical model of disease. The biomedical model assumes that disease can be explained in terms of measurable biological variables. Such a model requires that disease be considered separate from social behavior and, at its extreme, requires that abnormalities in behavior be reduced to "disordered somatic, biochemical or neurophysiological processes." This extreme biomedical model is reductionistic and maintains the concept of *mind–body dualism*, in which it is assumed that psychological and somatic processes are mutually exclusive, that is, the mind and the body are separate entities.

Engel argues that the biomedical model is, in fact, only a model or a shared set of assumptions and rules of conduct based upon the scientific method, not the unquestionably valid system that it was once commonly held to be. Engel suggests that the biomedical model is Western society's *folk model* of health and disease, no different from the culture-specific health models of American Indian or traditional Chinese medicine. The biomedical model has proved to be extremely useful in understanding and treating illness. Clearly, health psychologists would argue that this has been demonstrated numerous times. The issue under consideration is whether such a model should now be modified to incorporate rather than to exclude psychosocial and behavioral factors that often cannot be reduced to physiochemistry alone.

The alternative model Engel proposes is the *biopsychosocial model.* Although Engel makes a cogent argument for such an alternative, he does not describe the biopsychosocial model in detail. Simply stated, however, this model argues for the importance of psychological, social, and cultural factors in conjunction with biological factors when considering the determinants of disease and their treatment. Engel (1977) states that "the medical model must take into account the patient, the social context in which he lives, and the complementary system devised by society to deal with the disruptive effects of illness, that is, the physician role and the health care system" (p. 132).

A general model of health and disease that encompasses the biopsychosocial approach has been described more specifically by Brody (1973). This model is presented simply as an illustration of an attempt to integrate several variables proposed to effect health and illness. The validity of the specific components of the model remains to be determined. Brody's systems model is an early application of systems theory to health. He argues that health is best viewed within a hierarchy of natural systems in which certain requirements within the hierarchy must be met for proper functioning. Figure 2-1 illustrates a hierarchy of the various subsystems. These subsystems constitute the structural aspect of the system and are organized according to complexity, ranging from subatomic particles at the lowest level up through atoms, molecules, organelles, cells, tissues, the "person," family, community, subculture, culture, society–nation, species, and, lastly, the biosphere. The hierarchy is maintained in a state of dynamic equilibrium by the pattern of information flow of systems and subsystems. This interaction or information flow consists primarily of feedback loops as indicated by the arrows in Figure 2-1. It is possible to exchange information within a hierarchical level and between levels.

According to this model, the precondition for health is that each of the component systems or subsystems at each level be intact and functioning. All feedback loops must be intact and free from excessive noise or impedance to signal flow. Brody suggested that certain drugs and some types of surgery are factors that impede the flow. The hierarchy

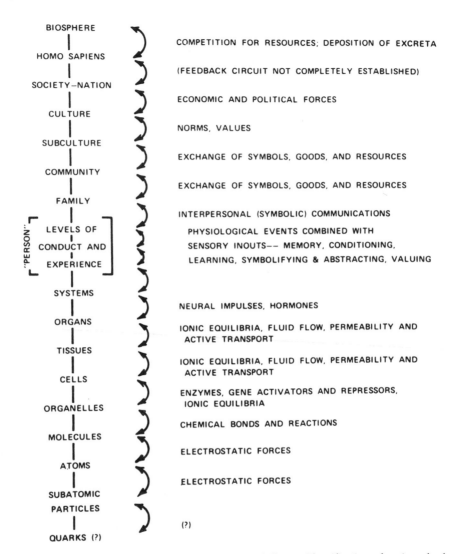

**FIGURE 2-1.** Brody's systems model of health and illness. Identification of various feedback loops in the system hierarchy. From "The Systems View of Man: Implications of Medicine, Science, and Ethics" by H. Brody, 1973, *Perspectives in Biology and Medicine*, 17(1), p. 77. Copyright 1973 by The University of Chicago Press. Reprinted by permission.

requires access to materials that are needed to produce the signals and access to an energy source (e.g., food). The sum of each of these components, in addition to the interactions that constitute the hierarchy's functional organization, produces a state of dynamic equilibrium. *Health* is this state of dynamic equilibrium.

Figure 2-2 illustrates the effects of a perturbation at a low level in the

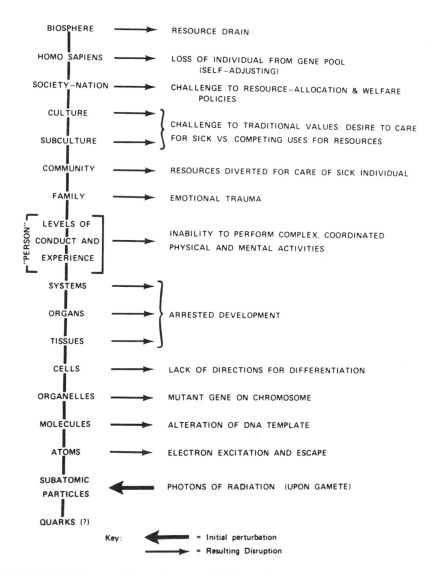

**FIGURE 2-2.** The impact of an environmental effect (radiation) on the health system of the individual. Severe physical and mental retardation caused by radiation-induced mutation in the gamete. Note spread of disruption upward through the hierarchy. From "The Systems View of Man: Implications of Medicine, Science, and Ethics" by H. Brody, 1973, *Perspectives in Biology and Medicine, 17*(1), p. 79. Copyright 1973 by The University of Chicago Press. Reprinted by permission.

hierarchy that results in a spread of disruption or disequilibrium upward through the hierarchy. The example is a radiation-induced mutation in a gamete resulting in severe physical and mental retardation. Such a perturbation may occur at any level initiating disregulation in a downward and/or upward direction. The closing of an aircraft plant as the result of a lost government contract is an example of a perturbation at a higher level that may have effects on several additional levels. Although models such as Brody's permit us to gain a perspective regarding the interdependence of several subsystems involved in health and illness, they are somewhat broad. At this stage in the validation of such models, it is perhaps more productive to keep these models in mind but to narrow the focus. Models that have attempted to explain the contribution of specific psychobiological factors in health and illness will be presented throughout this book.

A major shift in the conceptualization of the role psychobiological factors can play in physical illness is illustrated by the third edition of the *Diagnostic and Statistical Manual of Mental Disorders* (DSM-III)'s classification, "Psychological Factors Affecting Physical Condition" (American Psychiatric Association, 1980). This new category includes *any* physical disorder or, under certain circumstances, any sympton in which psychological factors play a role in *initiation* or *exacerbation*. In this context, *psychological* is defined as the "meaning ascribed to environmental stimuli by the individual." The patient may or may not be aware of the meaning of the stimuli or the effect of these stimuli on the physical condition. Clinical data suggesting a *temporal* relationship among environmental stimuli and their meaning and the initiation or exacerbation of the condition are required before this diagnostic category can be applied. In addition, the physical condition must involve either some demonstrable (organic) pathology, as, for example, in the case of rheumatoid arthritis, or some pathophysiological process, as in the case of migraine headache. The final criterion is the absence of a somatoform or other disorder, in which there are no demonstrable organic findings or known pathophysiological mechanism and for which there is positive evidence that the signs or symptoms are associated with psychological factors.

It is important to emphasize that this category can encompass any physical condition, sign, or symptom. The major limiting factor is the identification of a temporal relationship between environmental stimuli and physical disorder. The absence of a list of specific disorders in the DSM-III, as in the previous DSM-II's classification of disorders that most closely resembles the new category in type of problems (i.e., "Psychophysiological Disorders"), clearly represents a departure. In the DSM-II, the role of psychological factors was limited to the classic "Psychosomatic Disorders," which implied that psychological factors do not play a significant role in other disease states. In contrast, the DSM-III implies that psychological factors may affect *any* physical disorder or sign. Although support for such an approach is far from conclusive, the category does provide a heuristic model for pursuing the role psychological factors play in physical illness. The DSM-III provides a broader perspective regarding this point, but it does not specify which psychological factors affect which disorders or how psychological processes are linked to the pathophysiology of these disorders. Such knowledge will only be forthcoming following the development of rational psychobiological approaches to research on a variety of disorders.

## SUMMARY

A number of factors have contributed to the evolution of health psychology. Efforts by society to reduce the impact of chronic illness, coupled with advances in the behavioral sciences that can be directed toward achieving this goal, have played a significant role here. With greater recognition of the role of life-style in the development and continuation of chronic illness, the application of psychological principles to reduce the impact of psychological factors has become the focus of research and clinical activity. Despite this focus, further development of the field will require a firm integrative, conceptual, and empirical foundation. This foundation will form the basis for effective clinical intervention. Without such a scientific approach to the psychological study of health and illness, health psychology will not fulfill its potential.

## REFERENCES

Ader, R. (1981). *Psychoneuroimmunology.* New York: Academic Press.

American Psychiatric Association (1980). *Diagnostic and statistical manual of mental disorders* (3rd ed.). Washington, DC: Author.

Anisman, H., & Sklar, L. S. (1984). Psychological insults and pathology: Contributions of neurochemical, hormonal and immunological mechanisms. In A. Steptoe & A. Mathews (Eds.), *Health care and human behavior.* London: Academic Press.

Belar, C. D., Wilson, E., & Hughes, H. (1982). Health psychology training in doctoral psychology programs. *Health Psychology, 1*(3), 289–299.

Brody, H. (1973). The systems view of man: Implications of medicine, science, and ethics. *Perspectives in biology and medicine, 17*(1), 71–91.

Cannon, W. B. (1932). *The wisdom of the body.* New York/London: W. W. Norton.

Engel, G. L. (1977). The need for a new medical model: A challenge for biomedicine. *Science, 196* (4286), 129–136.

Fordyce, W. E. (1976). *Behavioral methods for chronic pain and illness.* St. Louis, MO: C. V. Mosby.

Gori, G. B., & Richter, B. J. (1978). Macroeconomics of disease prevention in the United States. *Science, 200* (4346), 1124–1130.

Kellner, R. (1975). Psychotherapy in psychosomatic disorders: A survey of controlled studies. *Archives of General Psychiatry, 32*(8), 1021–1028.

Matarazzo, J. D. (1979). Health psychology: APA's newest division. *The Health Psychologist, 1*(1), 1.

Melzack, R., & Wall, P. D. (1965). Pain mechanisms: A new theory. *Science, 150,* 971–979.

Plutchik, R. (1980). *Emotion: A psychoevolutionary synthesis.* New York: Harper & Row.

Schacter, S., & Singer, J. E. (1962). Cognitive, social and physiological determinants of emotional state. *Psychological Review, 69,* 379–399.

Schwartz, G. E. (1977). Psychosomatic disorders and biofeedback: A psychobiological model of disregulation. In J. D. Maser & M. E. P. Seligman (Eds.), *Psychopathology: Experimental models.* San Francisco: W. H. Freeman.

Schwartz, G. E. (1978). Psychobiological foundations of psychotherapy and behavior change. In S. L. Garfield & A. E. Bergin (Eds.), *Handbook of psychotherapy and behavior change: An empirical analysis* (2nd ed.). New York: Wiley.

Sternbach, R. A. (1978). *The psychology of pain.* New York: Raven Press.

Stone, G. C. (Ed.). (1983). National Working Conference on Education and Training in Health Psychology. *Health Psychology, 2*(Suppl. 5).

Strongman, K. T. (1978). *The psychology of emotion* (2nd ed.). Chichester: Wiley.

Weiner, H. (1977). *Psychobiology and human disease.* New York: Elsevier.

Weiss, S. M. (1982). Health psychology: The time is now. *Health Psychology, 1*(1), 81–90.

# RESEARCH STRATEGIES

The intent of this chapter is not to catalogue research methodologies in health psychology but rather to emphasize the areas most psychology students have not been exposed to, particularly, epidemiological research. General research issues in psychophysiology and clinical psychology will also be discussed to provide a foundation for later chapters, and issues of particular relevance to health psychology research will be delineated. Research using methodology from experimental and clinical psychology to investigate issues in health psychology will also be illustrated.

## ETIOLOGICAL INVESTIGATION

The goal of etiological research is to identify those factors that contribute in a causal manner to the development, exacerbation, and maintenance of a given disorder. The etiologist must realize that the factors that predispose an individual to a given disorder are not necessarily those that maintain or exacerbate it (Weiner, 1977). Also, it should be realized that etiological research is often conducted at different levels, from the molecular to the molar, and, as discussed in Chapter 1, the etiological factors investigated by health psychologists include behavioral, social, developmental, and physiological.

An example of such multilevel etiological research is found in pain studies. Early investigations have suggested that people in different subcultures respond to pain differently (Sternbach & Tursky, 1965). More recent work has been directed at attempting to explain the possible behavioral mechanisms responsible for these sociocultural differences. In a series of studies, Craig (1978) has suggested that processes involved in modeling or observational learning affect pain reports. Such modeling may be related to these cultural differences. Research at a biochemical level has indicated that endogenous morphinelike substances, the *endorphins*, may act in pain modulation. In theory, the release of endorphins may be affected by such culture-specific factors as social learning to modulate pain. Although speculative, it may be possible that the concentrations of endorphins can be influenced by environmental factors, such as learning, resulting in different basal levels of these substances in different subcultures. These environmental factors may also affect culture-specific endorphin release to painful stimulation. Even though some aspects of the above "etiological mechanism" are hypothetical, the example illustrates how an etiological analysis of a given phenomenon is undertaken at multiple levels.

## THE EPIDEMIOLOGICAL APPROACH

*Epidemiology* is a field of inquiry directed at determining the distribution and etiology of disease; it possesses a wealth of concepts and techniques useful for etiological research in health psychology (Palinkas & Hoiberg, 1982). The epidemiologist attempts to determine who develops a specific disease and why. For example, the epidemiologist asks such questions as Is the disease more frequent among men or women, young or old, rich or poor? Other questions include, Is the disease the consequence of a predisposing gene, occupational exposure, life-style, or some complex interaction among all three? The major question is, What characteristic is common to the sick but not to the well?

The terms *incidence* and *prevalence* are used to describe disease occurrences and form the bases of much epidemiological research. Incidence represents the number of people in a given population who contract a disease in a given time period; prevalence represents the total number of cases of a disease at a given time, in a given population. Incidence is equivalent to new cases, prevalence to all cases. The following formulas express the specific meaning of these terms. Incidence, therefore, re-

$$\text{Incidence rate} = \frac{\text{Number of new cases of a disease in a population over a specified time}}{\text{Number of people at risk over the same specified time}}$$

$$\text{Prevalence rate} = \frac{\text{Total number of cases of a disease in a population at a specified time}}{\text{Total population at the same specified time}}$$

flects the rate of disease occurrence, and a change in incidence may mean the balance of etiological factors has changed. This may result from some large-scale intervention, such as a prevention program (e.g., fluoridation of water reducing the incidence of dental cavities) or a naturally occurring fluctuation or secular trend (e.g., increased exercise by a population reducing cardiovascular disease). It is for these reasons that incidence rates are important to the researcher seeking to understand the etiology of a disease. Incidence rates are not unbiased values but rather are influenced by such factors as sociocultural trends (e.g., attitudes) and even inaccuracies of measurement. Figure 3-1 illustrates the variability in determining the presence of disease. This graph indicates considerable individual differences in the identification of postexercise ECG's revealing ischemia. Although it is commonly assumed that the determination of psychopathology is highly variable and problematic, the reliability of medical diagnoses can also be questioned (Koran, 1975).

Prevalence is a function of two factors, the incidence and the duration of a disease. A change in prevalence could reflect a change in incidence or treatment outcome (i.e., remission) or both. Also, better treatment may prevent death, but not produce complete recovery, which will, paradoxically, cause the prevalence rate of a disease to rise. Conversely, a decrease in prevalence may result from a decrease in

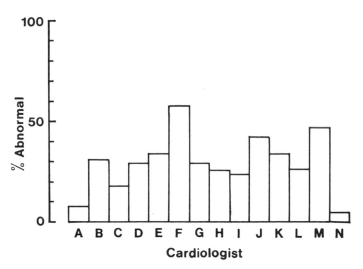

FIGURE 3-1. Example of variations in measurement of biological indicators of disease: Evaluation of 14 cardiologists of the abnormality of 38 post-exercise ECGs. From *Epidemiology in Medical Practice* (p. 22) by D. J. P. Barker and G. Rose. Copyright 1976 by Churchill Livingstone Inc. Reprinted by permission.

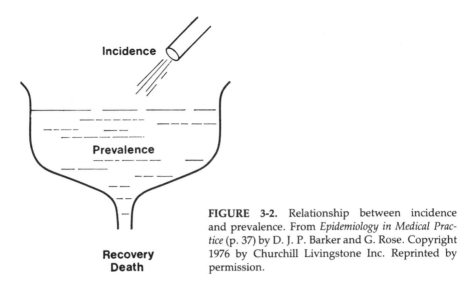

**FIGURE 3-2.** Relationship between incidence and prevalence. From *Epidemiology in Medical Practice* (p. 37) by D. J. P. Barker and G. Rose. Copyright 1976 by Churchill Livingstone Inc. Reprinted by permission.

incidence and a shortened duration of the disease through rapid recovery *or* earlier death. This can be seen in the funnel analogy in Figure 3-2. The prevalence rate increases as incidence increases and decreases with recovery or death.

The concepts of incidence and prevalence are explained here in such detail because they are important in understanding the concept of *risk.* Although the term *at risk,* or *risk factor,* has been used widely in psychology, for the most part such usage has been vague, with minimal understanding of the concept epidemiologically. Risk is an important concept in etiology. *Absolute risk* is the rate of occurrence of a condition or disease; it is equivalent to incidence. *Relative risk* is the ratio of the incidence of a group exposed to a particular etiological factor (e.g., cigarette smoke) to the incidence of the group not exposed to the factor (e.g., no cigarette smoke). It is not a rate itself, but rather a *ratio* that shows how much a risk is modulated (increased or reduced) through exposure. The relative risk is calculated as follows:

$$\text{Relative risk} = \frac{\text{Incidence rate of disease among exposed}}{\text{Incidence rate of disease among nonexposed}}$$

The relative risk is not the probability of an individual's getting a disease but rather a value that indicates that the probability of the disease occurring in a population exposed to the suspected factor or agent is $X$ times higher than in an unexposed population. Relative risk also measures the strength of an association between a factor and a particular health consequence. A high relative risk suggests a causal link between the two, providing additional, although not definitive evidence of an etiological contribution. A sample calculation is presented in Table 3-1.

Two major approaches used to identify risk factors and populations at risk are the *case control*, or retrospective study, and the *cohort*, or prospective study. The case control study involves the comparison of subjects with the "disease" with healthy controls for the purpose of demonstrating that the suspected factors or agents are present more frequently among those with the disease than among those without it. The cohort study involves the comparison of subjects exposed to the suspected causal agent and those not exposed for the purpose of demonstrating that a larger number of subjects exposed to the suspected factor develop the disease than their nonexposed cohorts.

Consider the following example. If one suspected that riding a bicycle to work during rush hour resulted in a higher risk of developing coronary heart disease (CHD), one might study individuals with CHD and those without CHD and determine whether those with CHD rode their bicycles to work more frequently during rush hour than those without CHD. Such an investigation represents a case-control study. In the cohort or prospective study, a group of subjects that typically rode bicycles to work during rush hour would be compared to a cohort or control group matched for other key factors (e.g., cigarette smoking, diet, other types of exercise, and health status) prior to the study who did not ride their bicycles to work during rush hour. All subjects would be followed over time (longitudinally), preferably for several years, to determine whether the incidence of CHD differed between the two groups.

These two types of studies are not mutually exclusive. Indeed, research in epidemiology generally incorporates both types. This is shown in Figure 3-3. In this figure, Steps 1 through 4 do not constitute controlled experiments in the classic sense of manipulation of independent

**TABLE 3-1**
Computation of Relative Risk

|  | Death rate from lung cancer[a] |
| --- | --- |
| Nonsmokers | 0.07 |
| Cigarette smokers | 0.96 |

Relative risk $= \dfrac{.96}{.07} = 13.8$

Conclusion: The probability of developing lung cancer is 13.8 times greater in cigarette smokers than in nonsmokers

[a]Per 1000 aged 35 or more years.

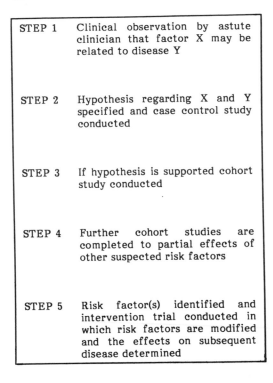

| STEP 1 | Clinical observation by astute clinician that factor X may be related to disease Y |
| STEP 2 | Hypothesis regarding X and Y specified and case control study conducted |
| STEP 3 | If hypothesis is supported cohort study conducted |
| STEP 4 | Further cohort studies are completed to partial effects of other suspected risk factors |
| STEP 5 | Risk factor(s) identified and intervention trial conducted in which risk factors are modified and the effects on subsequent disease determined |

FIGURE 3-3. Sequence of research for identifying etiological factors.

variables and, therefore, cannot definitively result in causal statements. These steps represent observational methods. The data are correlational (they coexist more frequently than chance). This is an important point. The exception to this is Step 5, or the clinical trial, which, if properly controlled, can be considered an experimental study. If the case control, or longitudinal study, only determines whether the disease in question and the suspected causal factor coexist more frequently than would be expected by chance alone, how can one evaluate the causal significance of an association between suspected risk factor and disease? Roberts (1977) lists a set of eight criteria (Table 3-2), none of which alone represents the *sine qua non* for judgment, although each one can assist in such an evaluation. These criteria should be considered when critically evaluating the role of suspected biopsychosocial risk factors in illness.

Although much useful information has been obtained through epidemiological research on various risk factors, contributions regarding the mechanisms of such risk factors in humans have been limited. Structural or fixed descriptions of blood pressure levels, for example, for individuals with certain personality types or in certain environmental settings (e.g., urban vs. rural) do not lead to an understanding of the dynamic psychobiological mechanisms involved in the development, exacerbation, and/or maintenance of hypertension (Lazarus, 1978; Linden & Feuerstein, 1981). A potentially more enlightening research strategy might involve an analysis of the interaction of physiological, psychological, and environmental factors in longitudinal or prospective research. Rose, Jenkins, and Hurst (1978) designed a comprehensive study of health changes in air traffic controllers that provides a model for such an integrative biopsychosocial research paradigm—the Air Traffic Controller Study.

In 1973, Rose and colleagues began a three-year prospective study of health changes in approximately 435 male air traffic controllers. The study was designed to determine the individual and combined effects of environmental sources of stress (job stress), psychological differences in stress responsivity, work attitudes, psychosocial support systems, and various personality attributes as predictors of health status over the three-year period. As Table 3-3 illustrates, nine general categories of variables, representing physiological, behavioral, psychological, social, and environmental domains, were investigated at several times throughout the study. Many of these variables, including the physiological, were recorded during actual exposure to the stressful environment. Table 3-4 illustrates the various indices of minor and major health changes recorded at points throughout the study. The methodology used in this research is state of the art epidemiological research. Such a research strategy should not only permit identification of biopsychosocial risk factors in this group but, perhaps more importantly, also provide data on the dynamic interactions among these variables to enhance our understanding of the mechanisms involved.

**TABLE 3-2**
Criteria for Evaluating the Validity of a Suspected Risk Factor

---

1. *Strength*—What is the value of the relative risk ratio?
2. *Consistency*—Has the association been repeatedly observed in different places at different times by different observers (i.e., reliability)?
3. *Specificity*—Is the association limited to a particular type of exposure and specific disease?
4. *Temporal relationship*—How confident can one be that the suspected cause antedated the observed effect?
5. *Dose response*—Is there sufficient evidence of increasing risk with increased dose?
6. *Plausibility*—Is the suggestion of causality biologically plausible?
7. *Coherence*—Does the suggestion of causality conflict with other known data on the natural history and etiology of disease?
8. *Experimental confirmation*—What is the effect of intervention?

---

**TABLE 3-3**
Health Measures Used in the Air Traffic Controller Study

| Source of information | Data collected | Visit 1 2 3 4 5 | Monthly | Per incident |
|---|---|---|---|---|
| | | **Frequency** | | |
| 1. Medical questionnaire | Past medical history | X | | |
| | Family history | X  X  X  X  X | | |
| | Smoking, eating, drinking habits, medications, and review of systems | X  X  X  X  X | | |
| 2. Physical examination | Physical findings, BP | X  X  X  X  X | | |
| | Timed vital capacity | X      X      X | | |
| | EKG | X      X      X | | |
| | Chest films | X             X | | |
| | Urinalysis, CBC | X  X  X  X  X | | |
| | SMA-12, Rd. 1, SMAC, Rd. 3 and 5 | X      X      X | | |
| | Audiological examination | X | | |
| 3. Psychiatric interview | Psychiatric Status Schedule | X  X  X  X  X | | |
| 4. Health checklist | Physical signs and symptoms as episodes, continuing problems, or isolated events | | X | |
| | Accidents and injuries | | X | |
| | Days lost from work and days below par | | X | |
| | Visits to physician or hospitalization | | X | |
| 5. Mood checklist | Zung anxiety and depression questionnaires | | X | |
| 6. Physician and hospital reports | Records of illnesses, diagnoses | | | X |
| 7. Special diagnostic tests and consultations | As required to make diagnosis | | | X |

TABLE 3-3 (*Continued*)

| Source of information | Data collected | Frequency | | | | | | | |
| --- | --- | --- | --- | --- | --- | --- | --- | --- |
| | | Visit | | | | | Monthly | Per incident |
| | | 1 | 2 | 3 | 4 | 5 | | |
| 8. Sleep questionnaire | Characteristics of sleep complaints | | | | | | | Once |
| 9. Headache questionnaire | Characteristics of headache complaints | | | | | | | Once |

*Note.* From "Health Change in Air Traffic Controller: A Prospective Study. I Background and Description" by R. M. Rose, C. D. Jenkins, and M. W. Hurst, 1978, *Psychosomatic Medicine, 40,* p. 150. Copyright by The American Psychosomatic Society, Inc. Reprinted by permission of Elsevier Science Publishing Co., Inc.

## CLINICAL RESEARCH METHODS

This section shifts from an etiological focus to the clinical research methodology available to health psychology. Designs actually implemented in health psychology research will be illustrated.

### Types of Experimental Strategies

Research design is all important in obtaining solid scientific data. The basic principle is that the experiment should be designed so that the effects of the independent variables can be evaluated unambiguously. Systematic manipulation of the independent variable, as well as an awareness of two basic types of research errors, are necessary (Campbell & Stanley, 1963). The first type involves the concept of *internal validity*, which means the degree to which plausible, rival hypotheses have been ruled out, and particularly those variables that may be confounded with the effects of the independent variable. For example, when studying the effects of a relaxation procedure on angina, one would control the medication prescribed by the patient's physician so as not to contribute to any reduction or increase of pain, which might then be erroneously attributed to the effects of the relaxation procedure. Table 3-5 lists eight different classes of extraneous variables that might produce effects confounded with the effect of the experimental variable, if not controlled for, and therefore affect the internal validity of the research design (Campbell & Stanley, 1963).

The second type of research error is related to *external validity*. External validity is the generalizability of data obtained in a given experiment.

**TABLE 3-4**
Process Variables Used in the Air Traffic Controller Study

| Generic variable | Instrument or technique | Visit 1 | 2 | 3 | 4 | 5 | Yearly Twice | Four times |
|---|---|---|---|---|---|---|---|---|
| 1. Physiological responsivity at work | | | | | | | | |
|   a. Endocrine | Cortisol and growth hormone levels each 20 min for 5 hr while working | | | | | | X | |
|   b. Cardiovascular | BP and HR responses each 20 min for 5 hr while working | | | | | | X | |
| 2. Behavioral responsivity at work | Behavioral rating scale, POMS | | | | | | | X |
| 3. Work environment | Measures of workload, subjective difficulty questionnaires (collected with endocrine and BP data) | | | | | | | X |
| 4. Sociodemographic background (e.g., education of self, parents, wife, status incongruity) | Biographical questionnaire | X | | | | | | |
| 5. Specific psychological attitudes and orientation (e.g., "burnout," investment in job, anxiety at work, bounceback, marital and social support, coping by physical activity, drinking) | ATC questionnaire | X | X | X | X | X | | |
| 6. Work morale and satisfaction | Job Description Inventory, Leadership Behavior Questionnaire, Kavanagh Life Attitude Profile, satisfaction with FAA policies | X | X | X | X | X | | |
| 7. Life change events | Review of Life Experiences (ROLE), life | X | X | X | X | X | | |

**TABLE 3-4** (*Continued*)

| Generic variable | Instrument or technique | Frequency of observation | | | | | | |
|---|---|---|---|---|---|---|---|---|
| | | Visit | | | | | Yearly | |
| | | 1 | 2 | 3 | 4 | 5 | Twice | Four times |
| | change inventory with standardized and individual adjustment and distress ratings | | | | | | | |
| 8. Work competence | Sociometric questionnaire—peer ratings of competence, amicability, ideal team choice | X | X | X | X | X | | |
| 9. General psychological assessment | CPI, JAS | X | | | | | | |
| | MMPI subscales, "connectedness" | | | X | | | | |
| | Cattell 16PF | | | | | X | | |

*Note.* From "Health Change in Air Traffic Controller: A Prospective Study. I Background and Description" by R. M. Rose, C. D. Jenkins, and M. W. Hurst, 1978, *Psychosomatic Medicine, 40*, p. 153. Copyright by The American Psychosomatic Society, Inc. Reprinted by permission of Elsevier Science Publishing Co., Inc.

An example of a potential problem with the external validity of an experiment would involve evaluating the effects of a behavioral weight reduction program on a group of 18- to 21-year-old college students and generalizing these findings to middle-aged, chronically obese women. The several factors jeopardizing the external validity of an experiment are described in Table 3-5.

Internal validity is crucial, because, without it, the results are meaningless. Certain statistical and methodological procedures, on the one hand, allow experimenters to establish a fair degree of internal validity. On the other hand, external validity can be established only with additional investigations of different populations or replications with similar populations. The problem of external validity is especially relevant when the utility of analogue "clinical" research studies is evaluated.

An *analogue study* generally focuses on a carefully defined research question using well-controlled conditions. These conditions usually only resemble or approximate the clinical situation; hence the term *analogue*. Analogue investigations are often undertaken for practical and ethical reasons. Practical reasons include limited access to a clinical set-

## TABLE 3-5
### Factors Affecting Validity

Internal Validity

  *History*. Specific events occurring between the first and second measurement in
    addition to the experimental variable

  *Maturation*. Process within the respondents operating as a function of the passage of
    time *per se* (not specific to the particular events), including growing older, or
    becoming bored with study

  *Testing*. Effects of taking a test upon the scores of a second testing

  *Instrumentation*. Changes in the calibration of a measuring instrument or changes in
    the observers or scorers used may change the obtained measurements

  *Statistical regression*. Tendency for measures to drift toward the mean or average often
    occurs when groups have been selected on the basis of their extreme scores

  *Selection*. Biases resulting in differential selection of respondents for the comparison
    groups

  *Experimental mortality*. Differential loss of respondents from the comparison groups

External Validity

  *Reactive or interactive effect of testing*. Pretest might increase or decrease the re-
    spondent's sensitivity or responsiveness to the experimental variable, therefore,
    results would be unrepresentative for a population not pretested

  *Interaction effects*. Selection biases interacting with the experimental variable

  *Reactive effects of experimental arrangements*. May preclude generalization about the
    effect of the experimental variable on persons exposed to treatment in nonexperi-
    mental settings

  *Multiple-treatment interference*. Likely to occur whenever multiple treatments are
    applied to the same respondents

ting, with such associated difficulties as obtaining an adequate number of subjects, controlling for competing factors or treatments, random assignment of patients to various treatment groups, and obtaining therapists who will meet the demands of controlled research. Ethical considerations include withholding treatment or using treatments that may be ineffective or harmful when other more effective treatments are available. The disadvantage of analogue research is the question of the applicability of the findings to relevant clinical populations. Kazdin (1978), a proponent of the analogue research design, points out that all treatment research, even in clinical settings, is an analogue of the situation to which an investigator wishes to generalize. He also questions the assumption that the greater the similarity of a treatment procedure to the clinical situation, the more generalizable the findings will be to the clinical situation. Kazdin suggests that research is needed to determine the various dimensions of departure from clinical situations and the effects of such departures for generalizing findings to the clinical situation. The issues of an analogue study versus clinical research are important in that the health psychologist should be cautious in assuming that the findings of a specific clinical or analogue study are generalizable to other populations, unless the intervention or findings have been demonstrated to be effective in the population of concern.

Four basic types of research designs used in clinical research in health psychology are (a) individual case study, (b) nonfactorial single group design, (c) nonfactorial group design with untreated controls, and (d) factorial design with untreated and nonspecifically treated controls (Mahoney, 1978). For each type of design, there are variations in strategy, some of which are designed to obtain greater experimental control. Table 3-6 lists examples of each type of design. In general, as one moves down the table, the designs become more complex and have a greater degree of internal validity. Each of these designs can be used for various purposes, each having advantages and disadvantages.

*Single case studies* are thought to have a low degree of experimental control over the physical and social environment or the "spontaneous" fluctuations of biological or psychological processes that may affect the findings. For rare clinical cases, however, or for running a pilot for a specific procedure, a controlled, single case study provides useful infor-

## TABLE 3-6
### Clinical Research Designs

| Design | Example | Symbol[a] | |
|---|---|---|---|
| 1. Individual case study | Multiple baseline across settings | Settings–OXOO<br>OOXO<br>OOOX | |
| | A-B-A reversal design | OXOXO | |
| 2. Nonfactorial single group design | Multiple baseline across subjects with a reversal | Subjects–OXOOXOO<br>OOXOOXO<br>OOOXOOX | |
| | Pre–post group design | OXO | |
| 3. Nonfactorial group design with untreated controls | Randomized posttest control group | (R)–XO<br>O | |
| | Solomon four group | OXO<br>(R)–O  O<br>XO<br>O | |
| 4. Factorial group design with untreated and nonspecific treatment controls | Attention and control groups | OXO<br>(R)–  XO or (R)–OYO<br>OYO<br>YO<br>O | OXO<br>OZO |

[a]O, observation of testing; X, treatment or intervention X; Y, treatment or intervention Y; Z, treatment or intervention Z.

mation that can be applied to more complex research strategies. Such single case studies as the multiple-baseline across settings or subjects design or the A-B-A reversal design result in a fair degree of confidence in the experimental manipulation, but the validity of generalizing the findings to other individuals and settings can still be questioned. To assure some degree of internal validity, when employing a single case design, the experimenter should obtain stable measures of the dependent variables during the baseline phase, that is, before manipulating the independent variable. Changes during the intervention, posttreatment, and follow-up are more likely to be *related* to the intervention since regression toward the mean, nonspecific attention–placebo variables, and the spontaneous fluctuations in the symptom or problem behavior are less likely to account for observed changes when a stable baseline is established. Note that one can make a statement about the probable *relationship*, but given the limitations of a single case study, one cannot make a definite cause–effect statement. An example of one type of single case design (A-B) employed by the authors in their clinical practice is presented below.

> *Systematic desensitization treatment for an 8-month avoidance of food ingestion secondary to $T_2N_2$ squamous cell carcinoma of the left tonsil was implemented in the case of a 49-year-old male admitted to a specialty behavior therapy unit. The target problem was identified as the absence of oral food ingestion due to postirradiation difficulties with swallowing necessitating nasogastric (NG) tube feeding. Baseline measures of oral food ingestion were obtained at each meal over a 6-day period. Intervention consisted of biofeedback-assisted relaxation training, using skin conductance feedback followed by in vivo desensitization to food. Results indicated that 2 days following in vivo desensitization, the patient gradually began to ingest greater quantities of food, which reduced NG feedings. Weight began to gradually increase and stabilize over a 14-day period, with the observed increase in oral ingestion. At treatment termination, all NG feedings were discontinued. This was accompanied by a reduction in noxious sensations during food ingestion. Follow-up at 3 and 12 months revealed maintenance of treatment gains and weight. This case illustrates the use of an A-B design consisting of baseline measures (A) and treatment (B). Such a design can be readily implemented in clinical health psychology.*

*Nonfactorial single group* designs have the same basic methodological problem as single case studies, because randomization of and comparison between groups are not involved. This type of design can be thought of as a replication of several single cases. Replication increases the confidence in the reliability of a finding, as the number of subjects increases, although, as with single case studies, no cause–effect statement can be made. Variations, however, of the single group design provide greater experimental control. For example, a multiple baseline-across-subjects design that includes a reversal for each subject controls extraexperimental events. With this type of design, intervention occurs at different times for each subject. When it is reliably demonstrated that changes in the dependent variable (clinical problem) across subjects is temporally contingent upon the manipulation of the independent variable (treatment), a cause–effect relationship between these variables may be established.

The *nonfactorial group design* with an untreated group or with a no treatment control represents the classic or true experiment. Equivalence between groups before treatment is assured through randomization. This design overcomes many internal validity errors that result from the inclusion of the equated untreated group. Extraenvironmental events, spontaneous fluctuations in biological or psychological processes over time, reactive effects of measurement, instrument calibration over time, and statistical regression should be similar for both groups. Two versions of this design are the Randomized Post-Test Only Design and the Solomon Four Group Design; both designs allow a cause–effect relationship between the intervention and the changes in dependent variables to be established. However, specific cause–effect relationships on what *aspects* of the treatment condition were responsible for the change cannot be stated.

*Factorial designs* with untreated and nonspecific treatment controls (i.e., placebo, attention) are the *only* type of designs that establish cause–effect relationships for the several complex variables assumed to contribute to the intervention. The basic design is a pre–post control group design, with additional groups representing various levels or components of the treatment procedure. Attention–placebo controls are employed to identify potent aspects of the treatment package. Overall levels of the treatment condition, nonspecific variables, and the interaction between classes of variables may be determined.

If an investigator were interested in determining the effects of aerobic exercise in the treatment of patients with mild hypertension, he or she would utilize a factorial design. The goal of this design would be to determine the specific effects of aerobic exercise on blood pressure. The design might include the following groups: (a) aerobic exercise only, (b) nonaerobic exercise (i.e., muscle endurance), (c) a no exercise control, and (d) an attention–placebo group. Subjects matched on a number of key variables would be randomly assigned to one of the four groups.

The advantage of using more complex designs is that researchers can state more confidently the cause–effect nature of their findings. The disadvantages include the time and the number of subjects necessary, the considerable homogeneity of groups, and randomization. With any of these designs, researchers can strengthen their findings by incorporating short- and long-term follow-up of results. This has been particularly lacking in clinical health psychology research. Even the better-designed study without follow-up indicates very little about the generalization and maintenance of treatment effects, which can only be evaluated with follow-up assessment. Given that many health psychology interventions have as a focus a long-term life-style change, which is indeed a complicated and difficult goal to achieve, such follow-up evaluations are particularly essential.

**Importance of Programmatic Research**

Reflecting on the previous discussion, one realizes that even with more complex and internally valid designs, one cannot answer all or even most of the questions regarding a particular mechanism or treatment effect. Theoretically, a grand factorial study may yield such answers, but a program of small studies is more feasible. Each study would deal with one set of research questions. Most laboratories, both basic and applied, function in a programmatic manner. Confidence is gained through replication over a series of studies, rather than from a single multifactorial study that controls for all possible rival hypotheses. Because of the tendency to perhaps go beyond the data, especially when a new field with clinical implications is being developed, it is particularly important that health psychology research be systematic. Gottman and Markman (1978) suggest that because there are different sets of research questions at different stages of program development and evaluation, a model such as the Program Development Model (PDM) that allows one to conceptualize the range of designs and analysis options at various stages be used. They strongly suggest developing an intervention program for a *specific target population*. A flowchart of such a program is depicted in Figure 3-4. The flowchart shows the eight phases of research activity. Different research designs are useful for different phases of the program. The program attempts to establish checks for internal and external validity and a feedback loop, which provides the option to redesign the program.

The first phase of the flowchart entails selecting a specific target population. The selection of target populations should involve some assessment of how the target population differs from individuals who would not be considered subjects. An example is, What is different about women with premenstrual tension syndrome (PMS) who sign up for a treatment study as compared to those women who have similar symptoms but who are not interested in treatment and may not even

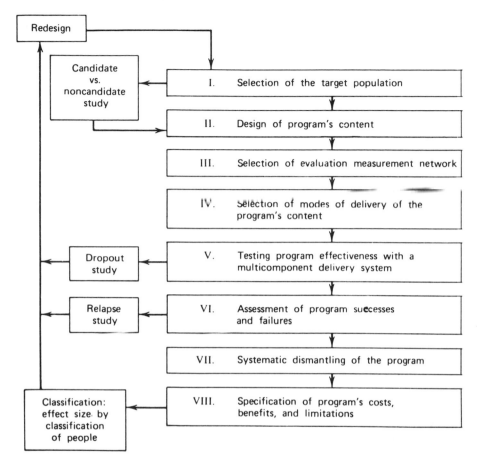

**FIGURE 3-4.** Program Development Model (PDM) for clinical outcome research. From "Experimental Designs in Psychopathology Research" by J. M. Gottman and J. H. Markman in *Handbook of Psychotherapy and Behavior Change* (p. 32), edited by S. L. Garfield and A. E. Bergin. Copyright 1978 by John Wiley & Sons, Ltd. Reprinted by permission.

consider PMS a problem? This type of question can be answered through a candidate versus a noncandidate study.

The second phase of the model involves designing the content of the program. The researchers should adequately understand how the subject should change in order to experience benefits. An example of a research question in health psychology might be, Do chronic back pain patients need to be more assertive, increase activity levels, and/or engage in relaxation procedures in order to cope better with pain? The third phase consists of the selection of assessment measures, which should be relevant to the treatment program. Multimodal and clinically meaningful measures are desirable. In the case of the low-back-pain patient, measures of assertiveness, activity, and relaxation levels would be obtained using a variety of techniques (e.g., behavioral observation, questionnaires, and family reports).

The fourth phase is the selection of modes of delivery. Treatment procedures should be specified in such a manner as to be reproducible by other investigators. Initially, a treatment package is outlined and utilized and is later dismantled during phase seven. Dismantling treatment procedures will help identify potent variables, that is, variables responsible for change and subsequent trimming of the treatment package. Phase five involves testing the treatment program's effectiveness. At this point, any of the aforementioned research designs are useful, particularly nonfactorial control group designs such as the Solomon Four Group Design. Phase six involves the evaluation of successes and failures of the program. During this phase, an assessment of the kinds of people who benefit from the program as well as a follow-up assessment are made. Determining what kinds of people failed and why is also important and may provide information necessary to redesign the program for future investigations. During phase seven, dismantling the program, researchers can utilize factorial group designs with attention, placebo, and nonspecific treatment groups, as well as groups experiencing various components of the treatment package. Dismantling designs can involve adding components of the treatment protocol until changes are established or comparing groups experiencing various components of the package. Phase eight entails specifying the program's cost, benefits, and limitations. These specifications can be used as input data for redesigning the treatment. The PDM can give health psychologists involved in clinical outcome research a perspective on how their work is contributing to the overall development of various treatment programs, as well as remind them that the potentially frustrating aspects of the research, such as information on drop-outs, provide pertinent data for enhancing a treatment program.

## Selected Examples of Research Designs in Health Psychology

An example of a single case design involves a 27-year-old female with chronic *bruxism* (teeth grinding, usually at night) (Finch & Gale, 1980). Bruxism may damage teeth and supporting structures, as well as the temporomandibular joint, and cause face and head pain. Bruxism was measured using (1) the total time of bruxism as indicated by taped-recorded electromyogram (EMG) (muscle) activity and (2) the number of bruxing incidents per night (EMG greater that a preset level), regardless of duration. The study consisted of five baseline periods and two treatment periods, each consisting of 10 days of recorded activity.

The first experimental condition consisted of auditory biofeedback to the subject through an earphone during sleep. The second experimental condition consisted of auditory feedback and the requirement that the subject get out of bed and note the quality of sleep and the time the signal went off. Table 3-7 summarizes the EMG data from the study. The results indicate that although bruxing behavior decreased during treatment as compared to baseline, during both follow-up periods and for the final baseline, bruxing was greater than before the treatment period. The authors concluded that the experimental treatment did result in a decrease in bruxing behavior. However, when the treatment phase was discontinued, bruxing not only returned to normal, but increased significantly. Note that two "reversals" occurred during the study; after treatment the intervention was discontinued, to assess the treatment effects. Also, this study is noteworthy in that the *negative* effects of removing treatment and a possible rebound effect are demonstrated and communicated to other professionals. Frequently, only interventions with positive results are published.

One interesting study applying methodology from experimental psychology (perception, sensation) demonstrates the use of a nonfactorial control group design. Murphy and Donderi (1980) hypothesized that postoperative recovery for cataract patients may involve the psychological process of perceptual learning. Using a healthy, age-matched control group and a group of patients with cataracts, they tested the subjects preoperatively, usually the day before the operation and 7 and 16 weeks, postoperatively. The evaluation battery included an adaptation questionnaire, an activity questionnaire, mirror drawing, path walking, reading tasks, and visual matching. Results of the study indicated that a greater amount of activity and the ability to learn new visuomotor skills predicted "satisfaction with surgery" as well as increased performance on the postoperative evaluation measures.

The effect of spouse involvement upon weight loss was studied by Murphy, Williamson, Buxton, Moody, Asher, and Warner (1982), using a factorial group design. This design is identified as a factorial group design because couples were *randomly* assigned to *four* experimental conditions and *two* control conditions. The four experimental conditions were subject with spouse, subject without spouse, contingency contract for subject alone, and contingency contract with spouse. The two control conditions included an attention–control (supportive) group and a

**TABLE 3-7**
Findings from a Research Study using a Single Case Design

| | First baseline | First experiment | First follow-up | Bruxism activity Second baseline | Second experiment | Second follow-up | Final baseline |
|---|---|---|---|---|---|---|---|
| Mean duration (sec) | 20.2 | 24.3 | 39.2 | 63.9 | 29.2 | 92.4 | 105.7 |
| SD | (8.5) | (8.0) | (9.1) | (18.2) | (12.2) | (50.3) | (54.0) |
| Mean count | 16.9 | 13.6 | 24.5 | 50.7 | 29.1 | 65.0 | 67.2 |
| SD | (9.0) | (4.9) | (5.3) | (12.6) | (8.5) | (29.4) | (27.4) |

*Note.* From "Factors Associated with Nocturnal Bruxism and Its Treatment" by D. P. Finch and E. N. Gale, 1980, *Journal of Behavioral Medicine, 3(4),* p. 391. Copyright 1980 by Plenum Publishing Corporation. Reprinted by permission.

waiting-list control group. The treatment consisted of 11 weekly sessions and 8 maintenance sessions over a 2-year follow-up period. Primary dependent variables were absolute weight loss, percentage excess weight loss, and a weight-reduction index. Based on an analysis of data from 78 couples, the results indicated that subjects in all conditions, except the waiting-list control, lost weight at the end of the 11-week phase, and that there was no significant difference between groups. However, as shown in Figure 3-5, at the 2-year follow-up, subjects in both couples' groups maintained weight loss to a greater degree than the individuals treated alone. It is interesting to note that the supportive control group did as well as the behavioral treatment groups during treatment, although weight loss was not maintained as well as it was for the groups in which spouses were involved. The authors report a high attrition rate, especially after the first session. High attrition can be a difficulty when working with clinical populations in research.

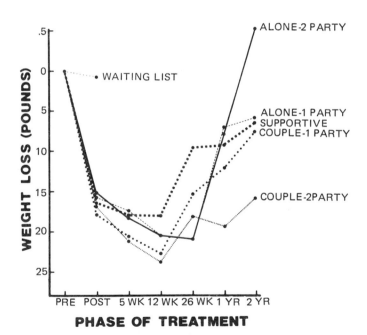

FIGURE 3-5. Example of outcome (weight loss) from long-term factorial group design. From "The Long-Term Effects of Spouse Involvement upon Weight Loss and Maintenance" by Joseph K. Murphy, Donald A. Williamson, Alfred E. Buxton, Sarah C. Moody, Nelea Absher, and Mark Warner, 1982, *Behavior Therapy, 13.* Copyright 1982 by the Association for the Advancement of Behavior Therapy. Reprinted by permission.

## METHODOLOGICAL AND CONCEPTUAL PROBLEMS IN
## HEALTH PSYCHOLOGY RESEARCH

The health psychology researcher is faced with a number of methodological and conceptual difficulties that must be addressed in order to increase the knowledge base in this field. Although these problems are illustrated throughout the book, a discussion of some of the more general concerns should help the reader place the findings discussed in the various chapters in perspective. Students often experience a sense of discouragement when "facts" are not presented in black and white, although it is a rare field that can provide such "facts." Given the early stage of development of health psychology, such definitive statements are even more difficult to make. The problems inherent in research in health psychology account for some of this.

Researchers in the field are faced with the problem of developing operational definitions of such broad concepts as health, illness, stress, coping, and pain. Measurement is an essential component of any research effort, and operational definitions represent an important first step. The development of valid and reliable instruments for measurement clearly represents an area of opportunity and difficulties.

A second problem area relates to the choice of appropriate control groups for etiological research on disease. Is it more valid for the researcher to compare his or her group of interest with "healthy controls" or with controls with other disorders? Of course the answer to this question relates to the specific research question. It is important that the research question be well phrased and that selection criteria, screening devices, and screening procedures be carefully prepared.

Clinical research in health psychology faces several other concerns. It is difficult to determine the *specific* effects of a health psychology intervention (i.e., effects relative to the efforts under study) when the patient/subject is undergoing multiple interventions. This problem is not specific to health psychology and represents a persistent problem in all health care research. The elimination of as many confounding treatments as possible is a reasonable compromise approach; however, it is important to remember, when considering the results of outcome research, that several additional variables are often contributing to treatment effects. Other related difficulties emerge in clinical research, in which the use of placebos are not ethical or when placebo treatments are not easily designed. This latter issue is discussed in more detail in subsequent chapters. Identification of clinically meaningfully and statistically valid multiple indices of outcome also is a source of concern. From a clinical perspective, statistically significant changes may have very little meaning. Patients with intractable pain and depression who experience a statistically significant drop in a Beck Depression Inventory following treatment, but who continue to display low levels of activity, high levels of narcotic analgesic use, and high levels of family conflict, have not improved clinically. Measures must be developed to reflect the complex nature of the clinical problems health psychology practitioners face that are also psychometrically, theoretically and clinically valid.

Many of the methodological problems encountered in the psychology and health fields can simply be generalized to the new discipline of health psychology. A careful consideration of general methodological issues will help the student differentiate "signal" from "noise" in this rapidly developing field.

## SUMMARY

This chapter has reviewed the research strategies used in health psychology. Etiological investigation designed to help identify factors that contribute causally to the development, exacerbation, and maintenance of specific problems have been discussed. The importance of a multilevel approach to etiological research was also illustrated.

Most students are not taught epidemiology, yet epidemiological concerns are important in research in health psychology. In this chapter we have reviewed such important concepts and issues in epidemiology as incidence, prevalence, absolute risk, relative risk, case control study, cohort or prospective study, and the process typically used in an epidemiological approach to a problem, as exemplified in the Air Traffic Controller Study.

Clinical research methods were discussed to illustrate various experimental strategies and problems of internal and external validity. The importance of programmatic research in developing treatment protocols was emphasized, and examples of actual clinical research designs in health psychology were given. Finally, this chapter concluded with a brief discussion of general methodological and conceptual problems in health psychology research.

## REFERENCES

Baker, D. J. P., & Rose, G. (1976). *Epidemiology in Medical Practice*. New York: Churchill Livingstone.

Campbell, D. T., & Stanley, J. C. (1963). *Experimental and quasi-experimental designs for research*. Chicago: Rand McNally.

Craig, K. D. (1978). Social modeling influences on pain. In R. A. Sternbach (Ed.), *The psychology of pain* (pp. 73–104). New York: Raven Press.

Finch, D. P., & Gale, E. N. (1980). Factors associated with nocturnal bruxism and its treatment. *Journal of Behavioral Medicine, 3*(4), 385–397.

Gottman, J., & Markman, H. J. (1978). Experimental designs in psychotherapy research. In S. L. Garfield & A. E. Bergin (Eds.), *Handbook of psychotherapy and behavior change: An empirical analysis* (2nd ed). New York: Wiley.

Kazdin, A. E. (1978). Evaluating the generality of findings in analogue therapy research. *Journal of Consulting and Clinical Psychology, 46*(4), 673–686.

Koran, L. M. (1975). The reliability of clinical methods, data, and judgments: Part I. *New England Journal of Medicine, 293*(13), 642–646.

Lazarus, R. S. (1978). A strategy for research on psychological and social factors in hypertension. *Journal of Human Stress, 4,* 35–40.

Linden, W., & Feuerstein, M. (1981). Essential hypertension and social coping behavior. *Journal of Human Stress, 7*(1), 28–34.

Mahoney, M. (1978). Experimental methods and outcome evaluation. *Journal of Consulting and Clinical Psychology, 46*(4), 660–672.

Marks, I. (1978). Behavioral psychotherapy of adult neurosis. In S. L. Garfield & A. E. Bergin (Eds.), *Handbook of psychotherapy and behavior change: An empirical analysis* (2nd ed.). New York: Wiley.

Murphy, J. K., Williamson, D. A., Buxton, A. E., Moody, S. C., Absher, N., & Warner, M. (1982). The long-term effects of spouse involvement upon weight loss and maintenance. *Behavior Therapy, 13,* 681–693.

Murphy, S. B., & Donderi, D. C. (1980). Predicting the success of cataract surgery. *Journal of Behavioral Medicine, 3*(1), 1–14.

Palinkas, L. A., & Hoiberg, A. (1982). An epidemiology primer: Bridging the gap between epidemiology and psychology. *Health Psychology, 1*(3), 269–287.

Roberts, C. J. (1977). *Epidemiology for clinicians.* England: Pitman Books.

Rose, R. M., Jenkins, C. D., & Hurst, M. W. (1978). Health change in air traffic controllers: A prospective study. I. Background and description. *Psychosomatic Medicine, 40*(2), 142–165.

Sternbach, R. A., & Tursky, B. (1965). Ethnic differences among housewives in psychophysical and skin potential responses to electric shock. *Psychophysiology, 1,* 241–246.

Weiner, H. (1977). *Psychobiology and human disease.* New York: Elsevier.

# PRINCIPLES OF PSYCHOPHYSIOLOGY

As discussed in Chapter 2, psychophysiological concepts and techniques have played an important role in the development of health psychology. The field of psychophysiology has contributed much to the understanding and treatment of a variety of health problems. Therefore, an understanding of the field is essential for an in-depth appreciation of health psychology. The purpose of this chapter is to review basic psychophysiological concepts and techniques. A review of principles of the nervous and endocrine systems is followed by an overview of the physiological response systems that are often the focus of study in the field. Finally, theoretical considerations in the field will be presented and their implications for understanding psychological mechanisms of health and illness discussed. Psychophysiological research relevant to health and illness will be discussed throughout this book. The material covered in this chapter will provide a basis for understanding such research.

## DEFINITION

Psychophysiology is not synonymous with physiological psychology. Both refer to the study of the relationships between psychological and bodily events; however, the methods for studying them and the types of relationships studied differ. Specifically, psychophysiology attempts to manipulate mental, emotional, or behavioral conditions while monitoring physiological events. Physiological psychology, on the other hand, manipulates some physiological variable (e.g., stimulation of or lesion production in brain structures) and observes the effect on behavior. Measuring the blood pressure during interpersonal conflict is psychophysiological, whereas producing a lesion in a rat's lateral hypothalamus and measuring changes in defecation rate in an open field test is physiological psychology. A definition of psychophysiology proposed by Sternbach (1966) is

> the study of the interrelationships between the physiological aspects of behavior. It typically employs *human* subjects whose physiological responses are usually recorded on a polygraph *while stimuli are presented which are designed to influence mental, emotional or motor behavior* and the investigator need not be a psychologist. (p. 3)

Although this chapter focuses on psychophysiology, the concepts and techniques in physiological psychology have also been used in an attempt to identify possible psychobiological mechanisms of health and illness. This is particularly true for pain and coronary heart disease, as will be discussed in later chapters.

## BASIC PRINCIPLES OF THE NERVOUS AND ENDOCRINE SYSTEMS

### Nervous System

The nervous system includes the central nervous system (CNS) and the peripheral or autonomic nervous system, comprising the cranial and spinal nerves. The CNS includes all the neural cells within the bony enclosure of the spinal cord and the skull, whereas the autonomic nervous system (ANS) includes the neurons outside these structures. The ANS is further differentiated into the sympathetic and parasympathetic divisions. Anatomically, the sympathetic division originates within the thoracic and lumbar regions of the spinal cord; the parasympathetic division originates in the cranial and sacral regions.

Functionally, the CNS is primarily responsible for receiving and processing sensory information and regulating bodily movement. The ANS, in general, regulates the viscera and glands. It is commonly argued that the sympathetic division of the ANS is associated with bodily responses that mobilize the organism. More specifically, the sympathetic division has a catabolic function, facilitating internal processes that affect muscular efficiency (Van Toller, 1979). The parasympathetic division, however, is assumed to play a role in conserving energy (an anabolic function) and generally functions to conserve, accumulate, and store energy (Van Toller, 1979). Although this dual function of the two divisions of the ANS has been argued by several investigators, there are several exceptions, and some researchers propose that there is no anatomical basis for such an antagonistic action between the sympathetic and parasympathetic divisions (cf. Van Toller, 1979).

As illustrated in Figure 4-1, the autonomic fibers innervate all the major organ systems in the body. A major anatomical difference between the sympathetic and parasympathetic divisions is the innervation pathway of fibers from each system. Most of the sympathetic fibers travel directly to the sympathetic chain or sympathetic ganglia, where they synapse with other nerves. These are the preganglionic fibers. Postganglionic fibers travel from the sympathetic chain to specific end organs. Parasympathetic fibers, however, synapse near their end organs rather than traveling first to the sympathetic chain. Figure 4-1 indicates that certain end organs are innervated by only one division of the ANS. The sweat glands, peripheral blood vessels, and adrenal glands are innervated exclusively by sympathetic fibers. However, as the figure illustrates, most end organs are innervated by both the sympathetic and parasympathetic divisions; the reaction produced by one is opposite to that produced by the other. Table 4-1 lists the different effects of each division and the main receptor types. These two types, alpha- and beta-receptors, are stimulated by the sympathetic branch but have opposite actions. The alpha-adrenergic receptors are associated with functions that are inhibited during sympathetic activation, whereas the beta-adrenergic receptors are associated with functions that are stimulated during sympathetic activation (Van Toller, 1979).

### Endocrine System

Claude Bernard argued that the fluid bathing the cells must be controlled by some complex regulatory system because of the stability of

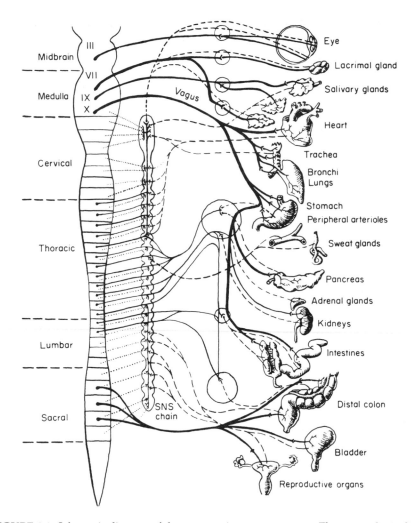

**FIGURE 4-1.** Schematic diagram of the autonomic nervous system. The sympathetic division is made of up those fibers that leave the spinal cord in the middle region (— — —) and (———). The parasympathetic division consists of those fibers originating from the upper and lower parts of the spinal cord (▬▬▬). From *Principles of Psychophysiology: An Introductory Text and Readings* (p. 16) by R. A. Sternbach. Copyright 1966 by Academic Press, Inc. Reprinted by permission.

this *milieu organique interieur,* or internal environment, relative to the fluctuations characteristic of the external environment. The stability observed by Bernard and others is indeed maintained by a complex system of feedback mechanisms within the CNS, endocrine system, and ANS.

Although these regulatory systems appear at first glance to be somewhat independent in that biological information is transmitted by nerve impulse in the CNS and ANS and by blood in the endocrine system, and in that CNS and ANS responses are more localized and rapid relative to hormonal responses, the three systems comprise an interdependent network responsible for the integration and coordination of the metabolic activities of the organism. We will briefly review the structure of this "system," along with the various hormones and their function while discussing regulation by hormonal activity. Given the critical role of neurohumoral activity in the psychobiological mechanisms of a number of psychological or behavioral processes relevant to health and illness (e.g., emotion, eating, motor activity, addiction, learning, perception), a basic understanding of the endocrine system is important.

As Figure 4-2 illustrates, the integrative center for autonomic-endocrine activity is the hypothalamus, although the amygdala and hippocampus are also important at a higher level within the central nervous system. Along with its nervous system functions, the hypothalamus is the site of synthesis for several polypeptide hormones. The nervous and endocrine systems interact most closely at the hypothalamus. At the upper portion of the figure, one can identify the neurons responsible for secreting hypothalamic-releasing factors (HRF), releasing factors or hormones that enter the portal circulation to regulate the activity of the anterior pituitary cells. Neurotransmitter substances such as norepinephrine (NE) and 5 hydroxytryptamine (5HT) are found in cell bodies in the brain stem and affect activity in the neurons which secrete the various releasing factors or hormones. Dopamine (the precursor of epinephrine and norepinephrine), acetylcholine (predominantly from parasympathetic neurons), and serotonin are also important regulatory neurotransmitters that are active in this region.

The supraoptic (SO) and paraventricular (PV) nuclei, two well-defined groups of hypothalamic cells, produce vasopressin and oxytocin. These hormones are not released into the general (systemic) circulation until they have reached the neurohypophysis. The SO nucleus, an "osmoreceptor," reacts to changes in osmolality of the fluid surrounding it. The osmoreceptor has a variable "set-point," which regulates its output. The concept of set-point is used to explain the regulation of many hormones.

The adenohypophysis contains several different types of cells. The hormone-producing cells include (1) somatotroph or growth hormone (GH); (2) lactotroph or prolactin (PR); (3) corticotroph or adrenocorticotropin (ACTH), and its precursor polypeptide-lipotropin, that give rise to a number of fragments, including endorphins and enkephalins; (4) thyrotroph, which produces thyroid-stimulating hormone (TSH);

**TABLE 4-1**
Effects of Stimulation on the Autonomic Nervous System

| | Parasympathetic effects | Main receptor type | Sympathetic effects |
|---|---|---|---|
| **Eye** | | | |
|   Iris | Contraction of sphincter pupillae; pupil size decreases | $\alpha$ | Contraction of dilator pupillae; pupil size increases |
|   Ciliary muscle | Contraction; accommodation for near vision | $\beta$ | Relaxation; accommodation for distant vision |
| Lacrimal gland | Secretion | | Excessive secretion |
| Salivary glands | Secretion of watery saliva in copious amounts | $\alpha$ | Scanty secretion of mucus-rich saliva |
| **Respiratory system** | | | |
|   Conducting division | Contraction of smooth muscle; decreased diameters and volumes | | Relaxation of smooth muscle; increased diameter and volumes |
|   Respiratory division | Effects same as on conducting division | | Effect same as on conducting division |
|   Blood vessels | Constriction | | Dilation |
| **Heart** | | | |
|   Stroke volume | Decreased | $\beta$ | Increased |
|   Stroke rate | Decreased | $\beta$ | Increased |
|   Cardiac output and blood pressure | Decreased | $\beta$ | Increased |
|   Coronary vessels | Constriction | | Dilation |
| **Peripheral blood vessels** | | | |
|   Skeletal muscle | Constriction | $\alpha,\beta$ | Dilation |
|   Skin | Dilation | $\alpha$ | Constriction |
|   Visceral organs (except heart and lungs) | Dilation | $\alpha,\beta$ | Constriction |
| **Stomach** | | | |
|   Wall | Increased motility | $\beta$ | Decreased motility |
|   Sphincters | Inhibited | $\alpha$ | Stimulated |
|   Glands | Secretion stimulated | | Secretion inhibited |
| **Intestines** | | | |
|   Wall | Increased motility | $\alpha,\beta$ | Decreased motility |
|   Sphincters | | | |
|     Pyloric, iliocoecal, | Inhibited | $\alpha$ | Stimulated |
|     internal anal | Inhibited | | Stimulated |

**TABLE 4-1** (*Continued*)

| | Parasympathetic effects | Main receptor type | Sympathetic effects |
|---|---|---|---|
| Liver | Promotes glycogenesis, promotes bile secretion | | Promotes glycogenolysis, decreases bile secretion |
| Pancreas (exocrine and endocrine) | Stimulates secretion | | Inhibits secretion |
| Spleen | Little effect | | Contraction and emptying of stored blood into circulation |
| Adrenal medulla | Little effect | | Epinephrine secretion |
| Urinary bladder | Stimulates wall, inhibits sphincter | $\alpha,\beta$ | Inhibits wall, stimulates sphincter |
| Uterus | Little effect | | Inhibits motility of nonpregnant organ; stimulates pregnant organ |
| Sweat glands | Normal function | $\alpha$ | Stimulates secretion (produces "cold sweat" when combined with cutaneous vaso-constriction) |

*Note.* From *The Nervous Body: An Introduction to the Autonomic Nervous System and Behavior* (pp. 30–31) by C. Van Toller. Copyright 1979 by C. Van Toller. Reprinted by permission of the author and John Wiley & Sons, Ltd.

and (5) gonadotroph, which produces follicle-stimulating (FSH) and luteinizing (LH) hormones.

For simplicity, let us consider the neuroendocrine system as comprised of five general subsystems: the *adrenal medullary axis*, the *adrenal cortical axis*, the *somatotrophic axis*, the *thyroid axis*, and the *posterior pituitary axis*.

The hypothalamus, through the spinal cord to the celiac ganglion and on to the adrenal medulla, regulates the release of two major substances into the circulation: epinephrine and norepinephrine. The effect of these catecholamines, in general, is similar to that of direct sympathetic stimulation, although it is delayed some 20 to 30 seconds. The

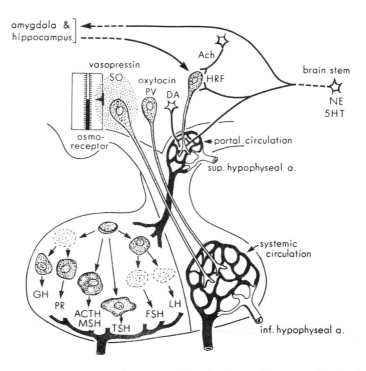

**FIGURE 4-2.** Integrative center for autonomic-endocrine activity. From *Systematic Endocrinology* edited by C. Ezrin, J. O. Godden, and R. Volpe. Copyright 1979 by Harper & Row Publishers, Inc. Reprinted by permission.

adrenergic sympathetic response, however, is prolonged by a factor of ten in contrast to direct neural stimulation (Usdin, Kretnansky, & Kopin, 1976). Cholinergic responses (electrodermal activity, bronchiole activity) are not affected by adrenal medulla hormones.

At the level of the adrenal cortical axis, neurosecretory cells release corticotropin-releasing factor (CRF) into the hypothalamic hypophyseal portal system to cells sensitive to CRF in the anterior pituitary. These cells release ACTH into the systemic circulation, which eventually reaches the adrenal cortex. Adrenocorticotropin is assumed to act at three distinct sites of the adrenal cortex to stimulate the release of glucocorticoids, including cortisol and cortiosterone, into the circulation to increase glucose production (gluconeogenesis), urea production, and free fatty acid production and possibly suppress immune mechanisms and stimulate keton synthesis (Everly & Rosenfeld, 1981). The secretion of mineralocorticoids, including aldosterone and deoxycorticosterone, is also triggered by ACTH to regulate electrolytes and blood pressure through sodium reabsorption (Guyton, 1979).

The somatotropic axis involves the release of somatotropin releasing factor (SRF), which stimulates the anterior pituitary to release GH. Growth hormone can be released in response to psychological stimuli (Selye, 1976) and may stimulate the release of mineralocorticoids; it has a diabeticlike insulin-resistant effect and mobilizes fats to increase free fatty acids and glucose in the blood (Yuwiler, 1976).

The thyroid axis involves thyrotropin releasing factor (TRF), which is transported to the anterior pituitary to effect the release of TSH into the systemic circulation, which, in turn, stimulates the thyroid gland to release thyroxine into the blood. Thyroxine increases the general metabolic rate, the heart rate, heart contractility, peripheral vascular resistance, and the sensitivity of some tissues to catecholamines (Levi, 1972). The final axis is the posterior pituitary or neurohypophysis, which releases vasopressin (antidiuretic hormone, ADH) and oxytocin to influence water retention and milk production during lactation, respectively.

Neuroendocrine activity is regulated by an intricate network of feedback loops to maintain homeostasis. We will discuss in detail the concept of feedback in Chapter 6. Let us simply indicate that in negative feedback, as factor A increases, factor B decreases, to effect a net balance. A thermostat is an example of such a feedback loop or interaction. As the temperature decreases, the thermostat registers that a threshold has been reached, at which point the heating system is activated until a preset level is reached. Deviations from that level initiate the negative feedback process. Positive feedback loops are also involved in endocrine regulation, when increases in factor A result in increases in factor B. These loops can suddenly increase hormone levels, and can lead to an unstable condition, but they are usually further regulated by negative feedback loops (Rasmussen, 1974). The constant interaction between the nervous system and endocrine system at multiple levels involves such feedback mechanisms.

## BIOLOGICAL RESPONSE SYSTEMS

Several responses can be monitored to determine activity in the CNS, the ANS, and the endocrine system. These responses have been broadly categorized as cardiovascular; skeletal muscle; electrodermal; electrocortical; biochemical; and miscellaneous, which includes respiration, temperature, salivation, pupillary activity, and gastric motility.

Mood and behavior are frequently recorded in psychophysiological research to monitor psychological concomitants or determinants of physiological state. It is important for the reader to realize that the response(s) chosen by the psychophysiologist is based upon a set of assumptions regarding the theoretical importance of that response (1) in the etiology, exacerbation, or maintenance of some illness; (2) as a representative measure of some biological activity, as in the case of a general index of sympathetic activity; and (3) as indicative of a specific end-organ response, such as vasoconstriction, which is important in understanding some psychobiological process. That is, the psychophysiologist does not simply record a response because it is simple to measure. The response(s) must relate to the problem studied. Because of the modern technological advances in electrophysiological and biochemical monitor-

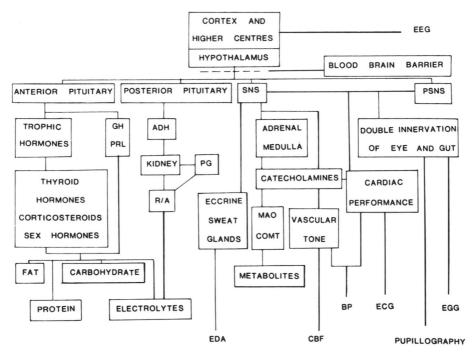

**FIGURE 4-3.** Physiological and biochemical measures and schematic representation of their anatomical basis. SNS, sympathetic nervous system; PSNS, parasympathetic nervous system; GH, growth hormone; PRL, prolactin; ADH, antidiuretic hormone; PG, prostaglandins; R/A, renin-angiotensin; MAO, monoamine oxidase; COMT, catecholamine-o-methyl transferase; EDA, electrodermal activity; CBF, capillary blood flow; BP, blood pressure; EEG, electroencephalogram; ECG, electrocardiogram; EGG, electrogastrogram. From *Techniques in Psychophysiology* (p. 461) edited by I. Martin and P. H. Venables. Copyright 1980 by John Wiley & Sons, Limited. Reprinted by permission.

ing, it is possible to use these measures as a sensitive window to intact human psychobiological functioning to obtain information that was previously unavailable. Figure 4-3 shows a complex set of the responses psychophysiologists measure and their underlying anatomical and/or physiological, electromechanical, and biochemical bases that provide an index of activity in a specific physiological system or set of systems. A general working knowledge of the physiological basis of such measures permits a greater appreciation of the biological significance of findings in human psychophysiological research.

We will briefly review the major response systems in terms of their characteristics, underlying physiological basis, and recording methodology. A more detailed presentation of these systems can be found in several textbooks in psychophysiology (Andreassi, 1980; Greenfield & Sternbach, 1972; Grings & Dawson, 1978; Hassett, 1978; Martin & Venables, 1980).

In general, most psychophysiological measures are monitored by a specialized recording device, the polygraph. In recent years, the polygraph is often interfaced with computerized data acquisition systems and miniaturized electronics, but the basic concept is the same. This concept can be best understood through an analogy with the common stereo component system, as discussed by Kallman and Feuerstein (1977):

> The record has a groove that has mechanical ridges pressed on it. The stylus converts the physical distortions on the surface of the record to an electrical signal that is amplified and converted back to a mechanical signal at the speaker. Physiological recording instrumentation works on a similar principle. The components are an input transducer (e.g., electrodes or specialized sensors), amplifier, and an output transducer for converting the amplified electrical signal into a usable visual or auditory form. (p. 331)

Figure 4-4 illustrates a typical recording system, schematically. At present, most systems interface with some type of computer that converts the fluctuating analogue signals to digital form and then plots the digital data.

## Cardiovascular System

Responses within the cardiovascular system that psychophysiologists most frequently measure include heart rate, blood pressure, and vasomotor activity. The cardiac muscle contains pacing cells that stimulate the muscle fibers to contract in a rhythmical manner. The rate of firing of these pacemaker cells can be excited by sympathetic fibers from the cervical and thoracic region of the spinal cord or inhibited by parasympathetic fibers of the vagus nerve. The firing rate is decreased by

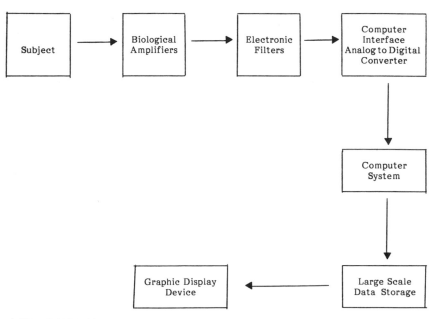

**FIGURE 4-4.** Schematic representation of physiological recording and signal processing system.

vagal stimulation, whereas blocking vagal input increases the firing rate. Heart rate, a common measure in psychophysiological research, represents the number of contractions or cycles of the heart rhythm per unit of time, usually expressed in beats per minute. Both the sympathetic and parasympathetic divisions of the ANS influence heart rate. Contractions of the heart are associated with large voltage changes or electrical potentials. The electrocardiogram (ECG) is a measure of these electrical potentials. Figure 4-5 illustrates the various components of the ECG and what they represent in terms of nerve conduction through the heart. For our present purposes, let us focus on the R wave. Heart rate is frequently computed by monitoring R waves over a period of time. Either the heart rate is measured directly from a tally of R waves by some electronic system, or hardware and/or software is used to measure the time between successive R waves in milliseconds; this time is the interbeat interval (IBI) or heart period (HP). Longer IBIs or HPs indicate a slower heart rate.

Each time the smooth (cardiac) muscle of the heart contracts and forces blood out of the heart, the pressure of the blood against the walls of the arteries increases. As the heart relaxes and fills with blood, this pressure decreases. The maximum pressure, which occurs when the heart contracts, is the *systolic blood pressure* (SBP). The *diastolic blood pressure* (DBP) is the minimum pressure when the heart relaxes. Blood pressure is determined by several factors, including viscosity of the blood, plasticity of the blood vessels, strength and rate of cardiac contractions, and volume of blood in the system relative to total volume. A formula for determining blood pressure is as follows:

blood pressure = cardiac output × peripheral resistance

Therefore, rises in blood pressure are influenced by cardiac output or the amount of blood being pumped and the resistance by the vascular system to the flow of blood (peripheral resistance). There are several areas in the cardiovascular system at which the sympathetic and the parasympathetic branches of the ANS exert influence. The CNS is also

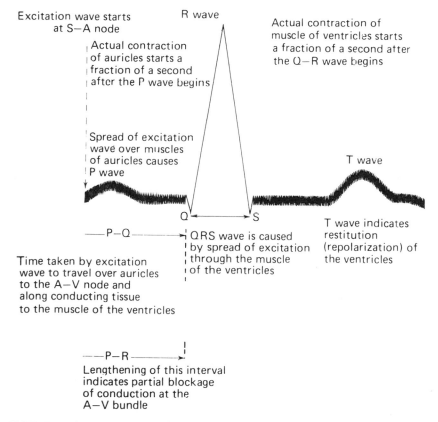

**FIGURE 4-5.** Components of the electrocardiogram. From *Structure and Function in Man* by S. W. Jacob and C. A. Francone (2nd ed.). Copyright 1970 by W. B. Saunders Co. Reprinted by permission.

involved in blood pressure regulation. Figure 4-6 illustrates the complex mechanisms involved.

Human blood pressure is measured with a *sphygmomanometer*, which is the instrument the physician uses in the office. Several modifications of this basic device automatically inflate and record pressure at set intervals and provide digital (numerical) displays of both systolic and diastolic blood pressure. There are also portable devices that can be used by patients to monitor blood pressure. The basic principle of all these devices is the occlusion of blood flow through the artery by an air-filled cuff; the air is gradually released until the sound of the blood flowing through the artery with each heart beat is heard, either through a stethoscope or by way of an electronic circuit. Systolic pressure is the

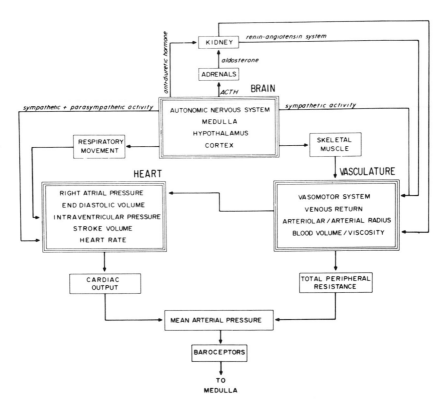

**FIGURE 4-6.** Physiological mechanisms of blood pressure regulation. From "Learned Control of Physiological Function and Disease" by D. Shapiro and R. S. Surwit in *Handbook of Behavior Modification and Behavior Therapy* edited by H. Leitenberg. Copyright 1976 by Prentice-Hall, Inc. Reprinted by permission.

point, expressed in millimeters of mercury (mm Hg), at which the sound of the blood (Korotkoff sounds) is first heard. The point at which the Korotkoff sounds disappear is the diastolic pressure. The sound of the blood flow is no longer perceptible at the diastolic point because the cuff no longer interferes with the blood flow. Blood pressure can fluctuate considerably with each heart beat; therefore, continuous noninvasive measurement of human blood pressure is important if one is interested in its fluctuations. Certain techniques have been developed, including an arterial pulse wave velocity measurement, that record relative changes in blood pressure on a beat-by-beat basis.

Vasomotor activity represents the distribution of blood to organs and muscles. Blood vessels constrict and dilate. When a blood vessel is constricted, blood flow decreases. When the vessels dilate, blood flow increases. The systemic distribution of blood varies as a function of demand at any given time. For example, blood volume may decrease in the periphery (hands, feet) and increase in the skeletal muscles of the forearm during situations requiring some manual act. The vessels in the periphery of the hands and toes are innervated by sympathetic fibers.

Blood volume can be recorded using a device known as a plethysmometer. Although there are several types of plethysmographic devices, a commonly used unit is the photoelectric plethysmograph which detects the amount of light transmitted through tissue at the skin surface, which is a function of the amount of blood in the tissue area. This transmitted light is converted to current and changes in voltage are recorded by specialized amplifiers. Vasomotor activity has two components: blood volume and blood volume pulse. Blood volume, the tonic or basal component, represents the absolute level of blood in the tissue. The blood volume pulse represents the blood flow through the tissue with each cardiac contraction and is assumed to be the sum of the tonic blood volume and the phasic pulse volume (Brown, 1967).

## Electrodermal Activity

The electrical properties of the skin are regulated by the ANS, and various responses recorded from the skin provide a sensitive index of electrodermal activity. Specifically, electrodermal activity, to a large degree, represents activity in the sweat glands (Edelberg, 1972). Sweat glands are innervated exclusively by sympathetic postganglionic fibers. This exclusive sympathetic innervation makes electrodermal activity a particularly useful response system, in that it acts as a unidirectional index of sympathetic arousal or excitation. That is, as arousal increases, certain measures of electrodermal activity also increase.

The skin resistance response is the most commonly recorded measure of electrodermal activity. Galvanic skin resistance (GSR) (an earlier name) has been widely studied in psychology, particularly in research on emotion. The basic principle is simple—two electrodes are placed on the skin and a minute current is transmitted from one electrode through the skin to the second electrode. A biological amplifier is used to measure the resistance the current meets in traveling from electrode to electrode. Sweat gland and vasomotor activity affect the resistance of the skin such that the greater the sweat gland activity (minute concentrations of moisture), the lower the resistance, since sweat lowers resistance. Skin conductance, which is the reciprocal of skin resistance, is also frequently used to measure electrodermal activity. Here, a positive linear relationship is observed between skin conductance and sympathetic arousal, with higher conductance associated with greater sympathetic arousal. A set of measures of electrodermal activity that represent bioelectric potentials of the skin in the absence of an external current, skin potential measures, are also frequently recorded. All electrodermal measures (resistance, conductance, potential) are reported as either *levels* that represent tonic or baseline indices or *responses* that represent the phasic or the reaction component. Therefore, it is possible to find such terms in the research literature as skin resistance level, skin resistance response, skin conductance level, skin conductance response, skin potential level, and skin potential response.

### Skeletal Muscle Activity

Many etiological and clinical studies include measurements of skeletal muscle activity. Recordings are usually made from the skin surface; such measurements reflect the electrical activity of motor units. Surface recording of this type is not similar to diagnostic electromyograph (EMG) measurements, in which the emphasis is on recording nerve conduction or needle electrode recordings when data from single motor fibers are required. Electrodes placed on the skin over an active muscle reflect the algebraic sum of a large number of neuromuscular junction depolarizations, which occur when a group of motor units are activated (Lippold, 1967). This summed activity across a number of individual muscle fibers generates a signal that can be recorded by sensitive amplifiers and is referred to as the surface electromyograph (EMG). An example of the raw surface EMG is shown in Figure 4-7. The signal is often integrated to smooth or average the spike activity over time. Figure 4-7 also shows an integrated EMG, which reflects the fluctuations of the continuous raw potentials. Skeletal muscle activity is not innervated by autonomic fibers, but rather by the CNS.

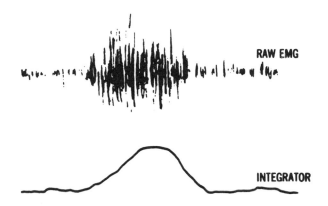

RAW EMG

INTEGRATOR

FIGURE 4-7. Representation of raw and integrated electromyographic recordings. From "Muscle Action Potentials—Raw Form and Integrated Form" in *Users Guide to: Operation, Specifications, Applications* (p. 45). Copyright 1984 by Coulbourn Instruments, Inc. Reprinted by permission.

## Electrocortical Activity

The electrical activity of the brain has been a focus of interest in psychophysiology since the development of the electroencephalographic recorder. Electrical activity is often recorded from surface electrodes on the scalp and is believed to represent activity from a group of cortical neurons in the area of the electrode. The electroencephalogram (EEG) represents a gross measure of the electrical activity of the cortex of the brain; EEG activity is classified in terms of frequency, or cycles per second (Hertz, Hz). Several frequency ranges have been identified, including delta waves (0.5–3.5 Hz), theta waves (4–7 Hz), alpha waves (8–13 Hz), and beta waves (14–30 Hz) (see Figure 4-8). Although controversial, certain investigations have suggested that the slower waveforms (i.e., delta and theta) are associated with a lower state of arousal, whereas the alpha wave is correlated with a "relaxed-alert" state. The beta wave is observed during extreme attentiveness or hyperalertness.

Although the percentage of total time of a given EEG frequency band (e.g., percent time alpha) is usually reported, more recent advances over the past decade have made power spectrum analysis available to a number of researchers. This technique is based upon the mathematical principles of the Fourier series, which argues that a complex waveform is "identical to the sum of a series of sine waves of varying amplitude and frequency" (Hassett, 1978, p. 113). Therefore, the complex waveforms of the EEG can be similarly reduced, using a Fourier transformation. The output of such an analysis graphically represents

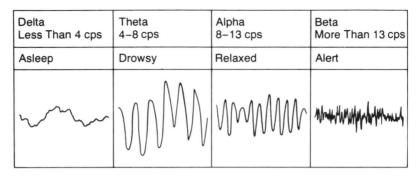

| Delta<br>Less Than 4 cps | Theta<br>4–8 cps | Alpha<br>8–13 cps | Beta<br>More Than 13 cps |
|---|---|---|---|
| Asleep | Drowsy | Relaxed | Alert |

FIGURE 4-8. Representation of electrocortical activity. Brain waves classified by frequency with behavioral labels for each frequency band representing the very gross distinctions typically discussed in arousal theory. From *A Primer of Psychophysiology* (p. 104) by J. Hassett. Copyright 1978 by W. H. Freeman & Co. Reprinted by permission.

the relative power or amplitude at different frequencies. This power spectrum analysis, in short, produces a graph indicating the amount of activity at given EEG frequencies for a large series of waves. The EMG (raw form) can also be analyzed using spectral analysis.

Other responses derived from the EEG, using a variety of recording and statistical procedures, have been developed. These, which include the sensory-evoked potential or response and contingent negative variation, are more promising as indices of cortical and subcortical responsivity than simple shifts in the frequencies of the EEG (Andreassi, 1980). A number of so-called event-related brain potentials (ERP) have been demonstrated to represent indices of the brain's response to both physical (i.e., intensity, sensory attributes) and psychological (i.e., meaning, significance) features of stimuli. These ERPs are stable in time for actual or anticipated environmental events. An excellent review of these brain potentials is found in Andreassi (1980). For our purposes, we will focus on the sensory-evoked potential or response or, more generally, the averaged evoked response (AER).

The AER can be triggered by sensory stimuli, including visual, auditory, somatosensory, and olfactory, or simply by the expectation that an event will occur at a given time. The AER is derived from the EEG according to the following principle. In the experimental paradigm for recording AERs, a stimulus event (e.g., visual, auditory) is presented to the subject at a set time for several hundred presentations while the EEG is continuously monitored. The event-related brain activity, or "response," is time-locked to the stimulus; the background EEG remains relatively constant over time. Therefore, through an averaging technique, the event-related potential or brain response can be extracted from the background "noise" of the EEG over several presentations.

The signal-to-noise ratio can be improved through additional trials or stimulus presentations. Figure 4-9 illustrates the outcome of such averaging. Although this procedure appears relatively simple, there are several theoretical and methodological complexities involved in such recordings that are beyond the scope of this book (see Picton, 1980).

As Figure 4-9 indicates, the AER has several components defined according to their time of occurrence (latencies), amplitude, and direction—negative (N) or positive (P). Each component is labeled in terms of direction and point of occurrence. For example, the first negative going wave is labeled N1, the second positive going wave, P2, and so on. In general, the earlier latency components reflect the brain's response to the sensory aspects of the stimulus (e.g., intensity), whereas the latter components (e.g., P300) reflect a variety of psychological processes, such as expectancy and attention (Andreassi, 1980). Researchers in pain perception have used the AER in an attempt to understand the differential input from sensory and psychological components of pain.

## Additional Responses

A number of other measures affected by the ANS have been used in psychophysiological research and treatment. These include respiration, peripheral temperature, salivation, sexual arousal (both sexes), pupil

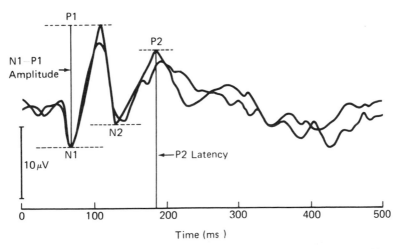

FIGURE 4-9. Averaged evoked response. Method for measuring amplitudes and latencies of AER components. The amplitude of the $N_1$-$P_1$ component (larger of the two traces) is 17.2μV based on the calibrated 10 μV signal. The $P_2$ latency is 190 msec. Each of these two ERPs was based on averaged responses to 100 light flashes on two different occasions. Negativity is downward. From *Psychophysiology: Human Behavior and Physiological Responses* (p. 78) by J. L. Andreassi. Copyright 1980 by W. B. Saunders Co. Reprinted by permission.

size, and gastric motility (Greenfield & Sternbach, 1972; Martin & Venables, 1980). In theory, any physiological response can be measured in psychophysiological research. The major limitations are the invasiveness of the technique and the availability of the instruments. With the recent rapid advances in biomedical recording technology, and the movement of psychophysiologists into relatively new areas of investigation (e.g., psychobiology of cancer and immune disorders), the area should witness an increase in the use of the newer medical technology in the next decade.

## Ambulatory Psychophysiology

Although the laboratory-based psychophysiological investigations, in general, have a significant degree of internal validity, many researchers and clinicians question the external validity or generalizability of such experiments, particularly with patient samples. Is exposure to a math stressor equivalent to an argument with the boss? Is role playing a marital argument with a female confederate equivalent to a typical argument with one's wife? The equivalence of such stimuli has not been resolved as yet, and many investigators have moved from the laboratory to the natural environment in an effort to measure the physiological effects of naturally occurring environmental events. Other issues prompt such shifts from the controlled laboratory to the relatively uncontrolled natural environment, especially for patients. That is, when there is an infrequent or periodic symptom, and one is trying to monitor psychophysiological changes before, during, and after the occurrence of the symptom, it is difficult to "trap" the symptom in order to record it in the laboratory. This observation may also suggest that the mechanism is not some characteristic trait, but rather an interaction of a trait and a situation, or that the symptom may vary according to some biological or chronobiological rhythm. These considerations require a methodology that can record continuous, 24-hour measures of the psychophysiological parameters of interest. A number of portable recording devices have been developed over the past decade to so measure heart rate, cardiac activity (the Holter Monitor), gross motor activity, blood pressure, skeletal muscle activity, and a variety of other responses.

One device that records up to 24 hours of continuous data was recently developed. It uses a commercially available recorder and adds specific amplifiers, transducers, and specialized circuitry (Feuerstein, Barr, & Ives, 1985). The system permits the recording of two channels of EMG, heart rate, gross motor activity, and self-reports of pain (pain onset, duration, severity) and mood. The unit is shown in Figure 4-10. Computer digitization and graphic display permit the identification of

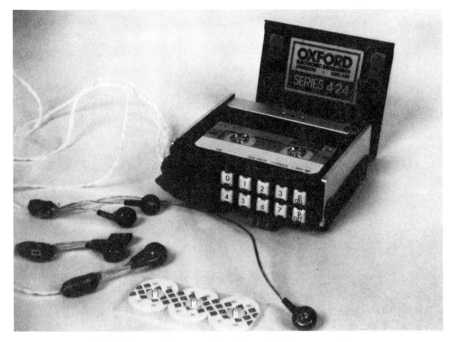

FIGURE 4-10. Photograph of the ambulatory recorder.

changes throughout the 12- or 24-hour recording period. Figure 4-11 illustrates such a graphic output from the system. The system is currently being used in psychophysiological research on naturally occurring stressors and recurrent abdominal pain in children and low back pain in adults.

## Biochemical Measures

As discussed in the section on the anatomy and physiology of the endocrine system, metabolic processes involved in normal biological functioning vary. In order to monitor these complex processes, samples of blood (plasma, serum, whole blood) or urine must be obtained. Although other body fluids, such as saliva and sweat, have been used in psychophysiological research (Christie & Woodman, 1980), their usefulness is limited. The measures that have been of most interest to psychophysiologists include catecholamines (epinephrine and norepinephrine) and adrenal cortical steroids.

Catecholamines are measured in either urine or plasma. Plasma permits the analysis of transient changes in secretion, although there are numerous complications associated with sampling from plasma

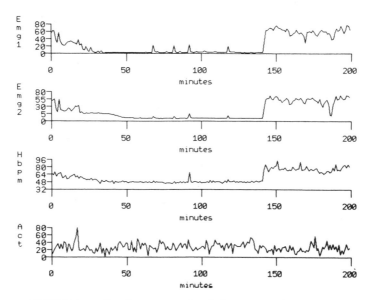

**FIGURE 4-11.** Graphic output of ambulatory recording system.

(Christie & Woodman, 1980). A variety of internal and external factors can affect catecholamine secretion and excretion; these include circadian rhythm, physical exertion, tea and coffee drinking, and cigarette smoking.

Adrenal cortical activity can be measured by determining the blood concentration of such substances as cortisol (Mason, 1972), which is a glucocorticoid; mineral corticoids, including aldosterone; and various androgens. The most common measure, and the major adrenocorticosteroid in human blood, is cortisol. Cortisol is a 17-hydroxy (−OH) corticosteroid (17-OHCS) compound. Cortisol is regulated via pituitary ACTH by circadian rhythm, the negative feedback system, and stress.

## BASIC CONCEPTS OF PSYCHOPHYSIOLOGY

This section will discuss the basic concepts of psychophysiology that are essential for understanding psychophysiological research, as well as health psychology. These concepts are especially relevant for studying the psychophysiology of emotion, motivation, learning, and stress. The psychophysiological measures and techniques described in the first section are used to define and validate some of the concepts to be discussed. There is no theoretical framework that organizes the following concepts, although psychophysiologists have attempted to show relationships between these concepts or have built major theories using these concepts.

## Orienting Response, Defensive Response, and Habituation

Imagine yourself walking down a school hallway and quite unexpectedly, a loud bell goes off. What would your initial response be? You might find that you would have "jumped" at the sound, your head and eyes shifted in the direction of the sound, your heart seemed to "stop," and other bodily changes may have occurred. Such a response to a novel stimulus is the *orienting response* (OR). A variety of simple environmental stimuli trigger or elicit this physiological response in humans and animals. Many physiological changes are involved in this seemingly simple response. Ongoing physical activity is arrested, muscle tone increases in preparation for action, sensory thresholds are lowered, pupils dilate, skin conductance increases, blood flow in the hands is reduced, superficial vessels in the head dilate, cortical activity increases, and heart rate decreases.

Sokolov (1963) has specified three conditions that must be met in order for a response to be characterized as an OR: The response must be (1) nonspecific with regard to the quality of the stimulus, (2) nonspecific with regard to the intensity of the stimulus, and (3) decrease in amplitude on repeated stimulation. A fourth criterion that the response must be locked to the onset of a "stimulus" has also been suggested. *Stimulus* is defined as a change in stimulation; therefore, onset as well as termination may be considered a stimulus. Generally, though, the response to onset is considered the OR if the response to stimulus termination habituates rapidly; a distinction has also been made between tonic and phasic OR. The OR as defined thus far is *phasic*, that is, a response produced on the presentation of a specific stimulus. *Tonic* ORs are responses observed over a relatively long period of time and are associated with an experimental paradigm. Decreases in tonic ORs are thought to be associated with a lowering of arousal or attention.

*Habituation* refers to the tendency of an OR to attenuate on repeated stimulation. In other words, the stimulus tends to lose its significance for the organism, and this is reflected by the decrease in magnitude of the OR, until there is very little or no response. An example of habituation follows: Suppose that while you are studying, you hear a loud noise that elicits an OR. After investigating the source of the noise, you discover that it is a carpenter hammering in your neighbor's house; you continue studying. The hammering sometimes startles you, but as you continue to study, you eventually do not notice it.

Psychophysiologists differentiate between the OR and the defensive response (DR). The *defensive response* is a complex physiological response to simple aversive or noxious environmental stimuli. Discrimination between the OR and DR is not validly made in all physiological systems. Note that the OR occurs with novel stimuli; the DR with intense, potentially painful stimuli. For example, in both responses there is generally a drop in skin resistance and a desynchronization of alpha (EEG) activity. Major differences between the OR and DR are found in (1) the heart, whereby the OR is associated with heart rate deceleration and the DR with heart rate acceleration and (2) the vascular system, whereby the arteries in the head dilate for the OR and constrict for the DR.

A classic study by Hare (1973) used psychophysiological measures to differentiate the OR from the DR. The heart rate and cephalic vasomotor activity of 10 female undergraduate students who feared spiders and 10 female undergraduate students who did not were recorded while they viewed various slides. Of the slides shown, 6 were slides of spiders and 24 were slides of neutral objects (such as landscapes). Hare found that the no fear group responded with an OR, that is, heart rate deceleration and cephalic vasodilation, when spider slides were shown. The fear group, however, responded with a DR, that is, increased heart rate and cephalic vasoconstriction. There was no appreciable cardiovascular response to the neutral stimuli. Figure 4-12 shows the results for heart rate.

## Modulators of Physiological Activitiy

*Cognitive Tasks, Response Requirement, and Implicit-Explicit Sets.* Researchers have found that physiological reactivity is observed during mental as well as physical activity. An example of a study that demonstrates this phenomenon is one in which college students were presented with arithmetic problems of varying difficulty (Kahneman, Tursky, Shapiro, & Crider, 1969). The subjects were asked to add a 0, 1, or 3 to a series of digits. While the students were solving the problem, heart rate, skin resistance, and pupil diameter were recorded. Each problem was paced so that a "ready" signal was given at second 1; at seconds 5 and 6, the instruction to add 0, 1, or 3 was given; at seconds 10 to 13, digits were given, and at seconds 15 to 18 the subjects solved the problem. It was found that all three physiological responses increased during problem solving, which indicated sympathetic arousal, and the responses decreased after the subjects finished. Also, all three responses increased to a greater degree when the subjects were solving the more difficult problem (adding 3). These results indicate that mental activity is associ-

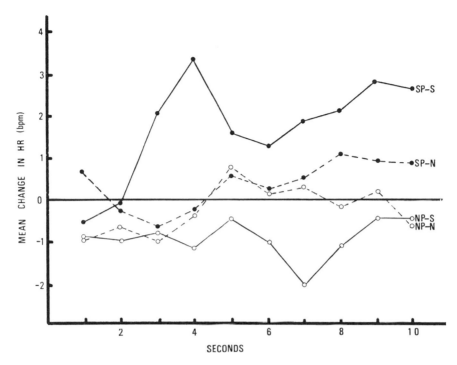

FIGURE 4-12. Example of heart rate changes to fearful and nonfearful stimuli. Mean second-by-second changes in HR shown by Groups SP and NP in response to the spider (S) and neutral (N) stimuli. From "Orienting and Defensive Responses to Visual Stimuli" by R. D. Hare, 1973, *Psychophysiology, 10,* 453–464. Copyright 1973 by the Society for Psychophysiological Research. Reprinted by permission.

ated with autonomic responses and that the responses are related to the degree of effort necessary to solve the problem.

A fairly consistent finding across studies of physiological reactivity during mental activity with response requirement is a pattern of physiological responses that generally includes increased heart rate and skin conductance. This response pattern is thought to occur when environmental *rejection* occurs and cognitive activity is the focus of attention. Recall Hare's study in which those students who feared spiders displayed a DR, with an increase in heart rate. Hare argues that when an aversive visual stimulus, such as those in the spider study, is used, the physiological changes that occur facilitate rejection of the stimulus to help the individual cope with it. It can be hypothesized that these women were "rejecting" the feared situation and engaging in some sort of cognitive process in order to cope with the feared stimulus. In general, then, when subjects are instructed to engage in problem solving or other mental activity, several convergent ANS responses occur, such as increases in heart rate and skin conductance.

It has also been found that a different pattern of physiological responses emerges when a subject is asked to only observe or attend to external stimuli. The pattern involves decreased heart rate and increased skin conductance and is thought to reflect a form of environmental intake as opposed to environmental rejection. Lacey (1959) suggested that cardiac deceleration facilitates the intake of environmental stimuli, whereas cardiac acceleration is associated with attempts to reject or exclude those stimuli that could disrupt the performance of some cognitive function. The divergent response of decreased heart rate and increased skin conductance is called *directional fractionation* of autonomic responses. Directional fractionation describes a stimulus situation in which the direction of change in physiological activity is contrary to the view that ANS responses must co-vary.

The subjects' attentional sets and attitude regarding the stimulus can also influence physiological reactivity. Set and attitude predispose to certain responses. Essentially, the *attitude* that is made *explicit* by the experimenter or that is *implicit* because of the attitudes and background of the subject or the characteristics of the experimental situation can influence physiological reactivity. Sternbach (1964) has studied the effect of explicit sets on physiological responding. Six subjects agreed to participate in a "drug" study involving three experimental sessions. Each subject was told that he would ingest three different pills that would have different effects on stomach activity. The effects would not last long and there would be no side effects. Each subject was given a placebo that contained a small magnet that recorded gastric activity. The pills were described as a relaxant, stimulant, or placebo. The results indicated that the overall effect of the instructions was statistically significant when four of the six subjects showed changes in the rate of stomach contractions according to their instructions (i.e., relaxant—stomach full and relaxed; stimulant—churning and some cramps; placebo—no change).

The research on *implicit sets* is best exemplified by a study by Sternbach and Tursky (1965) on ethnic differences regarding pain expression. The study was based on a report that behavioral expressions of pain differ among ethnic groups of patients in medical settings, in particular, Irish, Italian, Jewish, and Yankee (third-generation Americans). These differences were thought to occur because of implicit sets related to orientation in values of the ethnic groups. The Yankees tended to respond to pain in a matter-of-fact way and acted as if they should be good, noncomplaining patients. The Irish were similar in their pain expressions, because of their tight inhibition and control, yet their suffering comes through to the observer. On the other hand, the overt expression of pain is approved within their subcultures for Jews and Italians, and it elicits sympathetic responses from family and friends. For the Italians, pain is an evil to be avoided, and outer expressions are aimed at the elimination of pain. For the Jews, the concern is with the memory of pain and its implications. Housewives served as subjects for the study, with fifteen in each "ethnic" group. Electrical pain stimulation threshold was measured for all subjects and the skin potential on repeated brief shocks recorded. Figure 4-13 shows the skin potential habituation curves to electric shock for the four groups. The results indicate that the Yankee group habituated more rapidly and more completely than the other groups. These findings support the notion that implicit sets or attitudes can influence physiological reactivity significantly.

*Organismic Variables.* Much research in human psychophysiology is characterized by significant human variability in physiological response patterns. A number of sources for this variability have been identified; these include differences in time of day of recording, phase in menstrual cycle, and recording methodology. Although these and other

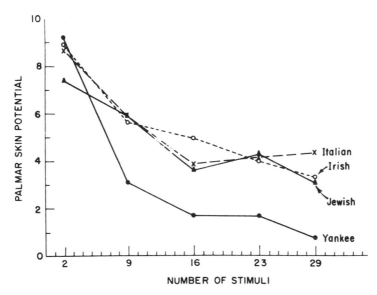

**FIGURE 4-13.** Habituation curves to electric shock in different subculture groups. From "Ethnic Differences among Housewives in Psychophysical and Skin Potential Responses to Electric Shock" by R. A. Sternbach and B. Tursky, 1965, *Psychophysiology, 1,* 241–246. Copyright 1965 by the Society for Psychophysiological Research. Reprinted by permission.

sources of variability have been identified, and attempts have been made to control them, it is increasingly evident that these so-called person variables, or characteristics of the individual, interact with the stimulus situation to influence physiological response patterns. The interaction of organismic variables with the stimuli and response pattern is depicted in Figure 4-14. Factors within the individual may include anxiety, hostility, extroversion–introversion, augmentation–reduction, field dependency, repression–sensitization, and sensation seeking. These factors will be briefly discussed and examples provided.

Anxiety is an often-studied phenomenon. A distinction is made between state and trait anxiety. *State anxiety* is thought of as situational, whereas *trait anxiety* is characteristic of the individual. The stereotypical person who is chronically anxious is described as having sweaty palms and a rapid heart rate and "shaky." Individuals with elevated scores on measures of anxiety, indicating anxiety as a trait, have been studied. High scorers on a Manifest Anxiety Scale were compared to low scorers (Haywood & Spielberger, 1966). Comparisons of sweat prints before and after the tasks indicated that trait anxiety tends to be associated with a higher palmar sweat index, which is suggestive of sympathetic arousal.

*Hostility,* as defined by a subscale of the Minnesota Multiphasic Personality Inventory (MMPI), may affect systolic blood pressure and skin conductance in a situation designed to increase frustration (Hokanson, 1961). The effects of anger and hostility on health have been a recent focus for health psychologists and will be discussed in later chapters.

Another concept relating to personality is extroversion–introversion. *Extroverts* are described as showing a strong interest in people, whereas *introverts* tend to withdraw from social contacts. Eysenck (1967) described a theory of personality that directly relates extroversion with the dimension of excitation and inhibition and predicts physiological reactions to environmental stimuli. Extroverts are assumed to have greater physiological inhibition or attenuation of physiological response to stimuli, whereas introverts display a heightened level of physiological excitation. Some psychophysiological evidence supports this theory, for

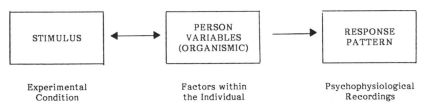

**FIGURE 4-14.** Interaction of stimulus and person variables.

example, one study observed that introverts had chronically larger pupil diameters and exhibited larger pupillary changes when "taboo" words were presented (Stelmack & Mandelzya, 1975).

A person's perceptual set (i.e., style in which stimulus information is processed) may also influence physiological reactivity. One type of perceptual style is characterized by individuals who overestimate the size of a stimulus (augmenters) as by those who underestimate the size of a stimulus (reducers). Another type of perceptual style involves individuals who are field dependent, that is, who are influenced by the context of a stimulus to such a degree that they cannot accurately position the stimulus without the surroundings, or who are field independent, that is, who are less influenced by contextual cues. Studies in both augmentation–reduction and field dependence–independence have shown that these organismic variables influence physiological reactivity. The concept of repression–sensitization suggests that individuals differ in the way they cognitively cope with threatening stimuli. Denying or repressing thoughts about a threatening stimulus characterize a *repressor*. Focusing on a threatening stimulus, conversely, characterizes a *sensitizer*. It has been shown that repressors "deny" their own negative feelings, and this is associated with an increase in physiological responsivity (Weinberger, Schwartz, & Davidson, 1979). In a classic study by Lazarus and Alfert (1964), in which subjects viewed a film that involved a primitive ritual found to induce sympathetic nervous system reactions, it was observed that, by presenting a narrative focusing on repression and denial before the film was shown, the repressors denied affective disturbance, although they showed a greater degree of autonomic reactivity (basal skin conductance and heart rate).

Another example of an organismic variable is *sensation seeking*. Individuals tend to differ in terms of their optimal level of stimulation, such that some individuals seek environmental variety and stimulation to a greater degree than others. Neary and Zuckerman (1976) found that high scorers on a sensation-seeking scale had larger initial ORs to novel stimuli than low scorers, although both groups habituated rapidly to repetitive presentations of the stimulus.

## Autonomic Balance

Since the beginning of recorded history, attempts have been made to classify individuals in regard to physiological disposition. In the early 1900s, individuals were characterized according to their tendency to respond in a sympathetic-like or a parasympathetic-like direction. The *sympatheticotonic* individual was characterized by a sympathetic response, such as a rapid heart rate, dilated pupils, and clammy hands, and described behaviorally as lively and excitable; the *vagatonic* individual was characterized by a parasympathetic response (involving the vagus nerve), such as a slow heart rate, constricted pupils, and dry skin, and described behaviorally as reserved and cold-blooded. Over the past 30 to 40 years, attempts to classify individuals with regard to psychophysiological dispositions have become more sophisticated. Although this work has lost its momentum, this type of research may prove important in advancing our knowledge of disease processes and developing diagnostic procedures.

The work of Wenger (1972) on *autonomic balance* represents the earliest sophisticated attempt at categorization. The concept of autonomic balance is used to describe human behavior and physiological reactivity within the context of the ANS. Imbalance is the extent to which the sympathetic or parasympathetic division is dominant in a given individual. Essentially, Wenger's approach was to measure 7 physiological responses (originally 20) under resting or tonic conditions. These responses included (1) palmar skin conductance, (2) forearm skin conductance, (3) salivation, (4) heart period, (5) pulse pressure, (6) respiration rate, and (7) red dermographia (persistance of red skin after stroking with a stimulator). Wenger combined these responses into a single composite score for each individual, the *autonomic balance score* or Ā. An evenly balanced ANS was represented by an average Ā score of 70; low Ā scores were less than 70 and indicated sympathetic dominance and high Ā scores were greater than 70 and indicated parasympathetic dominance.

Other studies by Wenger lend some validity to the concept of autonomic balance. The distribution of Ā scores were found to be normally distributed for a large sample of children and adults (Wenger, 1941, 1948). In a study with children, Wenger found that high Ā scorers were more emotionally inhibited, more patient, less excitable, and neater than low Ā scorers. Thus, children with parasympathetic dominance tended to be calmer, children with sympathetic dominance more excitable. A large-scale study in which 2,112 Air Force cadets were tested and assigned Ā scores found that 20 years following initial testing, those who developed high blood pressure, those who became apprehensive and anxious, and those who sweated excessively and had heart trouble had had low Ā scores. The Ā score also reflects phasic reactions to stimuli. Smith and Wenger (1965) measured Ā scores in a group of graduate students the day of an oral exam and found the scores to be lower, indicating sympathetic predominance, in contrast to scores measured one month before or after the exam. Although Wenger has obtained data supporting the sympathetic–parasympathetic dichotomy, such response styles are not observed as often as the Ā concept suggests. Many individuals demonstrate a *mixed pattern* of responses.

It is surprising that further work with the Ā score has not been reported. Research with infants conducted by developmental psychologists (Thomas, Chess, & Burch, 1970) is consistent with the notion of behavioral dispositions or temperaments that may be related to such physiological reactivity. Thomas *et al.* have found fairly consistent behavioral differences between infants and have described the "difficult to manage baby" (excitable and irritable), the "slow to warm up baby" (inhibited and less irritable), and the "easygoing baby" (a good balance between excitability and inhibition).

## Stimulus, Individual Response, and Symptom Stereotypy

More emphasis has been placed on the *pattern* of ANS responses than on a single level or measure, such as the Ā score (e.g., Ax 1953; Lacey, Kagan, Lacey, & Moss, 1963; Engel, 1972). Autonomic response patterns or stereotypes are thought of as clusterings of psychophysiological responses into specific patterns characteristic of individuals (individual-response stereotypy), stimulus situations (stimulus stereotypy), or a particular psychophysiological disorder (symptom stereotypy).

*Stimulus–response stereotypy*, sometimes called specificity, refers to a patterning of physiological responses associated with a particular stimulus situation. In essence, an individual's pattern of physiological activity will be constant in a given situation and the pattern of response will tend to vary as the stimulus situation changes. Stimuli that evoke various emotions have been studied, since researchers want to know whether a given emotion is associated with a specific physiological pattern and, if it is, whether different emotions have varying physiological patterns that may contribute to the emotion. Varying stimuli have been used, including pictures or slides assumed to elicit various emotions, experimental confederates and imagery, all designed to evoke a particular emotional state. Relationships between emotional imagery and physiological response have been reported by several investigators (e.g., Lang, Melamed, & Hart, 1970). Subjects in the Lang *et al.* study were spider phobic and socially anxious individuals as assessed by questionnaire and interview. These investigators found significantly greater sympathetic activation during imagined fearful scenes than neutral scenes. The fear ratings of imaginal scenes randomly chosen from a hierarchy of fearful situations constructed by the subject and experimenter and the heart rate were closely related.

In an early study, Ax (1953) used actual situations in which the experimenter attempted to induce fear in subjects by "accidentally shocking" them. Anger was produced by insulting and criticizing the same subjects. Ax reported greater increases in skin conductance levels and respiration rates in response to the fear rather than the anger situation. A different pattern for anger emerged, with increases in EMG, diastolic blood pressure, and greater decreases in heart rate.

Schwartz (1975) studied the relationship between emotions and facial muscle activity. The subjects were instructed to imagine happy, sad, and angry situations while EMG recordings were made from four facial muscle groups. Figure 4-15 shows the muscles of interest, including the frontalis, corrugator, massetor, and depressor. Schwartz found that imagined emotions were associated with different patterns of facial muscle activity, not generally observable by onlookers. A low corrugator EMG and a slight increase in depressor EMG were associated with happy thoughts. An increased corrugator EMG was related to sad thoughts. Angry thoughts were related to increased EMG in all four muscles. The studies described, although they are only a small sampling of the research on stimulus specificity, demonstrate the existence of the phenomenon.

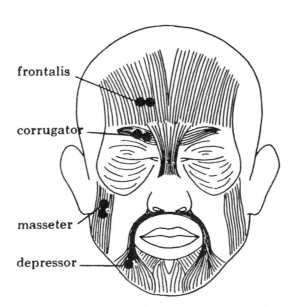

**FIGURE 4-15.** Muscles monitored in facial patterning. Location of electrodes used to measure electromyographic (EMG) activity of four facial muscles during different emotions. From "Biofeedback, Self-Regulation, and the Patterning of Physiological Processes" by G. E. Schwartz, 1975, *American Scientist, 62,* 314–324. Copyright 1975 by the American Scientist. Reprinted by permission.

*Individual-response stereotypy,* or specificity, refers to the concept that a particular *individual* will respond to a variety of stimulus situations with a characteristic pattern. For example, an individual may be a heart rate responder, skin conductance responder, muscle responder, or some combination of these. While stimulus-response stereotypy refers to the tendency of many individuals to respond to a specific or single stimulus, individual-response stereotypy refers to the consistency of an individual's response hierarchy in a variety of stimulus situations. Stimulus-response stereotypy and individual-response stereotypy are not necessarily incompatible.

Lacey *et al.* (1953) first formulated the concept of individual-response specificity. Their classic study demonstrated that individuals would respond maximally with a certain physiological pattern. Skin conductance, heart rate, and heart rate variability were among some of the responses determined under four "stressful" conditions (cold pressor, mental arithmetic, letter association, and hyperventilation). The results indicated that individuals respond maximally in the same physiological variable under the four stress situations. Lacey *et al.* also noted that some of the subjects responded with a fixed *pattern,* such as increased skin conductance, followed by heart rate, and then heart rate variability. Although other researchers have observed that most individuals display a consistent idiosyncratic pattern of responses, quantitative differences exist (Greenfield & Sternbach, 1972).

Moos and Engel's (1962) classic study of *symptom specificity* reported that the blood pressure in hypertensive subjects changed more than the blood pressure in arthritic patients in response to a stressful stimulus. The EMG increased more in muscles overlying (arthritic) joints in arthritic patients than in hypertensives. In a more recent study, Walker and Sandman (1977) reported both symptom and response stereotypy. Duodenal ulcer patients, rheumatoid arthritis patients, and healthy subjects were investigated using the electrogastrogram (EGG), heart rate, and tonic galvanic skin potential (GSP) during exposure to mildly stressful stimuli. They found that ulcer patients were physiologically less reactive to the stimuli than the other groups. With the exception of the ulcer patients' GSP response to an arithmetic stressor, these patients were responsive only to the stimulus of viewing slides of autopsies for which increases in EGGs and phasic GSPs were demonstrated. The EGG data are interesting in that they differentiate between groups (symptom) and task (response), since ulcer patients and healthy subjects showed increases in phasic EGG activity during affective, but not cognitive tasks; both patient groups differed from normals on tonic EGG. In sum, individual and symptom stereotypy have been observed in a variety of studies. These studies support a specificity view of physiological response to emotional stimuli and show that pattern, as well as level of physiological activity, must be considered in any attempt to understand the role of specific visceral/somatic input in symptoms experienced. The theoretical and experimental work in this area requires further elaboration, particularly in identifying the roles of explicit and implicit sets, the reliability over time of individual-response specificity, and the role of this specificity in various emotions and physical disorders.

## Activation or Arousal Theory

Activation, or arousal theory, attempts to correlate variations in level of physiological activity with changes in behavior. Proponents of this theory argue that peripheral autonomic responses to stimuli are undifferentiated and vary only in intensity and direction and that the generalized physiological state of the organism ranges from extreme excitement or activation at one end of a continuum to sleep and unconsciousness at the other end. Activation has been related to emotion and is important in understanding stress and stress-related symptoms and disorders.

In the section on specificity, different emotions were described as having different physiological response patterns. When activation theory is related to emotion, a diffuse sympathetic discharge, or arousal, which is similar for all emotions, is postulated (Cannon, 1927). Duffy (1962) contends that activation is controlled by the neurohumoral system and can be thought of as a physiological intervening variable between environmental and organismic variables and the psychophysiological response. She emphasized that the changes that occur in various physiological systems vary at different points of time and with different individuals. In general, however, the level of activation is thought to be related to the intensity of the emotional experience. Work by Schacter and Singer (1962) indicated that a person's cognitive set, or expectations, is important in defining an emotional state when aroused physiologically. In one experiment, subjects were led to believe that the experimenters were interested in the effects of a vitamin on vision; the "vitamin" was actually either epinephrine (which mimics sympathetic activation) or a placebo. One group was given a description of the effects of the vitamin that was an accurate, subjective description of the side effects of epinephrine. One group was given no description, and a third group was given a description of symptoms that were totally unrelated to the effects of epinephrine. Another aspect of the study involved exposing half of each group to a situation that should elicit anger and the other half to one that should elicit euphoria. Briefly, the results showed that subjects exposed to the euphoria condition were significantly more euphoric when they had no explanation of their bodily states. The epinephrine misinformed group was more euphoric than the placebo group, which was more euphoric than the epinephrine informed group. The findings were similar for the anger condition. As a result of this study and others, Schacter concluded that there may indeed be few physiological differences between emotional states. Although peripheral autonomic arousal is necessary to determine the emotional state, the *meaning* of the arousal is determined cognitively. Schacter assumed that emotions may involve an information search, such that the individual searches the environment (social and other) for an explanation, and a labeling process then occurs.

Roessler and Engel (1974) extended the theory of activation by integrating the concept of idiosyncratic response (IR) and stimulus response (SR) specificity within a framework of arousal. They define activation as "the patterns in the level of physiological variables relative to a stimulus of specifiable intensity and character and relative to a subject in a particular state." As Roessler and Engel (1974) pointed out, their definition takes into account (1) SR specificity and its intensity; (2) IR specificity; (3) the state of the organism, that is, the original temporal condition or level of activation; and (4) the interrelations of SR, IR, and the individual's state. Essentially, psychological, cognitive, and sociocultural factors are thought to effect the individual's idiosyncratic response to a stimulus, and determine how one would react and interpret environmental stimuli and label arousal. The theory of arousal, or activation, is also important in understanding the stress concept. Selye (1956) described a general, nonspecific pattern of biochemical responses to *prolonged* stress. Regardless of the type of stress (cold, injury, drugs, overwork), the response is the same and involves the discharge of adrenal cortical steroids, destruction of the thymus, and bleeding gastric ulcers. In Chapter 5, the stress response is discussed in more detail, but it should be noted that activation is a key concept in stress theory.

Although activation theory has played an important role in the psychophysiology of emotion, it has also been important in understanding the psychophysiology of performance. An inverted U-shaped relation has been observed for arousal and performance. Thus, the higher the activation, the better the performance, up to a point at which performance decreases. Frankenhaeuser, Nordheden, Myrsten, and Post (1971) showed that, although individuals who secrete relatively more epinephrine tend to perform better when working under conditions of low or moderate activation, they tend to perform poorly under conditions of high activation. Frankenhaeuser *et al.* (1971) compared performance efficiency under two contrasting conditions of work in subjects with different catecholamine excretion rates. Subjects who excreted relatively more epinephrine performed better under conditions of understimulation. In contrast, subjects with relatively lower excretion rates of epinephrine tended to perform better under conditions of overstimulation. This study may be interpreted in light of the inverted U-shaped relation between behavioral efficiency, or performance, and physiological arousal (Frankenhaeuser, 1975). Another approach to the study of the relationship between performance and activation involves the relationship between arousal manipulated by induced muscle tension (IMT) and task efficiency (Andreassi, 1980). An IMT level of one-fourth of maximum IMT was optimal for verbal learning, and higher degrees of tension were also superior to no tension. Learning efficiency fell below the no-tension condition at a level of three-fourths maximum IMT. Thus, an inverted U-shaped relationship was demonstrated between level of muscle tension and performance (cf. Andreassi, 1980).

## Cardiac-Somatic Decoupling

Most of the studies mentioned in the preceding discussions used heart rate (HR) as a dependent variable and reported increases as indicative of activation. Changes in cardiac activity in response to environmental stimuli suggest that the relationship between heart rate and behavior is more complex than previously assumed. The *cardiac-somatic theory*, an important theory in psychophysiology, postulates that cardiac responses facilitate preparation for and performance of a behavioral response. Obrist (1981) has reported consistent vagal control of HR and covariation between those HR effects and somatic activity. For example, there is an association between HR deceleration and ongoing somatic activity that is not related to performance. Deceleration in HR is considered to reflect a central mechanism that adjusts cardiac activity to metabolic requirements. The cardiovascular system maintains metabolic homeostasis so that the HR decelerates when the body is immobilized and accelerates in preparation for action (fight or flight). The "coupling" between cardiac-somatic responses occurs because both are controlled by brain processes concerned with preparatory activities.

Obrist has been concerned with identifying conditions that evoke sympathetic influences on the heart that result in the *decoupling* of cardiac-somatic activities (cf. Obrist, 1981). He suggests that evidence of cardiac-somatic decoupling would support the theory that behavioral events influence the course of cardiovascular disease. He assumes that environmental influences are mediated by the sympathetic division of the ANS and that the effects of such influences can be differentiated from the homeostatic-metabolic function of the cardiovascular system. An example of decoupling has been provided by Lawler, Obrist, and

Lawler (1976). Lawler *et al.* measured HR and somatic activity in 25 male college students and 25 fifth-grade boys while they performed a reaction-time task. The procedure involved manipulating attention by varying uncertainty (probability of a warning signal occurring) and motivation (money and feedback versus no money and no feedback). Variations in uncertainty resulted in systematic changes in HR before the reaction-time task, with HR acceleration increasing as uncertainty increased. The forearm EMG at this time differentiated variations in motivation, since increases in the EMG were associated with increases in motivation. The average level of HR and forearm EMG also increased as motivation increased. The results indicated that stimulus uncertainty is related to cardiac-somatic decoupling, since the HR increased with uncertainty during the pre-task period, whereas the EMG did not. Obrist concluded that when sympathetic influences are evoked experimentally, the sympathetic division functions *independently* of current somatic activities. Thus, sympathetic effects on the cardiovascular system are metabolically inappropriate and in excess of metabolic requirements. Cardiac-somatic decoupling is seen as nonadaptive, and possibly disruptive.

### Bio-Informational Theory of Emotional Imagery

Lang (1979) has proposed a theory of emotional imagery that integrates cognitive psychology and psychophysiology. The theory has implications for health psychology in a number of areas, and it has been applied in the area of fear reduction techniques in preparation for surgery or dental procedures, as well as sport psychology.

The theory integrates research on the psychophysiology of imagery with theory and research on information processing and behavior therapy. Psychophysiological research has indicated that imaginal activities are associated with efferent outflow or changes in ANS activity. This research has also noted that specific patterns of visceral and somatomotor activity are associated with the type of processing and the specific content of cognitive events. Information-processing models describing the mechanisms by which visual images are stored in and retrieved from the brain are also incorporated in the bio-informational theory. The hypothesis that visual images are stored as *propositional structures* or logical relationships between concepts represents a major aspect of the theory. This aspect of the theory is adopted from cognitive psychology. The image structure or propositional structure has an associated motor program that can act as a prototype or serve to influence the expression of overt behavior.

The theory suggests that an image in the brain represents a conceptual network or propositional structure that regulates specific soma-toviseral patterns (autonomic and skeletal muscle) consequently affecting overt behavior. Thus, the propositional structure is the basis for the emotional content and structure. Feedback from the somatovisceral and verbal report outputs to brain processes responsible for the initial propositional structure influence the emotional experience and associated behavior. An example of such a feedback system (Lang, 1979) might involve the following propositional structure or network: "You are walking alone. There is a snake about one meter long. It is very near. Your eyes move, following the snake as it crawls across your path. As you watch the snake, your heart begins to pound wildly. You feel afraid. You want to run away" (p. 502).

The theory would argue that modifying either the verbal report of fear or the efferent fiber response to the imagery influences subsequent evocations of the image, which modify its content and structure. Thus, by reducing the physiological response associated with the image, it is theoretically possible to modify the actual structure of the image. For example, the reduction of heart rate (i.e., heart pounding) might change the structure of the image to "As you watch the snake, your heart does not race at all and while you may be somewhat afraid you have no need to run away." Here the image content was modified to hypothetically reduce its impact on behavior. Lang (1979) presented a set of empirical findings that support the theory. The bio-informational theory of emotional imagery may prove to be a useful heuristic tool for understanding the role of emotions in health and illness, as well as explaining the effects of interventions (i.e., on health disorders modifying propositional structures). The theory delineates specific components, and Lang has devised a paradigm to test various aspects of the theory.

## SUMMARY

The field of psychophysiology provides the health psychologist with a wealth of techniques and concepts to explore certain physiological processes in the intact human while he or she is engaged in a complex cognitive and behavioral interchange with the environment. Psychophysiology has played a major role thus far in our understanding of the psychobiological bases of health and disease, and as it advances, technologically and theoretically, it should continue to be a valuable resource. This chapter was written with this assumption in mind.

The field of psychophysiology was defined and differentiated from physiological psychology, which also contributes significantly to health psychology. A review of the basic principles of the nervous and endocrine systems was then presented, followed by a general description of common biological response systems studied in psychophysiological research. Ambulatory psychophysiology was briefly discussed to illustrate a relatively new approach in psychophysiology that takes the laboratory out into the natural environment. Biochemical indices were then reviewed and their importance as a source of information regarding the effect of environmental, cognitive, and behavioral stimuli on physiological functioning in humans was discussed.

Such basic concepts and general observations as orienting response, defensive response, habituation, environmental rejection, environmental intake, role of implicit sets, and organismic variables were reviewed. Topics including autonomic balance, stimulus, individual-response and symptom stereotypy, activation or arousal theory, cardiac-somatic decoupling, and bio-informational theory of emotional imagery were presented to illustrate the evolution of theoretical considerations in psychophysiology. This chapter should provide a foundation for further considerations of the psychophysiological aspects of health and disease presented in the book.

## REFERENCES

Andreassi, J. L. (1980). *Psychophysiology: Human behavior and physiological response.* New York: Oxford University Press.

Ax, A. F. (1953). The physiological differentiation of fear and anger in humans. *Psychosomatic Medicine, 15,* 433–442.

Brown, C. C. (Ed.). (1967). *Methods in psychophysiology.* Baltimore, MD: Williams & Wilkins.

Cannon, W. B. (1927). The James–Lange theory of emotion: A critical examination and an alternative theory. *American Journal of Psychology, 39,* 106–124.

Christie, M. J., & Woodman, D. D. (1980). Biochemical methods. In I. Martin & P. H. Venables (Eds.), *Techniques in psychophysiology* (pp. 459–500). Chichester, England: Wiley.

Coulbourn Instruments. (1984). Muscle action potentials–Raw form and integrated form. In *Users Guide to: Operation, Specifications, Applications* (p. 45). Lehigh Valley, PA: Coulbourn Instruments.

Duffy, E. (1962). *Activation and behavior.* New York: Wiley.

Edelberg, R. (1972). Electrical activity of the skin. In N. S. Greenfield & R. A. Sternbach (Eds.), *Handbook of psychophysiology* (pp. 367–418). New York: Holt, Rinehart & Winston.

Engel, B. T. (1972). Response specficity. In N. S. Greenfield & R. A. Sternbach (Eds.), *Handbook of psychophysiology* (pp. 571–576). New York: Holt, Rinehart & Winston.

Eysenck, H. J. (1977). *The biological basis of personality.* Springfield, IL.: Charles C Thomas.

Feuerstein, M., Barr, R. G., & Iezzi, A. (1985). *The ambulatory psychophysiological monitoring system (APMS).* Manuscript submitted for publication.

Frankenhaeuser, M. (1975). Sympathetic–adrenomedullary activity, behaviour and the psychosocial environment. In P. H. Venables & M. J. Christie (Eds.), *Research in psychophysiology.* London: Wiley.

Frankenhaeuser, M., Northeden, B., Myrsten, A. L., & Post, B. (1971). Psychophysiological reactions to understimulation and overstimulation. *Acta Psychologica, 35,* 298–308.

Greenfield, N. S., & Sternbach, R. A. (Eds.). (1972). *Handbook of psychophysiology.* New York: Holt, Rinehart & Winston.

Grings, W. W., & Dawson, M. E. (1978). *Emotions and bodily responses: A psychophysiological approach.* New York: Academic Press.

Guyton, A. C. (1979). *Physiology of the human body* (5th ed.). Philadelphia: W. B. Saunders.

Hare, R. D. (1973). Orienting and defensive responses to visual stimuli. *Psychophysiology, 10*(5), 453–464.

Hassett, J. (1978). *A primer of psychophysiology.* San Francisco: W. H. Freeman.

Haywood, H. C., & Spielberger, C. D. (1966). Palmar sweating as a function of individual differences in manifest anxiety. *Journal of Personality and Social Psychology, 3,* 103–105.

Hokanson, J. E. (1961). Vascular and psychogalvanic effects of experimentally aroused anger. *Journal of Personality, 29,* 30–39.

Jacob, S. W., & Francore, C. A. (1970). *Structure and Function in Man* (2nd ed.). New York: W. B. Saunders.

Kahneman, D., Tursky, B., Shapiro, D., & Crider, A. (1969). Pupillary, heart rate and skin resistance changes during a mental task. *Journal of Experimental Psychology, 79,* 164–167.

Kallman, W., & Feuerstein, M. (1977). Psychophysiological procedures. In A. R. Ciminero, K. S. Calhoun, & H. E. Adams (Eds.), *Handbook of behavioral assessment* (pp. 329–364). New York: Wiley-Interscience.

Lacey, J. I. (1959). Psychophysiological approaches to the evaluation of psychotherapeutic process and outcome. In E. A. Rubenstein & M. B. Parloff (Eds.), *Research in psychotherapy.* Washington, DC: American Psychological Association.

Lacey, J. I., Kagan, J., Lacey, B. C., & Moss, H. A. (1963). The visceral level: Situational determinants and behavioral correlates of autonomic response patterns. In P. H. Knapp (Ed.), *Expression of the emotions in man.* New York: International Universities Press.

Lang, P. J. (1979). A bio-informational theory of emotional imagery. *Psychophysiology, 16,* 495–512.

Lang, P. J., Melamed, B. G., & Hart, J. E. (1970). A psychophysiological analysis of fear modification using an automated desensitization procedure. *Journal of Abnormal Psychology, 76,* 220–234.

Lawler, K. A., Obrist, P. A., & Lawler, J. E. (1976). Cardiac and somatic response patterns during a reaction time task in children and adults. *Psychophysiology, 13,* 448–455.

Lazarus, R. S., & Alfert, E. (1964). Short-circuiting of threat by experimentally altering cognitive appraisal. *Journal of Abnormal and Social Psychology, 69,* 195–205.

Levi, L. (1972). Psychosocial stimuli, psychophysiological reactions and disease. *Acta Medica Scandinavica* (Suppl. 528).

Lippold, O. C. J. (1967). Electromyography. In P. H. Venables & I. Martin (Eds.), *Manual of psychophysiological methods* (pp. 247–297). Amsterdam: North Holland.

Martin, I., & Venables, P. H. (Eds.). (1980). *Techniques in psychophysiology.* Chichester, England: Wiley.

Mason, J. W. (1972). Organization of psychoendocrine mechanism: A review and reconsideration of research. In N. S. Greenfield & R. A. Sternbach (Eds.), *Handbook of psychophysiology* (pp. 3–91). New York: Holt, Rinehart & Winston.

Moos, R. H., & Engel, B. T. (1962). Psychophysiological reactions in hypertensive and arthritic patients. *Journal of Psychosomatic Research, 6,* 227–241.

Neary, R. S., & Zuckerman, M. (1976). Sensation seeking, trait and state anxiety, and the electrodermal orienting response. *Psychophysiology, 13*(3), 205–211.

Obrist, P. A. (1981). *Cardiovascular psychophysiology: A perspective*. New York: Plenum Press.

Picton, T. W. (1980). The use of human event-related potentials in psychology. In I. Martin & P. H. Venables (Eds.), *Techniques in psychophysiology*. Chichester, England: Wiley.

Rasmussen, H. (1974). Organization and control of endocrine systems. In R. H. Williams (Ed.), *Textbook of endocrinology* (5th ed.). Philadelphia: Saunders.

Roessler, R., & Engel, B. T. (1974). The current status of the concepts of physiological response specificity and activation. *International Journal of Psychiatry in Medicine, 5*, 359–366.

Schwartz, G. E. (1975). Biofeedback, self-regulation, and the patterning of physiological processes. *The American Scientist, 63*(3), 314–324.

Selye, H. (1956). *The stress of life*. New York: McGraw-Hill.

Selye, H. (1976). *Stress in health and disease*. Reading, MA: Butterworth.

Smith, D. B. D., & Wenger, M. A. (1965). Changes in autonomic balance during phasic anxiety. *Psychophysiology, 1*, 267–271.

Sokolov, E. N. (1963). *Perception and the conditioned reflex*. Oxford: Pergamon Press.

Stelmack, C. M., & Mandelzya, N. (1975). Extraversion and pupillary response to affective and taboo words. *Psychophysiology, 12*, 536–540.

Sternbach, R. A. (1964). The effects of instructional sets on autonomic responsivity. *Psychophysiology, 1*, 67–72.

Sternbach, R. A. (1966). *Principles of psychophysiology: An introductory text and readings*. New York: Academic Press.

Sternbach, R. A., & Tursky, B. (1965). Ethnic differences among housewives in psychophysical and skin potential responses to electric shock. *Psychophysiology, 1*, 241–246.

Thomas, A., Chess, S., & Burch, H. G. (1970). The origin of personality. *Scientific American, 223*, 102–109.

Usdin, E., Kretnansky, R., & Kopin, I. (1976). *Catecholamines and stress*. Oxford: Pergamon Press.

Van Toller, C. (1979). *The nervous body: An introduction to the autonomic nervous system and behavior*. Chichester, England: Wiley.

Walker, B. B., & Sandman, C. A. (1977). Physiological response patterns in ulcer patients: Phasic and tonic components of the electrogastrogram. *Psychophysiology, 14*(4), 393–400.

Weinberger, D. A., Schwartz, G. E., & Davidson, R. J. (1979). Low-anxious, high-anxious, and repressive coping styles: Psychometric patterns and behavioral and physiological responses to stress. *Journal of Abnormal Psychology, 88*, 369–380.

Wenger, M. A. (1941). The measurement of individual differences in autonomic balance. *Psychosomatic Medicine, 3*, 427–434.

Wenger, M. A. (1948). Studies of autonomic balance in Army Air Forces personnel. *Comparative Psychology Monographs, 19* (4, Serial No. 101).

Wenger, M. A. (1972). Studies of autonomic balance: A summary. *Psychophysiology, 2*, 173–186.

Yuwiler, A. (1976). Stress, anxiety and endocrine function. In R. Grenell & S. Galay (Eds.), *Biological foundations of psychiatry*. New York: Raven Press.

# CURRENT CONCEPTS

*Part Two of the book presents core concepts in the field of health psychology. Chapter 5 reviews stress, a topic that cuts across several problem areas in health psychology. The relation of stress to illness is discussed in Chapter 6, and serves as a model for considering the role of other potential psychobiological factors in the development, exacerbation, and maintenance of illness. Chapter 7 reviews several techniques used to reduce the impact of stress on health and illness, as well as possible mechanisms of action. Chapter 8 presents another major concept in the field: health behavior. This chapter defines health behavior, reviews the factors that influence it, and considers clinical and educational approaches for modifying health behavior. Chapter 9 explores the area of illness behavior, a complex subject that represents a major challenge to the health care system. Definitions, etiological factors, and treatment approaches are considered.*

# STRESS

As Hans Selye (1980), a pioneer stress researcher, pointed out, "stress is a scientific concept which has suffered from the mixed blessing of being too well known and too little understood" (p. 127). Although stress is a difficult concept, or more accurately, construct, to define, as with anxiety or pain, much research has been directed at understanding the various phenomena associated with it. Whether or not stress is a useful construct depends to some degree on whether scientific investigation can unambiguously describe and measure it and whether factors that influence it can be isolated. A construct is only useful in terms of its organizing and explanatory power. The purpose of this chapter is to critically review the stress construct. A historical review, followed by a working or operational definition, will be presented. Models of stress will be reviewed, along with measurement techniques. Factors that influence or modulate the stress response will also be identified. One such factor is the coping process an individual engages in when confronted with a potentially threatening situation. Because of the recent emphasis on the role of cognitive modulation of the stress response, a detailed review of the research in this area will be presented.

## HISTORICAL REVIEW

*Stress* has been used in the English language to describe human experience and behavior for centuries. In the seventeenth century, the term was used to refer to "hardship, straits, adversity or affliction" (Onions, 1933). During the eighteenth and the nineteenth century, stress took on a somewhat different meaning. Rather than representing a negative experience, stress was defined as a "force, pressure, strain or strong effort" impinging upon an object or an individual or his or her "organs or mental powers" (Hinkle, 1974). In this definition, individuals were acted upon by external forces. In conjunction with this position, stress was viewed as distorting the individual, who resists in an attempt to maintain integrity and return to an original state (Hinkle, 1974).

Physics and engineering have contributed to the development of the stress concept and its current use in the biobehavioral sciences. Although developed during the early research of Boyle on the properties of gases and the study of the elasticity of springs in the late seventeenth century, stress was not defined until the early nineteenth century. Because of some similarities in its use in the biobehavioral sciences, the definition formulated in physics requires some elaboration. In physics, stress is applied to solid bodies and is defined as "an internal force generated within such a body by the action of any force which tends to distort the body" (Hinkle, 1974, p. 337). Three terms are used to define this concept from a physical perspective: stress, strain, and load. *Stress* represents the ratio of the internal force present when a solid is distorted to the area over which the force acts, and is quantifiable in dynes per square centimeter. *Strain,* or distortion, is the ratio of the change in size or shape to the original size or shape. *Load* is the external force producing the distortion. Although these three variables can be related mathematically, this relationship is applicable only to a small class of solid bodies, over a limited range, and under the assumption that these bodies are homogeneous. Thus, although a physical definition of *stress* is useful, such a definition has been somewhat restrictive even in the understanding of these forces on solid bodies. Despite this, the concepts of stress, strain, and load were adopted in the development of stress theories within the biobehavioral sciences.

Physicians in the nineteenth and the twentieth century hypothesized that such *stress* and *strain* could lead to certain physical illnesses.

Sir William Osler (1910) argued that the life-style of certain businessmen, which included, "living an intense life, absorbed in work, devoted to pleasures, passionately devoted to home" resulted in significant strain and predisposed them to angina pectoris. Later, the physiologist Walter Cannon (1932) used the term *stress* to describe his laboratory research on the "fight-or-flight" reaction, the complex response of the sympathetic adrenal medullary system of humans and animals to cold, lack of oxygen, low blood sugar, loss of blood or excitement. It has been suggested that the use of the stress concept seemed appropriate to Cannon because of the observed homeostatic characteristics of living organisms, since they tend to "bound back" and "resist distortion" in an effort to maintain the original state before exposure to some "external force" or disturbing stimulus (Hinkle, 1974).

During the late 1930s and early 1940s Selye reported a complex response in laboratory animals to a diverse set of damaging or "alarming" agents including bacterial infection, toxins, trauma, heat, cold, and psychological stimuli. The response includes heightened activity of the anterior pituitary and the adrenal cortex. A general adaptive response to such nonspecific agents was described as the *general adaptation syndrome* (GAS). Although the GAS will be discussed in a later section of this chapter and in Chapter 6, it is important to highlight certain features of Selye's conceptualization of stress here. Essentially, Selye viewed stress in terms of a nonspecific adaptive response of the body to any agent or situation. Although the response is relatively constant, regardless of type of stimulus, the degree of response may vary as a function of the intensity of the demand for adjustment. The same systemic reaction (general bodily response) can be triggered by stress-producing agents (stressors) that are pleasant or unpleasant (Selye, 1980). An often misunderstood aspect of Selye's theory is the term *nonspecific response*. The response is quite specific. Indeed, the GAS is a specific syndrome, a characteristic group of events. It is simply that the syndrome is associated with a set of general bodily reactions to nonspecific demands.

Around the time Selye was working on his formulation of stress, a group of physicians, spearheaded by H. G. Wolff, began describing a number of diseases that were thought to be influenced by *life stress*. Wolff defined stress as follows:

> that state within a living creature which results from the interaction of the organism with noxious stimuli or circumstances, i.e., it is a dynamic state within the organism; it is not a stimulus, assault, load, symbol, burden, or any aspect of environment, internal, external, social or otherwise. (Hinkle, 1974, p. 339)

Wolff further specified the types of noxious stimuli along a continuum ranging from "unconditional," or factors that directly damaged or distorted the structure and/or function of the organism (e.g., strong thermal or chemical agents), to "conditional," stimuli or factors with indirect effects because they can act as signals or symbols. The conditional stimuli are not necessarily closely linked in time with the response; they represent *psychological stressors*. Thus, both Selye and Wolff conceptualize *stress* as a state within the organism. According to Selye, this state could be inferred from the physiological and pathological changes observed. Although the definition is somewhat circular, both theoreticians implied that the stimulus itself is not necessarily stressful, but rather that it is the elaboration of the stimulus within the organism that identifies it as stressful. This, in turn, triggers physiological, and potentially pathological changes.

## OPERATIONAL DEFINITION

Although there are several definitions of the stress concept, some commonalities across them emerge. As with any construct, in order to pursue empirical research and develop interventions directed at modifying its potentially deleterious effects, some type of working definition is required. For purposes of simplicity, rather than generating yet another complex definition, let us conceptualize the *stress experience* as comprised of two major components: *stressors* and *stress response*. This dichotomy has been used in the stress literature and will serve to structure our discussion.

Stressors represent stimulus events requiring some form of adaptation or adjustment. Stressors usually evoke a relatively stereotypic set of responses, the stress response. The circular nature of this definition is intentional. It is believed that a complex feedback system exists between stressor and stress response, with each influencing the other. Thus, any definition of one requires reference to the other.

Stressors can be such external physical stimuli as heat, cold, crowding, loud noise, or interpersonal difficulties with a loved one or such internal stimuli as interoceptive stimuli (pain or cognitions including thoughts and feelings). Two important points can be made regarding stressors: (1) They may have positive as well as the more commonly assumed negative valence and (2) there is considerable variability as to what is considered a stressor across individuals. Positive events may require as much adjustment or adaptation as negative events. Simply because an event is associated with a negative consequence does not somehow identify it as a stressor. Positive experiences and their concomitant emotions can activate neurohumoral mechanisms characteristic of the stress response.

Not all potentially stressful stimuli evoke a stress response in all individuals, and this common observation has significant consequences for understanding the stress experience. At the most basic level, one cannot assume *a priori*, with absolute certainty, that exposure to a stimulus will result in a stress response in all individuals observed. Indeed, the stress–response-producing properties of a stimulus may also vary across time and situations for the same individual. At a broader level, these observations suggest that a number of factors can augment or attenuate (i.e., modulate) the stressor–stress response interaction, thus determining the ultimate stress experience. Such factors will be discussed in detail in a later section of this chapter.

Although stressors are somewhat specific to individuals, several studies have identified a number of general stressors. The life events identified by Holmes and Rahe (1967), based upon a large-scale sampling (the subjects indicated situations that required some form of adjustment), are examples of such stressors. Table 5-1 lists these stressors. Other examples of more general stressors are those reported in a large-scale study of coping in 2,300 individuals, aged 18–65, in the Chicago area (Pearlin & Schooler, 1978). The focus of this study was on individuals engaged in ordinary daily pursuits as they participate in multiple roles as marriage partners, financial managers, parents, and workers. A sampling of some of these stressors is presented in Table 5-2.

The *stress response* is a complex reaction pattern that often has physiological, cognitive, and behavioral components. As discussed in Chapter 4, the physiological component of the stress response activates the sympathetic and parasympathetic branches of the autonomic nervous system and also elicits a set of complex physiological reactions (see Figure 5-1).

The neurotransmitter norepinephrine from sympathetic telodendria is responsible for most of the changes in end-organ activity; however, acetylcholine is also released during exposure to "threatening" stimuli or stimuli requiring adaptation and is responsible for the parasympathetic postganglionic activity. This generalized sympathetic arousal has been termed the *ergotropic* response, whereas activation via the parasympathetic division has been termed the *trophotropic* response (Hess, 1957). Hess argued that the trophotropic response inhibits or slows certain end-organ responses. It is important to emphasize that sympathetic *and* parasympathetic activation have been observed in response to stressors (Gellhorn, 1968).

The autonomic neural activation by a stressor is rapid, but not chronic, since the sympathetic telodendria do not constantly release neurotransmitters during chronic high stimulation (LeBlanc, 1976). The neuroendocrine axis, primarily the adrenal medulla, however, does exert a slower effect. The release of epinephrine and norepinephrine into

## TABLE 5-1
### Life Events and Relative Stress Values

| Rank | Life event | Stress values |
|------|-----------|---------------|
| 1 | Death of spouse | 100 |
| 2 | Divorce | 73 |
| 3 | Marital separation | 65 |
| 4 | Jail term | 63 |
| 5 | Death of close family member | 63 |
| 6 | Personal injury or illness | 53 |
| 7 | Marriage | 50[a] |
| 8 | Fired at work | 47 |
| 9 | Marital reconciliation | 45 |
| 10 | Retirement | 45 |
| 11 | Change in health of family member | 44 |
| 12 | Pregnancy | 40 |
| 13 | Sex difficulties | 39 |
| 14 | Gain of new family member | 39 |
| 15 | Business readjustment | 39 |
| 16 | Change in financial state | 38 |
| 17 | Death of close friend | 37 |
| 18 | Change to different line of work | 36 |
| 19 | Change in number of arguments with spouse | 35 |
| 20 | Mortgage over $10,000 | 31 |
| 21 | Foreclosure of mortgage or loan | 30 |
| 22 | Change in responsibilities at work | 29 |
| 23 | Son or daughter leaving home | 29 |
| 24 | Trouble with in-laws | 29 |
| 25 | Outstanding personal achievement | 28 |
| 26 | Wife begins or stops work | 26 |
| 27 | Begin or end school | 26 |
| 28 | Change in living conditions | 25 |
| 29 | Revision of personal habits | 24 |
| 30 | Trouble with boss | 23 |
| 31 | Change in work hours or conditions | 20 |
| 32 | Change in residence | 20 |
| 33 | Change in schools | 20 |
| 34 | Change in recreation | 19 |
| 35 | Change in church activities | 19 |
| 36 | Change in social activities | 18 |
| 37 | Mortgage or loan less than $10,000 | 17 |
| 38 | Change in sleeping habits | 16 |
| 39 | Change in number of family get-togethers | 15 |
| 40 | Change in eating habits | 15 |
| 41 | Vacation | 13 |
| 42 | Christmas | 12 |
| 43 | Minor violations of the law | 11 |

*Note.* Adapted from "The Social Adjustment Rating Scale" by T. H. Holmes and R. H. Rahe, 1967, *Journal of Psychosomatic Research, 11,* 213–218. Copyright 1967 by Pergamon Press, Ltd. Reprinted by permission.
[a]Marriage was arbitrarily assigned a stress value of 500; no event was found to be any more than twice as stressful. Here the values are reduced proportionally and range up to 100.

the circulation on adrenal medullary stimulation results in epinephrine and norepinephrine activity in humans; the effects are identical to those of direct sympathetic stimulation. This activity, however, requires a 20- to 30-second delay of onset for measureable effect, and the effect lasts approximately 10 times longer than that of neural stimulation (Usdin, Kretnansky, & Kopin, 1976). A variety of physiological effects have been observed in response to stressors. These responses represent the physiological component of Cannon's fight-or-flight reaction.

The stress response has three physiological components: tonic, phasic, and recovery. The *tonic* component is defined as the resting or basal level of activity in the specific response, the *phasic* component represents the reaction to a given stressor, and *recovery* relates to the response following the stressor and is typically defined as the component associated with return to the resting or tonic level. Figure 5-2 illustrates these three components.

The endocrine axes (Mason, 1968) involved in the stress response are responsible for the relatively longer physiological response to stressors. The major endocrine axes involved include the adrenal cortical axis, the somatotropic axis, and the thyroid axis (Everly & Rosenfeld, 1981). These three axes can be stimulated in humans by a variety of psychosocial stressors, although they require a more intense level of stimulation (Levi, 1972). As discussed in Chapter 4, the release of adrenocorticotropic hormone (ACTH) by the anterior pituitary stimulates the adrenal cortex to release the glucocorticoids cortisol and corticosterone

TABLE 5-2
Stressors in a Normative Adult Sample[a]

Marital Strain Items
  Nonacceptance by spouse
  Nonreciprocity in give and take
  Frustration of role expectations
Parental Strain Items
  Deviations from parental standards of behavior
  Nonconformity to parental aspirations and values
  Disregard for parental status
Household Economics Strain Items
  Standard of living brinkmanship (insufficient money to purchase clothing should
    have, food should have, paying monthly bills)
Occupational Strain Items
  Inadequacy of reward
  Noxiousness of work environment
  Depersonalization in the work environment
  Role overload

[a]$N = 2,300$.

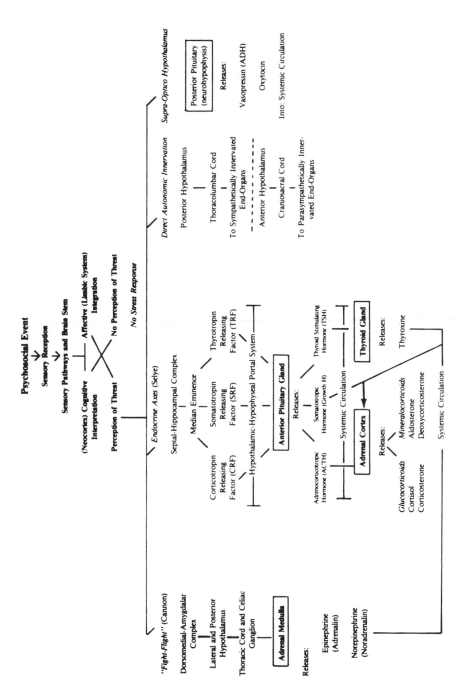

**FIGURE 5-1.** Potential pathways for stress reactivity to psychosocial stressors. From *The Nature and Treatment of the Stress Response: A Practical Guide for Clinicians* (p. 31) by G. S. Everly, Jr., and R. Rosenfeld. Copyright 1981 by Plenum Press. Reprinted by permission.

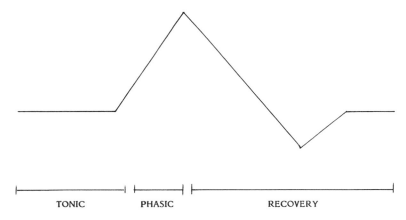

FIGURE 5-2. Phases of the physiological component of the stress response.

and the mineralocorticoids adolsterone and deoxycorticosterone into the circulation. These hormones exert a variety of effects, as indicated in Table 5-3. Release of growth hormone (somatotropic axis) and thyroxine (thyroid axis) have also been observed in response to psychosocial stressors (Levi, 1972; Selye, 1976). Although their role in the stress response is not as well delineated, some of their functions are listed in Table 5-3. Other physiological components of the stress response include the release of endogeneous morphine-like substances (endorphins), immunosuppressors, and cholesterol.

The cognitive components of the stress response include fluctuation in mood state, ranging from elation to tension, depression, difficulty in concentrating, vigor, and fatigue. The cognitive component generally represents the conscious appraisal of the stimulus, that is how the individual evaluates or perceives the situation. Coping styles also represent the cognitive component of the stress response. Examples of such cognitive coping responses include the use of *positive comparisons*, for example "We're all in the same boat" or "You must count your blessings— look at Joe Smith—he's really bad off," and *selective ignoring*. An example of selective ignoring is the devaluation of money in response to household economic strain (Pearlin & Schooler, 1978).

The behavioral component represents the actual overt behavioral response to the stressor(s). This response can vary from extreme violence to overt hostility to avoidance and withdrawal. Facial expressions are often important behavioral components of a stress response. Impatience, heightened competitiveness, and sexual dysfunction have all been reported as behavioral manifestations of a stress response.

TABLE 5-3
Some Effects of the Stress-Related Hormones

| Axis | Physiological effects |
|---|---|
| Adrenal medullary axis (Epinephrine/norepinephrine) | Increase arterial blood pressure |
| | Increase cardiac output |
| | Decrease blood flow to kidneys |
| | Vasoconstriction of skin vascular beds |
| | Increase plasma free fatty acid levels |
| | Increase muscle tension |
| | Increase plasma triglyceride levels |
| | Increase plasma cholesterol levels |
| Adrenocortical axis (Glucocorticoids: Cortisol/corticosterone) | Increase glucose production |
| | Increase urea production |
| | Increase free fatty acid release into circulation |
| | Potential suppression of immune mechanisms |
| | Increase ketone body production |
| Mineralocorticoids (Aldosterone/deoxycorticosterone) | Regulate electrolytes and blood pressure *via* volumetric adjustments |
| Somatotropic axis (Growth hormone) | Stimulates release of mineralocorticoids |
| | Results in diabetic-like insulin resistance |
| | Mobilizes fats |
| Thyroid axis (Thyroxine) | Increases general metabolism |
| | Increases heart rate |
| | Increases heart contractility |
| | Increases peripheral vascular resistance |
| | Increases sensitivity of some tissues to catecholamines |

Note. Adapted from *The Nature and Treatment of the Stress Response* (pp. 25, 27) by G. S. Everly, Jr., and R. Rosenfeld. Copyright 1981 by Plenum Press. Reprinted by permission.

## MEASUREMENT TECHNIQUES

Methods for studying stress vary in terms of type of setting, such as a laboratory or naturalistic environment, and mode of measurement, such as physiological, behavioral, or cognitive. Some of the methods have been quite innovative. Given the wide variety of assessment methods available, the health psychologist has an impressive array of devices with which to study stress. The following section will not attempt a detailed discusssion of the development and validity of each assessment device, but will illustrate a variety of current techniques for studying stress. First, the measurement of stressors will be discussed, followed by the measurement of various aspects of the stress response.

## Measurement of Stressors

In the laboratory, the stressor of interest is known by the experimenter, who manipulates its intensity, duration, or frequency. Examples include varying the intensity or duration of an electric shock or making a laboratory task (e.g., learning) more difficult by adding increasingly complex problems. However, there is also an interest in assessing stressors in the subject's past or stressors found in the natural environment. Efforts to identify these stressors involve measuring "life events" or experiences believed to be associated with significant adaptation. Self-report questionnaires, checklists, and rating scales are generally used for this purpose.

Studies on life events or experiences thought to be related to stress measure the frequency of major life changes assumed to require adjustment or situations that disrupt daily living. The Holmes and Rahe (1967) Social Readjustment Rating Scale (SRRS) was the first significant attempt to scale social and environmental changes that appear, mostly at face value, to require some type of adjustment or adaptation. An attempt was made to obtain a *quantitative* index of the degree of stress experienced following exposure to a situation requiring adjustment. This scale was used in research directed at determining whether a relationship between stressful life events and less obvious stress-related physical illnesses, such as bacterial or viral infection, exists. Table 5-1 lists the Social Readjustment Rating Scale items or life events considered important. There is limited empirical support relating accumulation of life change to *onset* of illness. The greater the magnitude of life change, the greater the risk of illness and, in addition, the greater the seriousness of a chronic illness (Holmes & Masuda, 1974; Wyler, Masuda, & Holmes, 1971).

The principle of scaling life stressors is quite interesting and similar to scaling in psychophysics (Henry & Stephens, 1977). Subjects were requested to rate the length of time to adjust to various life events, the intensity of these events, and the average degree of readjustment necessary. In the original sample, each subject rated 43 life events in reference to marriage, which was given an arbitrary value of 500. In other words, each event was rated as indicating more or less readjustment than marriage. Instructions were "is the adjustment more intense and prolonged; if so, choose a proportionately large number in the value section."

Early studies indicated that a significant degree of agreement between various subgroups (age, sex, marital status, education, social class, religion, race) was obtained in ratings of life change events. However, recent research indicates that significant variability exists among groups in the perception of life events, as well as reports of the frequency of occurrence of the events (Goldberg & Comstock, 1980). The following four factors have been found to influence the perception of stressful events:

1. *Age.* Younger populations tend to accumulate more life events than older populations, with younger people scoring almost three times more than people over 30 years.

2. *Sex.* Although results tend to be somewhat ambiguous, studies indicate that women accumulate greater life change scores than men.

3. *Marital status.* Single, separated, and divorced people accumulate a larger number of life events than married or widowed people.

4. *Social class.* Results on social class are less consistent; some studies suggest that the poor experience more life events than those with higher income, whereas other studies report no relationship between social class and number of life events.

What does appear clear from this research is that life events and physical illness are related and that this relationship must be evaluated within specific populations.

Initially, there was much enthusiasm over ratings of life events and changes. The public became familiar with such scales when versions of it were published in several popular magazines. Researchers are critical of these types of scales, and questions concerning methodological problems have been raised. Some issues regarding these scales include the identification of events that are truly stressful, the degree of stress that should be accorded a particular life event, and the importance of time elapsed since the event as it affects the current experience of stress. We have discussed differences in subgroups (sex, age, socioeconomic status) and life events. The effect of life events on various subgroups or individuals may differ significantly. Another problem is determining whether positive life events are stressful, and if they are, to what degree, compared to negative life events. The current utility of life event schedules, especially in determining an individual's stress level is uncertain. Modifications of early forms may prove more useful. Johnson and McCutchen (1980) have used the Life Events Checklist (LEC) in studying life stress in older children and adolescents. These investigators required that the subject check life events, but also state whether the event was perceived as negative or positive and the degree of impact the event had on the subject's life. Johnson and McCutchen (1980) provide interesting data regarding the validity of the LEC in that subjects who had experienced higher levels of negative change were found to be more anxious and more depressed and perceived themselves as having less control over environmental events and generally less well adjusted.

Another approach to studying stressors in a person's natural environment focuses on relatively minor events, rather than on dramatic events or traumatic situations. The minor stressors and pleasures of everyday life, "hassles and uplifts," may be significant in health outcomes and the study of stress in general. The Hassles and Uplifts Scale was recently developed to assess the daily and cumulative impact of everyday demands (Kanner, Coyne, Schaefer, & Lazarus, 1981). An example of the 10 most frequent hassles and uplifts reported in a study on the Hassles and Uplift Checklist are presented in Table 5-4 (Kanner *et al.*, 1981). The checklist was administered once a month for 10 consecutive months to a community sample of 100 middle-aged adults. The Hassles Scale was found to be a better predictor of concurrent and subsequent psychological symptoms than were life events scores. Scores on the Uplift Scale were positively related to symptoms for women only. Hassles and Uplifts tended to be modestly related to negative and

**TABLE 5-4**
Frequent Hassles and Uplifts (N = 100)[a]

| Item | % of times checked |
|---|---|
| Hassles | |
| 1. Concerns about weight | 52.4 |
| 2. Health of a family member | 48.1 |
| 3. Rising prices of common goods | 43.7 |
| 4. Home maintenance | 42.8 |
| 5. Too many things to do | 38.6 |
| 6. Misplacing or losing things | 38.1 |
| 7. Yard work or outside home maintenance | 38.1 |
| 8. Property, investment, or taxes | 37.6 |
| 9. Crime | 37.1 |
| 10. Physical appearance | 35.9 |
| Uplifts | |
| 1. Relating well with your spouse or lover | 76.3 |
| 2. Relating well with friends | 74.4 |
| 3. Completing a task | 73.3 |
| 4. Feeling healthy | 72.7 |
| 5. Getting enough sleep | 69.7 |
| 6. Eating out | 68.4 |
| 7. Meeting your responsibilities | 68.1 |
| 8. Visiting, phoning, or writing someone | 67.7 |
| 9. Spending time with family | 66.7 |
| 10. Home (inside) pleasing to you | 65.5 |

*Note.* From "Comparison of Two Modes of Stress Measurement: Daily Hassels and Uplifts versus Major Life Events" by A. D. Kanner, J. C. Coyne, C. Schaefer, and R. S. Lazarus, 1981, *Journal of Behavioral Medicine*, 4, 1–39. Copyright 1981 by Plenum Press. Reprinted by permission.
[a]Items are those most frequently checked over a period of 9 months. The "% of times checked" figures represent the mean percentage of people checking the item each month averaged over the nine monthly administrations.

positive affect, respectively, indicating discrimination between events in comparison to measures of emotion. The initial research indicates that the measurement of daily hassles and uplifts may be a useful assessment of stressors. We can also speculate that ongoing daily stressors may be more directly related to the elicitation of daily stress responses than major life events, since the individual has to respond and expend energy to cope continually. The Hassles and Uplifts Scale provides a tool to evaluate such a hypothesis.

Considerable effort has been directed at measuring social stimuli or, more specifically, the *social environment* or *social climate* (e.g., Moos & Moos, 1981). Moos argues that environments, like people, have unique "personalities," some felt to be more supportive while others more controlling. Also, all environments will have physiological, behavioral, and

**TABLE 5-5A**
Family Environment Subscales and Dimension Descriptions

| | | |
|---|---|---|
| | | Relationship dimensions |
| 1. | Cohesion | The degree of commitment, help, and support family members provide for one another |
| 2. | Expressiveness | The extent to which family members are encouraged to act openly and to express their feelings directly |
| 3. | Conflict | The amount of openly expressed anger, aggression, and conflict among family members |
| | | Personal growth dimensions |
| 4. | Independence | The extent to which family members are assertive, are self-sufficient, and make their own decisions |
| 5. | Achievement orientation | The extent to which activities (such as school and work) are cast into an achievement-oriented or competitive framework |
| 6. | Intellectual–cultural orientation | The degree of interest in political, social, intellectual, and cultural activities |
| 7. | Active–recreational orientation | The extent of participation in social and recreational activities |
| 8. | Moral–religious emphasis | The degree of emphasis on ethical and religious issues and values |
| | | System maintenance dimensions |
| 9. | Organization | The degree of importance of clear organization and structure in planning family activities and responsibilities |
| 10. | Control | The extent to which set rules and procedures are used to run family life |

*Note.* From *Family Environment Scale Manual* (p. 2) by R. H. Moos and B. S. Moos. Copyright 1981 by Consulting Psychologists Press. Reprinted by permission.

psychological effects on the persons interacting within it. Moos and Moos discuss three aspects that discriminate and characterize the following types of environments: psychiatric wards, community-oriented treatment programs, correctional institutions, military basic training companies, college dormitories, junior and senior high school environments, primary work groups, therapeutic and task-oriented groups, and families. Scales have been developed for each environment. The three basic general dimensions characteristic of social climates include relationships, personal development, and system maintenance and change. The Family and Work Environment Scales are examples of social climate scales. Tables 5-5A and 5-5B list the subscales and dimensions of these scales. The *relationship* dimensions assess the degree of an individual's involvement in the environment and with other members in terms of social support. Specific examples include scores on involvement, affiliation, staff support, and expressiveness. The *personal development* dimen-

## TABLE 5-5B
### Work Environment Subscales and Dimension Descriptions

| | Relationship dimensions |
|---|---|
| 1. Involvement | The extent to which employees are concerned about and committed to their jobs |
| 2. Peer cohesion | The extent to which employees are friendly and supportive of one another |
| 3. Supervisor support | The extent to which management is supportive of employees and encourages employees to be supportive of one another |
| | Personal growth dimensions |
| 4. Autonomy | The extent to which employees are encouraged to be self-sufficient and to make their own decisions |
| 5. Task orientation | The degree of emphasis on good planning, efficiency, and getting the job done |
| 6. Work pressure | The degree to which the press of work and time urgency dominate the job milieu |
| | System maintenance and systems change dimensions |
| 7. Clarity | The extent to which employees know what to expect in their daily routine and how explicitly rules and policies are communicated |
| 8. Control | The extent to which management uses rules and pressures to keep employees under control |
| 9. Innovation | The degree of emphasis on variety, change, and new approaches |
| 10. Physical comfort | The extent to which the physical surroundings contribute to a pleasant work environment |

*Note.* From *Work Environment Scale Manual* (p. 2) by R. H. Moos. Copyright 1981 by Consulting Psychologists Press. Reprinted by permission.

sions examine basic directions of self-enhancement and personal development within an environment, although dimensions vary according to the type of environment. For example, practical applications appear on the scale for psychiatric workers, but not for military companies. The third category includes *systems maintenance and system change* dimensions that involve order and organization, clarity and control. Kiritz and Moos (1974) cite several studies that support the hypothesis that the dimensions within the three categories have important effects on physiological processes. Thus, it has been shown that social stimuli associated with support, cohesiveness, and affiliation dimensions generally have positive effects, such as enhancing normal development and reducing recovery time from illness. But responsibility, work pressure, and change can increase the likelihood of illness, disease, or subjective distress. Given the potential importance of the perception of one's social environment, further research on the relationship between social climate and the stress response, as well as on the potential utility of social climate scales for clinical purposes, is warranted.

An approach somewhat similar to the social climate strategy of Moos is the identification of specific groups of individuals commonly exposed to a set of stressors in order to develop a method of defining and quantifying these stressors. An example of this type of approach is the Nursing Stress Scale (NSS), in which situations that may cause stress for nurses in the performance of their duties were identified (Gray-Taft & Anderson, 1981). Gray-Taft and Anderson argue that despite the recognition of stress experienced by nursing staff, which may be related to burn-out, job satisfaction, and patient care, few measures are available to assess such stress. Items on the NSS were based on 34 potentially stressful situations identified from the literature and from interviews with nurses, physicians, and hospital chaplains. A sample of 122 nurses in five units of a large, private general hospital were asked to rate how frequently the items on the scale were stressful for them. Six factors or subscales were identified; they included work load, death and dying, inadequate preparation to deal with the emotional needs of patients, lack of staff support, uncertainty concerning treatment, conflict with physicians, and conflict with other nurses and supervisors. The NSS was found to be acceptably reliable on test–retest and internal consistency and correlated with trait anxiety, job satisfaction, and nursing turnover. Although still in the experimental stage, the NSS measures stressors relevant to nurses. Given the problems discussed earlier with the various general life events scales, it is likely that such devices as the NSS will be developed for assessing stressors in specific groups or subpopulations.

In summary, attempts to measure stressors fall into several categories; these include life events, daily stressors, and social climate for particular environments and/or subgroups. In the laboratory, the experimenter usually identifies and manipulates the stressor; therefore, he or she does not assess the stressor, but rather the stress response. In the following section, the measurement of the stress response in the laboratory, as well as in the natural environment, will be discussed.

## Measurement of Coping/Appraisal Processes

Cognitive coping responses have been postulated as moderating or intervening variables between stressors and the stress response. Cognitive coping responses may include (1) active cognitive attempts to manage one's appraisal of the stressfulness of the event, "tried to see the positive side of the situation"; (2) cognitive attempt to avoid actively confronting the problem, "keep my feelings to myself"; and (3) cognitive responses, the primary function of which is to manage the emotional consequences of stressors or to help maintain emotional equilibrium (Billings & Moos, 1981). Attempts to assess coping responses are exemplified by two large-scale surveys (Billings and Moos, 1981; Ilfeld, 1980).

Billings and Moos (1981) focused on both coping responses and social resources as intervening variables mediating the effect of life events on personal functioning among a representative adult community sample in the San Francisco Bay Area. They mailed surveys to 360 families; 82 percent (294) were completed. Their results are based on a subsample of 194 families in which both partners responded to items on social resources and coping responses. Measures in the survey were designed to assess a broad range of personal, social, and health-related information; the family setting; negative life change events; coping responses; and mood and symptom measures.

Coping responses were assessed by requesting that respondents indicate a recent personal crisis or stressful life event and then indicate yes/no to 19 items to determine how they handled the situation. Items were selected from a review of the coping response literature and another inventory. Items were grouped both in terms of problem focused (active-cognitive, active-behavioral, and avoidance) and emotion focused; these groupings were based on cluster analysis, judges ratings, and the conceptual and empirical literature. Table 5-6 lists the various coping response categories. The percentage of items answered "yes" was the score for each coping measure.

The respondents endorsed all categories of coping responses. Active-behavioral and active-cognitive coping strategies were more frequently used (60.9% and 62.7%, respectively), with less use of avoid-

**TABLE 5-6**
Coping Response Categories

| Coping items | Method of coping | | | Focus of coping | |
|---|---|---|---|---|---|
| | Active cognitive | Active behavioral | Avoidance | Problem focused | Emotion focused |
| Tried to see the positive side | X | | | | X |
| Tried to step back from the situation and be more objective | X | | | | X |
| Prayed for guidance or strength | X | | | | X |
| Took things one step at a time | X | | | X | |
| Considered several alternatives for handling the problem | X | | | X | |
| Drew on my past experiences; I was in a similar situation before | X | | | X | |
| Tried to find out more about the situation | | X | | X | |
| Talked with professional person (e.g., doctor, clergy, lawyer) about the situation | | X | | X | |
| Took some positive action | | X | | X | |
| Talked with spouse or other relative about the situation | | X | | X | |
| Talked with friend about the situation | | X | | | |
| Exercised more | | X | | | X |
| Prepared for the worst | | | X | | X |
| Sometimes took it out on other people when I felt angry or depressed | | | X | | X |
| Tried to reduce the tension by eating more | | | X | | X |
| Tried to reduce the tension by smoking more | | | X | | X |
| Kept my feelings to myself | | | X | | X |
| Got busy with other things in order to keep my mind off the problem | | | | | X |
| Didn't worry about it; figured everything would probably work out fine | | | | | X |

*Note.* From ''The Role of Coping Responses and Social Resources in Attenuating the Stress of Life Events'' by A. G. Billings and R. H. Moos, 1981, *Journal of Behavioral Medicine, 4,* 146. Copyright 1981 by Plenum Press. Reprinted by permission.

ance strategies (24%). Problem-focused (49.9%) responses were used more frequently than emotion-focused responses. Small but significant sex differences were found, with men reporting less frequent use of active-behavioral, avoidance, and emotion-focused strategies than women. Higher levels of education were related to active-cognitive and problem-focused coping and less to avoidance coping. A positive relationship was reported for higher income individuals and active-behavioral, active-cognitive, and problem-focused coping.

No significant correlations were found between severity and type of life event and measure of coping. The results indicated a reduction in the impact of life events as coping responses and social resources were sequentially entered into a regression equation. It was also found that coping measures added significant power to the prediction of stress levels. Avoidance coping tended to be more highly related to the criteria than active-cognitive or behavioral. Billings and Moos (1981) conclude that clustering coping responses into method and focus of coping resulted in an assessment device of psychometric adequacy and utility in examining the role of coping responses as moderator/variables between stressful life events and stress response, as indicated by negative mood and physical symptoms.

Ilfeld (1980) used a 90-minute structured interview that was designed to assess (1) demographic and background information; (2) sources of stress in marriage, parenting, finances, and job; (3) coping responses; and (4) psychological status. The interview section that assessed coping responses was initially developed by asking respondents both to identify problems of everyday life and to describe how they dealt with those problems. The final form of the interview focused on stressors relating to marriage, parenting, finances, and job and coping patterns. Interviewers probed in a structured way, but did not ask the same number of questions for each of the four role areas. Examples of the interview include asking about different things people do to "help them get along on their jobs" and asking about "different things parents do when they find something in their children's behavior that is troublesome."

Answers to the interview by 2,299 Chicago families were factor-analyzed and three patterns emerged:

1. *Action strategy.* Concrete active steps are taken toward the source of stress.

2. *Rationalization/avoidance.* The efforts made include minimizing, excusing, ignoring, and avoiding the stress.

3. *Acceptance.* Problems are recognized, but not minimized and respondents seem resigned to accept the circumstances rather than to change them.

**TABLE 5-7**
Coping Response Rates

| Response | Rate (%) |
| --- | --- |
| Distraction | 27 |
| Situation redefinition | 25 |
| Direct action | 46 |
| Catharsis | 25 |
| Acceptance | 30 |
| Social support | 15 |
| Relaxation | 17 |
| Religion | 6 |
| Other methods | 7 |

Respondents did not use only one style of coping response for all role areas. As with the Billings and Moos questionnaire, this study reports a potentially useful measure of cognitive and behavioral coping responses. Initial results with a large sample indicate that the types of cognitive coping responses used in dealing with stressors can be identified.

Because a brief measure sensitive to the dynamic process of change in coping over time was not available, Stone and Neale (1984) developed a questionnaire to measure various coping categories longitudinally. The coping categories included distraction, situation redefinition, direct action, catharsis, acceptance, seeking social support, relaxation, and religion. Preliminary results using the measure indicated the following: (1) coping styles were used with reasonable frequency, (2) women reported slightly more styles than males, (3) type of appraisal (e.g., desirable, meaningful, stabilizing) was associated with type of coping style, and (4) some degree of consistency in use of coping style is seen across days. Coping response rates are illustrated in Table 5-7.

## MEASUREMENT OF STRESS RESPONSE

An assessment of the stress response can be made using physiological, behavioral, or cognitive measures. Currently, there is more variety in the types of measures for the stress response than for the stressors themselves. Part of the reason for this is that the stress response is often thought of as the dependent variable in studies and, therefore, must be measured. We will examine examples of measurement devices for different components of the stress response and discuss current areas of concern.

## Biological Component

*Psychophysiological.* The psychophysiological responses are generally thought to be an important component of the stress response. Psychophysiological response is conceptualized as either a nonspecific or specific response to physical as well as to psychological stressors (e.g., Selye, 1956). Various models of stress directly or indirectly elude to the connection between stressors, stress response, and illness outcome. The psychophysiological response is frequently conceptualized as a peripheral index of the transduction process between stressor and illness. The electrical activity of muscle, heart rate, electrodermal response, and blood pressure are widely used in the measurement of the stress response. Blood pressure and muscle activity have been implicated in the establishment or maintenance of such health-related problems as hypertension and pain disorders, respectively. Psychophysiological responses are used to assess the impact of a stressor, as well as to compare the psychophysiological responses for different stressors or groups of individuals to a stressor. Chapter 4 provided a general description of these types of psychophysiological responses. Although psychophysiological measurement has been often used in studies of stress, there is much that is still unknown regarding these peripheral response systems. Future research should examine the relationship between psychophysiological indices and other components of the stress response. Perhaps the pattern of responses will permit a more comprehensive understanding of the interaction among stressors, stress response, adaptation, and illness. Most studies obtain one or two measurements in an acute stressor situation. It would be useful to examine these variables over time relative to other indicators of stress.

*Biochemical.* The assessment of biochemical factors relating to stress is becoming more sophisticated and is used more often. The availability of portable methods for obtaining blood samples from ambulatory subjects (Dimsdale & Moss, 1980) and the development of highly sensitive hormonal assays have allowed researchers to study the biochemical response to stressful situations more readily in the laboratory and the natural environment. Adrenocorticotropic hormone (ACTH), catecholamines, and endorphins are some of the biochemical variables studied. Several physiological systems have been implicated in active and passive coping with stress. These include the central nervous system, catecholamine, immune, endorphin-enkephalin, hypothalamico-pituitary-adrenocortical and the sympatho-adrenomedullary systems (McCabe & Schneiderman, 1984; Baum, Grunberg, & Singer, 1982).

The sympatho-adrenomedullary system (SAS) is activated during active coping (flight or fight), which generally, but not always, involves physical exertion. This system increases metabolic activity in response to stressful situations. Measures of norepinephrine and epinephrine are typically used to indicate the activity of the SAS (Frankenhaeuser, 1975a). Because of its importance in coping, the SAS has been studied in the stress literature and has been implicated in such physical disorders as hypertension, atherosclerosis, angina pectoris, cardiac arrhythmias, and myocardial ischemia, to name a few.

The hypothalamico-pituitary-adrenocortical (HPAC) system plays a role in the organism's response to emotionally stressful situations in which active coping is not possible. Other stressors that activate this system are heat, cold, infection, sympathomimetic drugs, and surgery. The HPAC system is associated with a "conservation-withdrawal" pattern characterized by vigilance, sympathetic nervous system activation, inhibition of movement, and bradycardia associated with the parasympathetic nervous system. Various cardiovascular diseases, peptic ulceration, suppression of the immune system, and clinical depression have been associated with this conservation-withdrawal pattern. Adrenocorticotropic hormone and corticosteroids are often measured, as they are thought to be involved in negative feedback loops of the HPAC system.

Brain catecholamines are thought to be involved in stress (Dunn & Kramarty, 1984) and depression (Sachar, Asnis, Halbreich, Nathan, & Halpern, 1980). The work reported by Sachar et al. (1980) is consistent with the view that norepinephrine depletion in the central nervous system (CNS) disinhibits cortisol releasing factor secretion in the hypothalamus, which contributes to cortisol releasing factor secretion in the hypothalamus and, thus, to the hypersecretion of cortisol seen in certain cases of clinical depression. It has also been discovered that animals in situations involving uncontrollable shock demonstrate disturbances similar to depression (Weiss, 1972). Regional changes of norepinephrine in the brainstem have been reported to correlate with stress or induced depression of motor activity (Weiss, Bailey, Pohorecky, Korzeniowski, & Grillione, 1980). Thus, one approach to studying stress is by assessment of brain catecholamines.

The endorphin-enkephalin system may also be involved in aversive situations requiring active coping (Jaffe & Martin, 1980). Endorphins and enkephalins may help reduce fear, inhibit pain-related withdrawal behaviors, and reduce pain during coping responses. The measurement of the endogenous opiates provides another avenue for measuring the physiological component of the stress response.

Intense, unavoidable stress, may influence susceptability to illness by affecting the immune system (McCabe & Schneiderman, 1984). In a review of the literature on stress and the immune system, McCabe and Schneiderman (1984) conclude that acute stress increases the steroid hormones known to be lymphalytic, which suppresses the immune response. This has been associated with increased susceptibility to infection and to a greater likelihood of tumor growth, although the mechanisms are both complex and unclear. The immune system is affected by the HPAC system, as well as the CNS, and stress has also been associated with an enhancement of immune function (Ader & Cohen, 1985).

Physiological markers of stress cannot be used as the sole indicators of the stress response; they measure only one aspect of the stressor–stress response and may be sensitive to other factors as well. In addition to stressors, level of activity, sex, age, and weight can affect the physiological responses in humans.

## Behavioral Component

Behavioral assessment, in general, includes both direct observations made by the experimenter and self-reports by the subject.

*Behavioral Observation.* There are two types of observational methods. The first includes recording such specific behaviors as facial expressions, and rate of speech, usually in an interview setting. A structured interview procedure that assesses Type A behavior, which has received considerable attention, appears to be a reliable and valid indicator of a behavior pattern associated with coronary heart disease (Chesney, Eagleston, & Rosenman, 1980). In a global assessment of Type A, specific behaviors such as voice volume, speech rate, posture, and competing for control of the interview, as well as patient attitudes and affect, are measured. Similar assessment procedures to assess stress-related behaviors for other types of problems may prove worthwhile, although such observational methods in stress studies have been limited because it is often difficult to construct reliable and valid measures of behavior. There is the problem of observer bias and reactivity of observational assessment techniques (Kent & Foster, 1977). Reliability coefficients should range between .80 and .90 for inter-rater reliability. The choice of what types of behavior to observe is often complicated. Should basic facial expressions, movement, or verbal responses be recorded, or more complex behaviors reflecting attitudes or emotions?

The second type of behavioral-observation method is used most often in stress research and has to do with performance ability or adaptive functioning. A wide range of tasks or tests have been used to assess changes in several aspects of a person's performance in such areas as memory, attention, learning, problem solving, and visual-motor skills. Performance tasks are useful in that distress, activation, or arousal can affect a person's ability to perform by decreasing motivation, attention, concentration, or other factors and that these factors determine the quality of performance before, during, and after exposure to stressors. Sometimes arousal is associated with improved performance, but on other tasks, it is associated with poorer performance (Evans, 1978). Performance tasks can be used to distinguish between people who are not stressed and those who are or to determine conditions in which tasks are made increasingly stressful while the subject's performance is compared under different conditions. It is important to choose tasks that distinguish stressed from nonstressed subjects or tasks that are potentially stressful and tasks that are not. Performance measures that assess aspects of the individual's response to stress have usually been obtained in a laboratory setting. The generalizability of laboratory based performance-stress studies to performance-stress in the natural environment is questionable, since experimental conditions are often quite contrived. Over the past two decades, for example, the most frequently used method for manipulating physical stimuli and recording the stress response has been with the use of electric shock (Patkai, 1974). Electric shock is easily quantified and manipulated in the laboratory, but how often is an individual's performance in the natural environment influenced by the knowledge that an electric shock may be subsequently administered? This is not to say analogue studies are not useful; they can provide data in well-controlled situations and test hypotheses that can later be evaluated in the natural environment.

*Self-Report Measures.*   Self-report questionnaires, rating scales, or checklists are used by the subject to indicate behavior that may not be observable in the experimental setting or to provide additional information on behavior. Activity schedules, marital satisfaction questionnaires, sexual behavior questionnaires, or ratings of such specific behaviors as nail biting, frequency of urination, or avoidance of certain stressors are only a few examples of *behavioral* self-reports. No comprehensive source of data is available on the use of self-report of behavior in studying stress. This is unfortunate, since many aspects of an individual's activity relative to stress could be important. For instance, what happens to a severely stressed person's sexual activity and sexual desire? Frequency of sexual activity may influence self-concept, and if frequency is at an undesirable level, it could become a source of distress itself. Although these are common clinical assumptions, there is little empirical support for such hypotheses.

## Cognitive Component

The cognitive component of the stress response represents an important variable in several stress models. Measuring cognition can only be by indirect means of observation, subject to inaccuracy and reactivity (Hollon & Bemis, 1981). But given the major role cognition may play in the phenomenon of stress, attempts to measure it are warranted. Hollan and Bemis delineate several dimensions in which cognitive processes can be assessed; these include *process-content, occurrence-nonoccurrence, conscious-nonconscious, meaning,* and *validity*. The difficulties in discussing cognitive assessment are that the concepts of *cognition* and *cognitive process* are not easily defined and operationalized; their meaning will often be based on a particular theoretical position. Different theories may focus on different aspects of the dimensions described by Hollan and Bemis. Thus, one researcher may be interested in the content or product of cognitive processes and may utilize introspection and self-report of "thoughts" or checklists of attitudes held or emotions experienced. Other researchers may be interested in cognitive processes that may or may not be consciously accessible to the subject. Nisbett and Wilson (1977) discuss how subjects frequently are unable to verbalize cognitive processes thought to mediate associations among stimuli, cognitive processes, change in evaluative and motivational state, and behavior. Researchers have found that subjects can accurately perform a task, yet be unable to explain how they did it. For example, Nisbet and Wilson found that subjects were consistently unable to detect the role that left-to-right position preference played in their evaluation of articles of clothing.

Cognitive assessment, then, can refer to a wide variety of measures designed to measure thoughts, beliefs, attitudes, and mood, to name a few. It is important to emphasize that cognitive processes do not only represent components of the stress response, but also that they can actually influence the stress response (i.e., serve as mediating variables). This concept will become clearer when transactional models of stress are discussed in the next section. Of particular relevance to the measurement of the cognitive component of the stress response is an assessment of perceived control, mood, and perceived autonomic arousal. A survey of the research literature shows that these concepts are often examined relative to behavioral and physiological variables that may be associated with stress, health, and disease. Measures of the cognitive components of the stress response are usually in the form of self-report questionnaire, checklist, or interview.

Eckenrode (1984) provides an example of an approach to measuring the cognitive component of the response to both acute and chronic stressors. In a time series analysis, Eckenrode requested female subjects to keep daily diaries for 28 days following an initial interview. The information obtained in the diary included daily stressful events, symptoms, and overall mood (Lickert-type scale—extremely poor to extremely good) or general feeling of well-being over the day. Interview data were collected on acute stressors (acute life changes in preceding 12 months), chronic stressors (low levels of socioeconomic status and persistent major social role conflict), psychological well-being (affect balance—positive/negative emotional state), and additional sociodemographic and health status measures. The findings indicated that concurrent daily stressors and physical symptoms, in addition to previous levels of psychological well-being, were the most important direct determinants of mood. Life events and chronic stressors indirectly affected mood through the influence of daily stressors, physical symptoms, and psychological well-being. This study illustrates the relative importance of daily stressors on mood in contrast to the more chronic stressors.

Cognitive and/or perceived control has been thought to reduce stress responses (Miller, 1978). Averill (1973) distinguishes two components to cognitive control: (1) *information gain,* predictability of a stressor and the anticipation of an aversive event, and (2) *anticipatory response,* cognitive preparation for an event, involving interpretation and evaluation of an event. The specific role of perceived control in stress will be discussed in the next section. At present, the reader should simply be aware that cognitive measures are often used to study these phenomena. Self-report ratings of anxiety, tension, and thoughts of anticipation, as well as self-reports of pain or aversiveness of an experimental condition are used. The subject is also asked to indicate whether they prefer controllable or uncontrollable aversive stimuli.

Self-report of autonomic nervous system (ANS) activity also represents a cognitive measure of the stress reaction. Inventories are used to assess an individual's ability to perceive ANS activity or as a means of assessing or predicting a specific ANS response. Both types of questionnaires can be helpful in the evaluation of cognitive aspects of the stress response. A number of self-report measures of ANS activity exist. An early self-report device is the Autonomic Perception Questionnaire (APQ) (Mandler, Mandler, & Uviller, 1958). The APQ includes 30 items, 28 of which represent ANS responses. The subject rates the items with end point anchoring statements (e.g., always–never), and 7 items are rated for pleasure and 21 for anxiety. The midpoints of the scales are not defined numerically or by anchoring statements. Basic psychometric data on reliability and norms are not reported, although some indices of validity are available. Research on the relationship of APQ scores and psychophysiological activity reports nonsignificant correlations between APQ scores and physiological activity. However, Mandler *et al.* (1958) observed a correlation between the APQ and a measure of anxiety. These data indicate that the APQ maybe useful in assessing an individual's ability to preceive ANS activity, but not in describing or predicting actual ANS activity.

A recent effort to develop a more comprehensive and multidimensional measure of perceived autonomic responsiveness resulted in the Perceived Somatic Response Inventory (Meadow, Kochever, Tellegen, & Roberts, 1978). A research inventory was given to 525 subjects 299 of which were female; median age over 20. Three scales were developed, based on the initial research instrument. The Autonomic Response Frequency scale represents a measure of the subject's experience of spontaneous fluctuations in autonomic reactivity. The second scale, Autonomic Response to Stress Scale, reflects a subject's perceived autonomic reactions when subjected to stress. The third scale, Somatic Response Control, indicates the autonomic functions over which the subject is believed to have voluntary control. Results indicate that the three scales are relatively independent of each other and of general personality variables. Also, all three demonstrate good internal consistency and reliability. The Perceived Somatic Response Inventory can be useful in a variety of research endeavors, including evaluating predictive utility and relationships among stress reactions and perceived autonomic reaction and somatic control. The Inventory can be readily included in an assessment procedure, since it is inexpensive and easy to use. However, as with all the above assessment devices, the exclusive use of a perceived somatic questionnaire is not a sufficient measure of stress. The next section will illustrate why this is so.

## Multimodal Measurement of the Stress Response

We have discussed physiological, behavioral, and cognitive assessment of the stress response. The question now arises as to what kinds of responses are to be regarded as indices of stress? The answer depends on the theoretical orientation of the researcher and the technical limitations of measurement. The use of several responses, that is, *multimodal measurement*, offers the greatest degree of information and allows comparisons of types of responses, as well as an assessment of the *patterning* of response. Several models of stress emphasize the occurrence of multiple responses in reaction to a stressor, including cognitive, behavioral, and physiological responses. Therefore, multimodal assessment as a means of evaluating such models would be useful. A well-designed study on stage fright in musicians exemplifies such a multimodal ap-

proach to the assessment of stress (Neftel, Adler, Kappelli, Rossi, Dolder, Kaser, Bruggesser, & Vor Kauf, 1982).

The action of beta-blockers on stage fright and on the technical
motor performance of 22 performing string players were assessed. Half
the subjects received 100 mg of atenolol and the other half a placebo $6\frac{1}{2}$
hours before performing with and then without an audience. Cognitive,
physiological, and behavioral measures of stage fright (considered a
stress response) were used before and after each performance. Physiological measures included *continuous* electrocardiogram (ECG) and urine
catecholamine levels. The cognitive measure used was a self-report rating scale of stage fright. The stage-fright scale consisted of six bipolar
statements chosen from 60 different statements reported regularly by
performing string players based on their experience of stage fright. The
six statements and their antitheses marked the two ends of a visual
analogue scale for each statement. Examples of the statements are (1) If I
could, I would give up; (2) I feel that my physical health is extremely
poor/I feel very well; (3) I could not sound better today/I have the feeling
I do not at all sound the way I would like to today. A behavioral measure
consisted of an analysis of technical motor performance by means of a
sonograph. The sonograph provides a graphic analysis of the frequencies of sound as a function of time recorded during the performance.
Analysis of these data can provide an index of the musical quality of the
performance.

Results of the study showed that the placebo group's technical
motor performance was significantly impaired in the presence of an
audience as compared to performance with no audience; however, the
beta-blocker group's performance was slightly but statistically significantly improved. The beta-blocker group did not experience a reduction
in stage fright *before* performing in the presence of an audience (i.e.,
anticipatory stress), but reported reduced stage fright *during* the concert.
Urine catecholamine analyses showed levels to be *increased* twice as
much under beta-blockade as under placebo in the presence of the audience. The authors conclude that the drug was somewhat effective in
the sense that it improved technical motor performance (behavioral response) and that the beta-blockade only involves a peripheral site of
action. Again, the significance of this study for the present discussion is
the illustration of several modes of assessment. It is interesting to note
that only the behavioral response was affected by the drug. With such a
multimodal assessment, it is possible for the authors to conclude with a
specific statement, that is the *behavioral* component of the stress response was influenced, rather than making a global and relatively meaningless statement of the effect of beta-blockade on stress.

As will be discussed in the next section, more recent models of
stress emphasize the importance of a dynamic evaluation of stressors

and cognitive appraisal processes and their outcome, that is, the stress response (Cox, 1978). These models hypothesize that environmental factors (i.e., potential stressors) may influence the pattern of coping efforts that are set into motion during a stressful transaction and also that coping may influence which environmental factors will be involved and what form they will take (Coyne & Lazarus, 1980). Therefore, rather than a fixed entity that impinges on the person, environmental stimuli are only potentially important, becoming more salient by their interaction or *transaction* with coping efforts. This transactional perspective, to be discussed in greater detail in the next section, hypothesizes reciprocal feedback loops. Such a model necessitates a dynamic assessment of the reciprocal interactions of environmental contexts, cognitive appraisals, and coping behaviors and their concomitant biological, behavioral, and cognitive consequences (i.e., the stress response).

## MODELS OF STRESS

As indicated earlier, reaching a generally accepted definition of stress is difficult, since there are several approaches to understanding stress. This section will discuss the major models of stress, and each model provides its own definition. They can be best divided into *response-based, stimulus-based, transactional,* and *information-processing* models.

### Response-Based Models

Response-based models tend to emphasize the determination of a particular response, or pattern of responses, that reflects a situation in which the person is under strain from a stressor. As depicted in Figure 5-3, the actual psychological and physiological responses are considered stress responses. Studies investigating this model view stress as a dependent variable. Selye's (1956) general adaptation syndrome (GAS) is an example of the response-based concept of stress.

The GAS model explicitly defines stress as a nonspecific physiological response of the organism to all types of demanding environmental stimuli. Selye emphasized that the stress response is nonspecific, that is, it is elicited by any stressor, and it can be thought of as a universal pattern of defense responses that serves to protect and preserve the biological integrity of the person. Thus, stress is a nonspecific and universal response. The second basic idea is that the stress response progresses through three identifiable phases as the individual is exposed to continual or repeated stressors. On an initial exposure to the stressor, an alarm reaction occurs and the level of resistance is reduced. During the

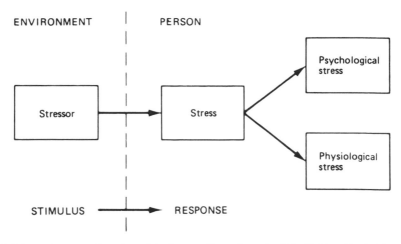

**FIGURE 5-3.** Response-based model of stress. From *Stress* (p. 4) by T. Cox. Copyright 1978 by Macmillan Press, Ltd. London. Reprinted by permission.

first phase, if the stressor is severe enough, resistance may collapse and death result. If not, the individual enters into the second stage in which continued exposure to stimulation is compatible with adaptation. During the second phase, the response characteristics of the alarm reaction diminish and resistance rises above normal. The third phase is one of exhaustion and possible death if the body's energy for adaptation is depleted from continued exposure. A final point regarding Selye's model is that the stress response, although initially adaptive, if severe and prolonged may result in disease states. Thus, a decline in resistance to stress below normal levels is associated with the development of disease and with physical trauma. A detailed explanation of the role of stress in the development of illness, according to the GAS model, will be discussed in Chapter 6.

### Stimulus-Based Models

The "person on the street" most often thinks of stress according to a stimulus-based model. As he or she might say, "that was a stressful situation, or he was surely stressed by that meeting." Figure 5-4 illustrates the stimulus-based model, which is essentially based on engineering principles. Stress is defined in terms of the stimulus characteristics of the environment that are disruptive to the individual. In other words, stress arises from the individual's environment and the reaction to external stressors is *strain*.

A physics concept, Hooke's Law of Elasticity, can be used to illustrate the stimulus-based model. Hooke's Law describes how loads produce deformation in metals. The stress or load is placed on the metal and deformation (strain) of the metal may result. Essentially, if the strain produced by a given load or stress is within the "elastic limit" of the material, when the load or stress is removed, the metal will return to its original shape. If the load pushes beyond the elastic limit, the metal will become deformed. Individuals vary in their ability to tolerate stress, which can be tolerated up to a point. However, when stress becomes intolerable, physical or psychological damage may result. The task for proponents of stimulus-based models is to delineate the conditions or characteristics of stressful situations.

Holmes and Rahe (1967) have attempted to identify stressful situations or life events and to determine the impact of these life events on individuals. According to Holmes and Rahe, stressful life events include a variety of situations, such as divorce, death of a significant other, job promotion, or vacation. The Holmes and Rahe model of stress will be discussed at greater length in Chapter 6, although it is important to note here that these researchers initially focused on environmental events as the "stress." In addition to the general group of stressful life events, specific stimuli that are considered "stressful" have been studied, usually in an experimental setting. These include the effect of shock, situations in which the experimenter attempts to elicit anger, isolation and confinement, group pressure, and situations in which the subject has no control over an aversive stimuli (Frankenhaeuser, 1975b; Lazarus, 1976;

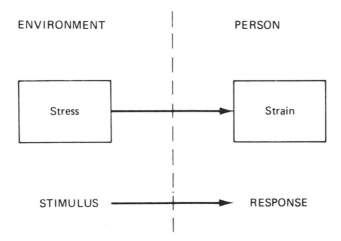

**FIGURE 5-4.** Stimulus-based model of stress. From *Stress* (p. 12) by T. Cox. Copyright 1978 by Macmillan Press, Ltd. London. Reprinted by permission.

Weitz, 1970). As with response-based definitions, stimulus-based definitions appear to focus on only one aspect of the stress experience, that is,
stimulus as opposed to response. The problems with such an approach
include the identification of a stressful stimulus, its measurement, and
how to account for the individual variability in response to it. An integration of the stimulus- and response-based models is provided by interactional models of stress.

## Interactional Models

Interaction models go beyond considering both stimulus and response aspects of stress and propose that stress occurs through a particular relationship between the person and the environment. The
individual is thought of as an active agent in the stress process, and it is
postulated that self-regulation of cognitive, behavioral, and emotional
coping strategies influence the impact of a stressor. Roskies and Lazarus
(1980) and Cox and Mckay (1978) propose models that focus on the
transactional and ecological nature of stress as well as the importance of
the individual's cognitive and psychological sets in evaluating the
stressors. Their models also specify the existence of feedback components, therefore describing a cyclical rather than linear system.

The transactional model, as described by Cox and Mackay and illustrated in Figure 5-5, has five discernible stages. The first stage identifies
the existence of demands or stressors placed on the individual. The
model identifies two types of demands: internal and external. The internal demands relate to the physical and psychological needs of the individual and can be potent factors in determining subsequent behavior.
The external demands represent potential sources of stress that are a
function of environmental factors, such as excessive work load provided
by a supervisor, a physically uncomfortable work area, or a family member who constantly requires one's involvement. The second stage consists of a person's perception of internal and external demands and of
his or her ability to meet these important needs. Stress occurs when an
imbalance between perceived demand and perceived coping ability exists. Such organismic variables as personality, ego strength, and intelligence account for individual variations in the cognitive appraisal of
stress. If a situation is more than an individual can handle, and this is
not recognized, the individual will continue working until it becomes
obvious that coping is no longer possible. This imbalance will result in
the experience of stress. The third stage of the model represents the
stress response, which is a method of coping with the stressor. The
subjective emotional experience of stress is accompanied by cognitive,
behavioral, and physiological changes that attempt to reduce the de-

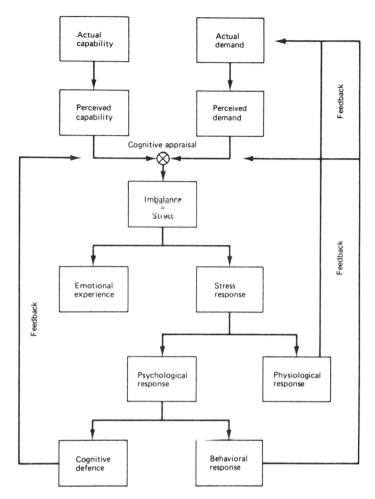

**FIGURE 5-5.** Transactional model of stress. From *Stress* (p. 19) by T. Cox. Copyright 1978 by Macmillan Press, Ltd. London. Reprinted by permission.

mand. Although in other models the stress response is often thought of as the final phase of the stress reaction, Cox and Mackay delineate a fourth stage. This fourth stage is concerned with both the actual and perceived consequences of the coping responses. Stress may continue to occur when the individual fails to meet demand or when negative consequences resulting from failure are anticipated. The fifth stage consists of the feedback that occurs throughout the system and may shape events at any point in the system. Feedback of appropriate responses can enhance the individual's ability to adapt. Feedback of inappropriate responses may intensify the stress response and cause greater damage or may alert the individual to change a response, if possible, or to seek intervention. Feedback occurs at many different levels, including the physiological, psychological, and social.

The person–environment transaction model explicitly states that stress is a function of the relationship between the person and environment. Thus, specific stimuli or responses cannot necessarily be labeled as stressful or not stressful without evaluating the person–environment relationship. The environment includes the social background of the individual (i.e., cultural factors). Social support systems also play a role in the individual experience of stress. Let us now consider a model of stress that utilizes concepts of information processing.

### Information-Processing Model

This model distinguishes among psychological, physiological, and biochemical stress (Hamilton, 1980). The stressors and stress response are both considered, but the information-processing model emphasizes that neither can be recognized without an interpretation of the stimuli as stressful. Thus, the information-processing approach relies heavily on cognitive appraisal and attention. The individual's interpretation of stress requires selective attention, as well as decisions on which stimuli to process, via short-term working memory, and which to ignore. Also, the processing of information involves long-term memory structures, that is, cognitive predisposition, which allows the individual to interpret some stimuli as pleasurable and others as aversive. In other words, perceptions of incoming stimuli are compared to perceptions the individual has had experience with and remembers. Attention, short- and long-term memory, and decision-making processes are involved in the cognitive appraisal of stimuli and responses as stressful. In addition to the cognitive labeling of stressors, these processes elicit such conditioned affective-emotive responses as anxiety, fear, anger, or sadness. Affective-emotive responses are important in activating the processes of cognitive appraisal. Figure 5-6 illustrates the information processing model, which postulates that the greater the number of stressors appraised by the individual, the greater the strain on the system. In general, the greater the strain, the greater the informational load on an individual's cognitive and biological processes. Hamilton points out that, although the model resembles Hooke's Law of Elasticity, it is considerably more complex, and a nonlinear relationship between load and strain is more likely to exist.

According to this model, three general types of stressors have been proposed: (1) anticipation of physical pain or danger, (2) situations that

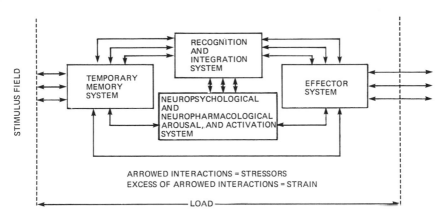

**FIGURE 5-6.** Information processing model of stress. From "An Information Processing Analysis of Environmental Stress and Life Crisis" by V. Hamilton in *Stress and Anxiety* (Vol. 7), edited by I. G. Sarason and C. D. Spielberger. Copyright 1980 by Hemisphere Publishing Corp. Reprinted by permission.

threaten social isolation or rejection, and (3) stimulus complexity involving either concurrent response demands or novelty and complexity. The information processing model of load, stressors, and strain is relatively new, and initial research has provided some support for the model (Hamilton, 1980).

## FACTORS THAT INFLUENCE RESPONSE TO STRESS

### Cognitive Modulators

A discussion of cognitive modulators of stress is important, since researchers are becoming increasingly concerned with their definition, existence, and function in the stress response. The transactional model of stress discussed earlier emphasizes the person's cognitive appraisal of the stressor as well as his or her response to the stressors as being important in the overall effects of stress and future responses. Concepts to be discussed in this section are *cognitive coping skills, perceived control,* and *defensiveness.*

In order to understand the meaning of *cognitive coping skills,* we must first define *coping skills.* There are many definitions of coping; two examples are (1) an individual's attempt to resolve life stressors and emotional pain (Ilfeld, 1980) and (2) self-regulation either by direct action, that is by attempting to control the environment, or by palliative modes, that is by reducing affective, visceral, or motor disturbances related to the stressful environment (Lazarus, 1974). Billings and Moos (1981) provide a framework for operationally defining coping responses and identify several potential behavioral and cognitive coping responses available to a person. *Coping* can be thought of as having two components: the *methods* used and the *focus* of the coping response. Table 5-8 illustrates eight types of potential coping responses, each defined by a particular combination of method and focus of coping. In terms of the method of coping, the individual can utilize either an *active* response to resolve the stressful event or choose to *avoid* the stressor. The focus of the coping response may be directed at the problem itself (problem focused) or the emotional consequences of the stressor (emotion focused).

Utilizing this framework to understand cognitive coping skills, we can refer to a wide variety of cognitive processes that focus on either the problem itself or its emotional consequences. Active cognitive coping responses are those responses designed to manage one's appraisal of the stressfulness of the problem itself or its emotional consequences. An example of an active cognitive coping response that focuses on reducing the emotional consequences of a stressor would be the utilization of a self-hypnosis procedure to decrease anxiety by a cancer patient who is about to receive chemotherapy. Avoidance cognitive coping responses include those attempts to avoid having to confront the problem or emotional tension actively. An example of an avoidance cognitive coping response would be a patient who is denying that he has experienced a heart attack, claiming that it was really just a severe case of indigestion.

Research on Type A personality and cognitive coping strategies provides further examples of how different types of people utilize different styles of coping in stressful situations. In one study, the Type A subjects demonstrated active cognitive coping responses. Subjects were

TABLE 5-8
Classification of Coping Responses

|  |  | METHOD | |
| --- | --- | --- | --- |
|  |  | Active | Avoidance |
| FOCUS | Problem oriented | Cognitive / Behavioral | Cognitive / Behavioral |
|  | Emotion oriented | Cognitive / Behavioral | Cognitive / Behavioral |

assigned a set of trials in which a difficult concept formation task was presented. Post-assessment indicated that Type A subjects were more active or involved and resisted feelings of helplessness to a greater degree than Type B subjects (Manuck & Garland, 1979). In another study, Type A subjects expended more physical effort on a treadmill test, but reported less fatigue than the Type B subjects (Carver, Coleman, & Glass, 1976). These preliminary findings suggest that Type A subjects tend to use cognitive coping responses of suppression and denial of negative symptoms to a greater extent than Type B subjects. Chesney and Rosenman (1983) attempt to link Type A coping strategies to coronary heart disease. They hypothesize that Type A persons deny fatigue and continue the struggle to achieve. Initially, this response style is rewarded and they are successful. However, their success is accompanied by increasing demands and more responsibility. The continued effort to do more and more in less time creates a situation that eventually leads to exhaustion and ill-health, often manifested as coronary heart disease. The Type A behavior pattern will be discussed in detail in Chapter 11.

As described in the section on cognitive assessment, some investigators attempt to gather self-report information regarding cognitive coping responses on large samples of individuals (Billings & Moos, 1981; Ilfeld, 1980). Other approaches hypothesize various personality traits, coping styles, or specific areas of cognitive appraisal that help predict an individual's response to a stressor, based on the degree that person possesses the trait, coping style, or type of cognitive appraisal.

One type of cognitive modulator of the stress response that has received considerable attention is *perceived control*. Perceived control refers to the extent events or the environment are interpreted by the individual as under personal control. Several studies by Glass, Singer, and colleagues (Glass & Singer, 1972) suggest that people prefer activities in which they are given control, whether or not they actually use that control. Aftereffects of stress are thought to occur following uncontrollable stressors, not controllable ones (Cohen, 1980). Studies investigating the relationship between control and the aftereffects of stress, generally involve placing half the subjects in a situation in which they have control over an aversive stimuli. In general, subjects tend to do better in the perceived control situation. An example of such a study is one by Greer, Davison, and Gatchel (1970) in which they examined control and the stressor of electric shock. One group of subjects was instructed that they could reduce the duration of shock they would be receiving if they quickly responded to a signal before the shock occurred. The other group of subjects was not given such instructions. Subjects in the situation in which the shock could be controlled had significantly lower levels of skin conductance than subjects in the no-control group, even though subjects in both groups received the same duration and intensity of shock.

It has been argued that the illusion of control rather than actual control over the aversive stimulus reduces the impact of the stressor (Johnson & Sarason, 1979). Johnson and Sarason were interested in whether individuals who perceive themselves as having little control over events are more adversely affected by life stress than individuals who feel they can control life events. They predicted that anxiety and depression would correlate with life stress among subjects who demonstrated an external locus of control orientation. Fifty-five college students identified as "internals" and sixty-six college students identified as "externals," using the Rotter Locus of Control Scale, were also given the Beck Depression Inventory, the State-Trait Anxiety Inventory, and the Life Experience Survey. They found that negative life changes (as measured by the Life Experience Survey) were significantly related to both trait anxiety and depression, but this relationship held only for external subjects. This study supports the notion that a cognitive modulator, that is, internal versus external locus of control, may be an intermediate variable between stressful events and the cognitive component of the stress response.

Another cognitive modulator of the stress response with a long history in psychology is *defensiveness*. Defensiveness is thought to occur when the person's appraisal of the stressor involves self-deception or distortion of reality or in situations that are sufficiently ambiguous, so that the person uses selective attention. Traditionally, defensive self-deception, such as denial or rationalization, was thought to be used by individuals with rigid and psychologically unhealthy personalities. Lazarus (1966), however, suggests that the research on stress and coping indicates that defensiveness can, at times, be a healthy and effective means of coping with stressors. For example, the coronary heart patient in an intensive care unit who denies the diagnosis and the possibility of sudden death may respond better, both physically and psychologically (Gentry, Foster, & Harvey, 1972). Valliant (1977) reported that men judged to be healthy and successful reliably and adaptively employed "immature defense mechanisms," whereas those men who were least adjusted overall did not have access to such defense strategies. A final example is a study in which the urinary excretion of 17-hydroxycorticosteroids were measured in parents of terminally ill leukemic children. Parents who responded with defensive coping by displacing their unpleasant affects and presumably utilizing a high degree of rationalization and intellectualization showed no elevation in 17-hydroxycorticosteroids. The parents who did not employ defensive strategies showed significantly elevated urinary 17-hydroxycorticosteroid excretion rates (Wolff, Friedman, Hofer, & Mason, 1964).

Although defensiveness may be helpful in many stressful situations, there may be other occasions when it is not adaptive. Repressors, who were prone to physical disorder, may not seek medical treatment when they should (e.g., Cochrane, 1969). Determining the condition when defensiveness is a successful coping response and when it is not is an important research problem that would allow one to predict when a person should employ such a coping strategy.

In summary, a framework for illustrating the different types of cognitive coping responses has been presented. Perceived control and defensiveness are two types of cognitive coping responses that have received considerable attention in stress research. Problems arise, however, when one attempts to summarize the current knowledge on cognitive coping responses. Some of the problems include different terms for similar, but not equivalent definitions of the coping response and actually determining whether the subject employed the particular cognitive response under study, particularly outside the laboratory setting. Suggestions for future research include use of operational and standard definitions and measurement methods of various coping responses and assessment of physiological and behavioral correlates of the response. The Neftel et al. (1982) study, discussed in the section on stress measurement, provides a model of such research, although a greater emphasis on the cognitive coping responses themselves would have led to a greater understanding of the cognitive modulation of the stress response in that particular investigation.

## Social/Behavioral Modulators

Social support is the primary "social modulator" variable studied and is thought to be important in the mediation of life stressors. Researchers have employed a variety of definitions of social support in their studies, ranging from simple operational definitions of presence of a spouse to the use of measures designed to assess various aspects of the social environment, such as cohesion, affiliation, and independence. At present, no widely agreed-upon definition or index of social support exists. Social support is difficult to define because it is a dynamic phenomenon, and as Broadhead, Kaplan, James, Wagner, Schoenboch, Grimson, Heyden, Tibblin, and Gehlbach (1983) note, determinants of social support are both internal and external or environmental. Internal determinants involve the individual's temperment, perception of the social environment, and pattern of interacting with others, particularly interactions utilizing social skills. External determinants include the quality and quantity of interactions with those available, as well as the social roles placed on the individual. Social support, in a general sense, can be thought of as the degree the individual has access to social resources, in the form of relationships with others. Ideally, these relationships should be reliable, especially when the individual is experiencing a greater degree of stress, and might include the spouse, friends, neighbors, community groups, and institutions. A frequently referred-to definition of social support is one by Cobb (1976), in which social support is described in terms of benefits associated with feelings of being loved and valued and belonging to a network of communications and mutual obligations to others. Cobb's definition emphasizes that the quality or kind of social support is more important than the quantity (Cobb, 1976; Tinbergen, 1974).

In distinguishing quantity versus quality of social support, Schaefer, Coyne, and Lazarus (1981) suggest using the terms *social network* and *perceived social support*, respectively. A *social network* can be thought of as the set of relationships of one individual and defined in "terms of its composition and structure (e.g., the number of people involved and the number who know each other) or by the content of particular relationships (e.g., friendship and kinship)" (Schaefer *et al.*, 1981). *Perceived social support* involves the individual's feelings and thoughts of how helpful the interactions or relationships are within his social network. A comparison of social network size and three types of perceived social support (tangible, emotional, and informational) relative to physical health status, stressful life events, depression, and morale was made in a sample of 100 persons, 45 to 65 years old (Schaefer *et al.*, 1981). The comparison indicated that social network size was empirically separable from perceived social support. Also, social network had a weaker overall relationship to outcomes than perceived social support. Low tangible and emotional support were related to depression and negative morale, and informational support was associated with positive morale. Results of the study indicate the importance of considering the type of support more specifically.

Determining what constitutes perceived social support has been difficult, but attempts have been made and possible determinants suggested. These hypothesized determinants include modeling of significant others who effectively cope with stressful events, assistance in solving problems, guidance, predictability, security and provision of information, and reassurance of the person's self-adequacy (Wills & Langner, 1980; Sarason, 1980). One problem in assessing the quality versus the quantity of social support is that the person's perception of social support is of interest, and thus, self-report measures are often used. There are problems with self-report measures of social support;

these include a person's unwillingness to admit to inadequate social support, loneliness, and feelings of rejection.

Although there is no general agreement on what constitutes social support, there is considerable evidence that an individual's interactions with others play an important role in that person's response to stress. Effects of the social environment on children's physical and social development have been reported frequently. For example, Powell, Brasel, and Blizzard (1967) studied 13 children thought to have idiopathic hypopituitarianism. All children were short for their age, had polydipsia, polyphagia, and retardation of speech and a majority of the cases had ACTH and growth hormone deficiencies. Interviews with the children's parents showed that the children had inadequate social support from their families. Half of the parents were divorced or separated, and almost all the children had very little contact with their father. The children were removed from their homes and placed in a convalescent home. All the children's physical symptoms and hormonal deficiencies were reversed in this more supportive social environment. MacCarthy and Booth (1970) report on 10 children with similar abnormalities. Seven of the mothers were described as providing inadequate social support or had "rejecting attitudes" toward the child and two other mothers were described as having significant emotional problems and thus were not able to provide adequate social support. Most of the children's symptoms reversed when they were removed from their homes and placed in the hospital.

The mediating influence of social support on stress associated with the nuclear power plant accident at Three Mile Island (TMI) was studied comprehensively by Fleming, Baum, Gisriel, and Gatchel (1982). They conceptualized the TMI event as stressful because the residents reported a number of stress symptoms after the accident (Flynn & Chalmer, 1980). Fleming *et al.* studied a random sample of this group soon after the accident, in an effort to determine the relationship between social support and stress, as measured by behavioral, psychological, and biochemical functioning. The groups studied included TMI residents with low social support, moderate social support, and high social support and three control groups with low, moderate, and high social support. The measure of social support used was a 6-item scale assessing an individual's perception of social support. Psychological functioning was assessed with the Beck Depression Inventory and the Symptom Checklist - 90 (SCL-90), a multidimensional symptom inventory. The behavioral effects of stress were based on two performance tasks, one required that the person proofread and correct errors in a passage, the other was a variant of the Embedded Figures Test. Finally, a biochemical assessment of the stress response was completed, using subjects' urine to measure catecholamine (epinephrine and norepinephrine) levels. Results indicated that all three TMI groups demonstrated greater evidence of stress across psychological, behavioral, and biochemical measures than did the control groups. Also, minimal social support was associated with a greater frequency of stress-relevant problems for TMI residents, whereas TMI residents with moderate or high levels of social support reported fewer stress-relevant problems. However, the moderating effect of social support was not uniform across all components of the stress response, since *all* TMI residents had high catecholamine levels. Fleming *et al.* conclude that perceived support serves to facilitate coping (psychologically and behaviorally), but does not protect individuals from a greater degree of physiological arousal, as indicated by high catecholamine levels.

The results of these studies exemplify the effects of social support on the stress response. The effects of the social environment on the stress response and physical and psychological health have been observed in other studies. However, because of varying definitions of social support and the observational or correlational methodologies used in these studies, it is impossible to determine whether the effect is direct, a moderating effect, or the result of a third factor. For instance, epidemiological studies of social support and mortality indicate that poor social support precedes mortality even when controlling baseline health status (e.g., Berkman & Syme 1979). The casual relationship may be weakened by considering that social support and health are independent consequences of a third factor, such as socioeconomic status. Another issue often raised is that loss of social support is in itself a stressor. Persons who live alone and have few social contacts often report greater degrees of symptomology even when experiencing few stressors. Furthermore, Wills and Langner (1980) point out that subjects with low social support were not randomly assigned to groups. Perception of the need for social support and type of support needed, along with availability, accessibility, and whether or not such support is used, are influenced by developmental or life cycle changes (Broadhead *et al.*, 1983). Figure 5-7 illustrates the fluctuating nature of social support throughout the life cycle, as proposed by Bruhn and Philips (1984). As the figure illustrates, need/availability of support tends to take the form of a curvilinear function over the time when peak support is needed or available, at middle age; lower levels are apparent during earlier and later years. Clearly, social support is a dynamic process.

Prospective, cohort studies, as well as controlled intervention studies, can help clarify the relationship between social support, stress, and health. Another avenue for investigating the effect of social support on the stress response is utilizing analogue studies, as suggested by

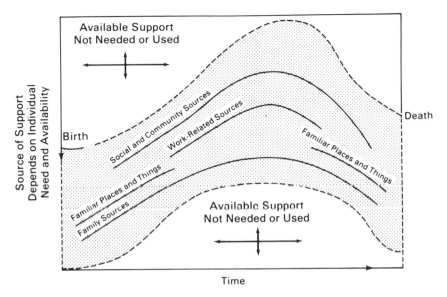

Available Support
Not Needed or Used

Source of Support
Depends on Individual
Need and Availability

Birth

Social and Community Sources

Work-Related Sources

Familiar Places and Things

Familiar Places and Things

Family Sources

Available Support
Not Needed or Used

Death

Time

**FIGURE 5-7.** Fluctuations in social support across the life cycle. From "Measuring Social Support: A Synthesis of Current Approaches" by J. G. Bruhn and B. U. Philips, 1984, *Journal of Behavioral Medicine, 7*(2), 158. Copyright 1984 by Plenum Press. Reprinted by permission.

Sarason (1980). Sarason described experimental studies in which varying levels of social support were provided for test-anxious college students. Results indicated that social support as defined in terms of group association served as a moderator variable to counteract the maladaptive consequences of high anxiety. The maladaptive consequences were conceptualized as self-preoccupation, which would, in turn, interfere with test performance.

As illustrated, the concept of social support is quite complex. In a review of the concept, Bruhn and Philips (1984) conclude the following: (1) Social support is dynamic, with its form and quantity varying over time; (2) social support has interactive, qualitative, and quantitative dimensions that should be simultaneously addressed; (3) perception of availability and need of support are important factors for use of such support; (4) the need for support varies across life situations and life cycle; (5) social support is an aspect of daily living, although the need for such support may vary in times of stress; (6) change in physical, psychological, and social functioning can influence perception of need and availability of social support; (7) individuals, groups, institutions, and communities must be considered, from a systems perspective, to define social support adequately; (8) social support can exert positive and negative effects; (9) social support can vary as a function of culture and sociocultural factors must be considered when attempting to measure it; (10) research should focus on the mechanisms of action of social support (i.e., how it works) in addition to its effects; and (11) longitudinal studies that incorporate psychosocial and biological measures on cohorts over long periods of time are needed.

## SUMMARY

As this chapter has illustrated, stress is a multifaceted concept that is not easily understood, despite its ubiquitous nature. The chapter provided a historical review with a discussion of the concept from the perspective of physics to the broader psychobiological position. A working definition that emphasizes stressors and stress response was presented. Measurement techniques were discussed in some detail to illustrate the problems and issues encountered in measuring a general construct such as stress. Various models of stress, including response based, stimulus based, transactional, and information processing, were reviewed and, lastly, a discussion of specific factors that influence response to stress, including cognitive and social modulators, were presented.

## REFERENCES

Ader, R., & Cohen, N. (1985). CNS-immune system interactions: Conditioning phenomena. *The Behavioral and Brain Sciences, 8,* 379–426.

Averill, J. R. (1973). Personal control over aversive stimuli and its relationship to stress. *Psychological Bulletin, 80,* 286–303.

Baum, A., Grunberg, N. E., & Singer, J. E. (1982). The use of psychological and neuroendocrinological measurements in the study of stress. *Health Psychology, 1*(3), 217–236.

Berkman, L. F., & Syme, S. L. (1979). Social networks, host resistance, and mortality: A nine-year follow-up study of Alameda County residents. *American Journal of Epidemiology, 109*(2), 186–204.

Billings, A. G., & Moos, R. H. (1981). The role of coping responses and social resources in attenuating the stress of life events. *Journal of Behavioral Medicine, 4,* 139–157.

Broadhead, W. E., Kaplan, B. H., James, S. A., Wagner, E. H., Schoenbach, V. J., Grimson, R., Heyden, S., Tibblin, G., & Gehlbach, S. H. (1983). The epidemiologic evidence for a relationship between social support and health. *American Journal of Epidemiology, 117*(5), 521–537.

Bruhn, J. G., & Philips, B. U. (1984). Measuring social support: A synthesis of current approaches. *Journal of Behavioral Medicine, 7*(2), 151–169.

Cannon, W. B. (1932). *The wisdom of the body.* New York: Norton.

Carver, C. S., Coleman, A. E., & Glass, D. C. (1976). The coronary-prone behavior pattern and the suppression of fatigue on a treadmill test. *Journal of Personality and Social Psychology, 33*(4), 460–466.

Chesney, M. A., Eagleston, J. R., & Rosenman, R. H. (1980). The Type A structured interview: A behavioral assessment in the rough. *Journal of Behavioral Assessment, 2,* 255–272.

Chesney, M. A., & Rosenman, R. H. (1983). Specificity in stress models: Examples drawn from Type A behaviour. In C. L. Cooper (Ed.), *Stress research* (pp. 21–34). New York: Wiley.

Cobb, S. (1976). Social support as a modulator of life stress. *Psychosomatic Medicine, 38,* 300–314.

Cochrane, R. (1969). Neuroticism and the discovery of high blood pressure. *Journal of Psychosomatic Research, 13,* 21–25.

Cohen, S. (1980). Aftereffects of stress on human performance and social behavior: A review of research and theory. *Psychological Bulletin, 88*(1), 82–108.

Cox, T. (1978). *Stress.* Baltimore, MD: University Park Press.

Cox, T., & McKay, C. (1978). Stress at work. In T. Cox (Ed.), *Stress.* Baltimore, MD: University Park Press.

Coyne, J. C., & Lazarus, R. S. (1980). Cognitive style, stress perspective, and coping: In I. L. Kutash & L. B. Schlesinger (Eds.), *Handbook on stress and anxiety.* San Francisco: Jossey-Bass.

Dimsdale, J. E., & Moss, J. (1980). Plasma catecholamines in stress and exercise. *Journal of the American Medical Association, 243*(4), 340–342.

Dunn, A. J., & Kramarcy, N. R. (1984). Neurochemical responses in stress: Relationships between the hypothalamic-pituitary-adrenal and catecholamine systems. In L. L. Iversen, S. D. Iversen & S. H. Snyder (Eds.), *Handbook of psychopharmacology* (Vol. 18). New York: Plenum Press.

Eckenrode, J. (1984). Impact of chronic and acute stressors on daily reports of mood. *Journal of Personality and Social Psychology, 46*(4), 907–918.

Evans, G. W. (1978). Human spacial behavior. In A. Baum & Y. Epstein (Eds.), *Human response to crowding.* Hillsdale, NJ: Lawrence Erlbaum.

Everly, G. S., Jr., & Rosenfeld, R. (1981). *The nature and treatment of the stress response: A practical guide for clinicians.* New York: Plenum Press.

Fleming, R., Baum, A., Gisriel, M. M., & Gatchel, R. J. (1982). Mediating influences on social support on stress at Three Mile Island. *Journal of Human Stress, 8,* 14–22.

Flynn, C., & Chalmas, J. (1980). *The social and economic effects of the accident at Three Mile Island* (NUREG/CR-1215). Washington, DC: U.S. Nuclear Regulatory Commission.

Frankenhaeuser, M. (1975a). Experimental approach to the study of catecholamines and emotion. In R. Levi (Ed.), *Emotions, their parameters and measurement* (pp. 209–234). New York: Raven Press.

Frankenhaeuser, M. (1975b). Sympathetic-adrenomedullary activity, behavior and the psychosocial environment. In P. H. Venables & M. J. Christie (Eds.), *Research in psychophysiology.* New York: Wiley.

Gellhorn, E. (1968). Central nervous system tuning and its implications for neuropsychiatry. *Journal of Nervous and Mental Disorders, 147,* 148–162.

Gentry, W. D., Foster, S., & Haney, T. (1972). Denial as a determinant of anxiety and perceived health status in the coronary care unit. *Psychosomatic Medicine, 34,* 39–44.

Glass, D. C. & Singer, J. E. (1972). *Urban stress: Experiments on noise and social stresses.* New York: Academic Press.

Goldberg, E. L., & Comstock, G. W. (1980). Epidemiology of life events: Frequency in general populations. *American Journal of Epidemiology, 111*(6), 736–752.

Gray-Taft, P., & Anderson, J. G. (1981). The nursing stress scale: Development of an instrument. *Journal of Behavioral Assessment, 3,* 11–23.

Greer, J. H., Davison, D. C., & Gatchel, R. I. (1970). Reduction of stress in humans through nonveridical perceived control of aversive stimulation. *Journal of Personality and Social Psychology, 16,* 731–738.

Hamilton, V. (1980). An information processing analysis of environmental stress and life crisis. In I. G. Sarason & C. D. Spielberger (Eds.), *Stress and Anxiety* (Vol. 7). New York: Hemisphere Publishing.

Henry, J. P., & Stephens, P. M. (1977). *Stress, health, and the social environment: A sociobiological approach to medicine.* New York: Springer-Verlag.

Hess, W. (1957). *The functional organization of the diencephalon.* New York: Grune & Stratton.

Hinkle, L. E. (1974). The concept of "stress" in the biological and social sciences. *International Journal of Psychiatry in Medicine, 5*(4), 335–357.

Hollon, S. D., & Bemis, K. M. (1981). Self-report and the assessment of cognitive functions. In M. Hersen & A. S. Bellack (Eds.), *Behavioral assessment: A practical handbook* (2nd ed.). New York: Pergamon Press.

Holmes, T. H., & Masuda, M. (1974). Life change and illness susceptibility. In B. S. Dohrenwend & B. P. Dohrenwend (Eds.), *Stressful life events: Their nature and effects.* New York: Wiley.

Holmes, T. H., & Rahe, R. H. (1967). The social readjustment rating scale. *Journal of Psychosomatic Research, 11,* 213–218.

Ilfeld, F. W., Jr. (1980). Coping styles of Chicago adults: Description. *Journal of Human Stress, 6*(2), 2–10.

Jaffe, J. H., & Martin, W. R. (1980). Opoid analgesics and antagonists. In A. G. Gilman, L. S. Goodman, & A. Gilman (Eds.), *The pharmacological basis of therapeutics.* New York: Macmillan.

Johnson, J. H., & McCutchen, S. M. (1980). Assessing life stress in older children and adolescents: Preliminary findings with the life events checklist. In I. G. Sarason & C. D. Spielberger (Eds.), *Stress and anxiety.* Washington, DC: Hemisphere Publishing.

Johnson, J. H., & Sarason, I. G. (1979). Moderator variables in life stress research. In I. G. Sarason & C. D. Spielberger (Eds.), *Stress and anxiety.* Washington, DC: Hemisphere Publishing.

Kagan, A., & Levi, L. (1971). Adaptation of the psychosocial environment to man's abilities and needs. In L. Levi (Ed.), *Society, stress and disease.* London: Oxford University Press.

Kanner, A. D., Coyne, J. C., Schaefer, C., & Lazarus, R. S. (1981). Comparison of two modes of stress measurement: Daily hassles and uplifts versus major life events. *Journal of Behavioral Medicine, 4,* 1–39.

Kent, R. N., & Foster, S. L. (1977). Direct observational procedures: Methodological issues in naturalistic settings. In A. R. Ciminero, K. S. Calhoun, & H. E. Adams (Eds.), *Handbook of behavioral assessment.* New York: Wiley.

Kiritz, S., & Moos, R. H. (1974). Physiological effects of social environments. *Psychosomatic Medicine, 36,* 96–114.

Lazarus, R. S. (1966). *Psychological stress and the coping process.* New York: McGraw-Hill.

Lazarus, R. S. (1974). Psychological stress and coping in adaptation and illness. *International Journal of Psychiatry in Medicine, 5,* 321–333.

Lazarus, R. S. (1976). *Patterns of adjustment.* New York: McGraw-Hill.

LeBlanc, J. (1976, July). *The role of catecholamines in adaptation to chronic and acute stress.* Paper presented at the proceedings of the International Symposium on Catecholamines and Stress, Bratislava, Czechoslovakia.

Levi, L. (1972). Introduction: Psychosocial stimuli, psychophysiological reactions, and disease. In L. Levi (Ed.), *Stress and distress in response to psychosocial stimuli* (pp. 11–27). Oxford: Pergamon Press.

MacCarthy, D., & Booth, E. M. (1970). Parental rejection and stunting of growth. *Journal of Psychosomatic Research, 14,* 259–265.

Mandler, G., Mandler, J. M., & Uviller, E. T. (1958). Autonomic feedback: The perception of autonomic activity. *Journal of Abnormal and Social Psychology, 56,* 367–373.

Manuck, S. B., & Garland, F. N. (1979). Coronary-prone behavior pattern, task incentive, and cardiovascular response. *Psychophysiology, 16*(2), 136–142.

Mason, J. W. (1968). A review of psychoendocrine research on the pituitary–adrenal cortical system. *Psychosomatic Medicine, 30,* 631–653.

McCabe, P., & Schneiderman, N. (1984). Psychophysiologic reactions to stress. In N. S. Schneiderman & J. J. Tapp (Eds.), *Behavioral medicine: The biopsychosocial approach.* Hillsdale, NJ: Lawrence Erlbaum.

Meadow, M. J., Kochevar, J., Tellegen, A., & Roberts, A. H. (1978). Perceived somatic response inventory: Three scales developed by factor analysis. *Journal of Behavioral Medicine, 1,* 413 426.

Miller, N. E. (1978). Biofeedback and visceral learning. *Annual Review of Psychology, 29,* 373–404.

Moos, R. H. (1973). Conceptualizations of human environments. *American Psychologist, 28,* 652–665.

Moos, R. H., & Moos, B. S. (1981). *Family environment scale manual.* Palo Alto, CA: Consulting Psychologists Press.

Neftel, K. A., Adler, R. H., Kappeli, L., Rossi, M., Dolder, M., Kaser, H. E., Bruggesser, H. H., & Vorkauf, H. (1982). Stage fright in musicians: A model illustrating the effect of beta blockers. *Psychosomatic Medicine, 44,* 461–469.

Nisbett, R. E., & Wilson, T. D. (1977). Telling more than we can know: Verbal reports on mental processes. *Psychological Review, 84,* 231–259.

Onions, T. (1933). *Shorter oxford english dictionary.* Oxford: Clarendon Press.

Osler, W. (1910). The lumleian lectures on angina pectoris. *Lancet, 1,* 696–700, 838–844, 974–977.

Patkai, P. (1974). Laboratory studies of psychological stress. *International Journal of Psychiatry in Medicine, 5,* 575–585.

Pearlin, L. I., & Schooler, (1978). The structure of coping. *Journal of Health and Social Behavior, 19*(1), 2–21.

Powell, G. F., Brasel, J. A., & Blizzard, R. M. (1967). Emotional deprivation and growth retardation simulating idiopathic hypopituitarism. I. Clinical evaluation of the syndrome. *New England Journal of Medicine, 276,* 1271–1278.

Roskies, E., & Lazarus, R. S. (1980). Coping theory and the teaching of coping skills. In P. O. Davidson & S. M. Davidson (Eds.), *Behavioral medicine: Changing health lifestyles* (pp. 38–69). New York: Brunner/Mazel.

Sachar, E. J., Asnis, G., Halbreich, U., Nathan, R. S., & Halpern, F. (1980). Recent studies in the neuroendocrinology of major depressive disorder. *Psychiatric Clinics of North America, 3,* 313–326.

Sarason, I. G. (1980). Life stress, self-preoccupation, and social supports. In I. G. Sarason & C. D. Spielberger (Eds.), *Stress and anxiety* (pp. 73–94). New York: Hemisphere Publishing.

Schaefer, C., Coyne, J. C., & Lazarus, R. S. (1981). The health-related functions of social support. *Journal of Behavioral Medicine, 4,* 381–406.

Selye, H. (1956). *The stress of life.* New York: McGraw-Hill.

Selye, H. (1976). *Stress in health and disease.* Reading, MA: Butterworth.

Selye, H. (1980). The stress concept today. In I. L. Kutash & L. B. Schlesinger *et al.* (Eds.), *Handbook on stress and anxiety* (pp. 127–129). San Francisco: Josey-Bass.

Stone, A. A., & Neale, J. M. (1984). New measure of daily coping: Development of preliminary results. *Journal of Personality and Social Psychology, 46*(4), 892–906.

Tinbergen, N. (1974). Ethology and stress disease. *Science, 185,* 20–27.

Usdin, E., Kretnansky, R., & Kopin, I. (1976). *Catecholamines and stress.* Oxford: Pergamon Press.

Vaillant, G. E. (1977). *Adaptation to life.* Boston: Little, Brown.

Weiss, J. M. (1972). Influences of psychological variables on stress-induced pathology. *Physiology emotion, and psychosomatic illness, Ciba Foundation symposium, 8,* 253–265.

Weiss, J. M., Bailey, W. H., Pohorecky, L. A., Korzeniowski, D., & Grillione, G. (1980). Stress-induced depression of motor activity correlates with regional changes in brain norepinephrine but not in dopamine. *Neurochemical Research, 5*(1), 9–22.

Weitz, J. (1970). Psychosocial research needs on the problems of human stress. In J. E. McGrath (Ed.), *Social and psychological factors in stress.* New York: Holt, Rinehart & Winston.

Wills, T. A., & Langner, T. S. (1980). Socioeconomic status and stress. In I. L. Kutash, L. B. Schlesinger *et al.* (Eds.), *Handbook of stress and anxiety: Contemporary knowledge, theory and treatment* (pp. 159–173). San Francisco: Josey-Bass.

Wolff, C. T., Friedman, S. B., Hofer, M. A., & Mason, J. W. (1964). Relationship between psychological defenses and mean urinary 17-hydroxycorticosteroid excretion rates: I. A predictive study of parents of fatally ill children. *Psychosomatic Medicine, 26,* 575–591.

Wolff, H. G. (1953). *Stress and disease.* Springfield, IL: Charles C Thomas.

Wyler, A. R., Masuda, M., & Holmes, T. H. (1971). Magnitude of life events and seriousness of illness. *Psychosomatic Medicine, 33,* 115–122.

CHAPTER 6

# STRESS AND ILLNESS

As discussed in Chapter 5, stress is a complex construct. Despite problems with a commonly accepted definition and model of stress, researchers and clinicians in a variety of fields have attempted to relate stress to the development, exacerbation, and maintenance of a number of health problems. The following article was excerpted from the *Manchester Guardian* to provide an example of the type of reasoning that characterizes some of the work in this controversial field.

> Excess Stress in Women—Hairy Chests and Lust
> London: Career women in modern Britain—under the added stress of looking after husbands and children—are developing hairy chests and hairy stomachs. They sometimes become lustful as well.
> These startling assertions are attributed to Ivor Mills, professor of medicine at Cambridge University and a respectable, 56-year-old endocrinologist with 22 lines in *Who's Who*.
> The findings are sensational, says the current issue of *Women's Own* magazine, which carries the story.
> Mills finds that strain on a woman's brain is related to hormonal changes that include the production of excess male hormones.
> He has begun to see patients in their 20's who have suddenly started growing excess facial hair. "It can be very distressing. Some women have to shave every day, others start growing hair on their breasts and abdomens."

Sometimes they develop aggressive drives, and heightened sex drives. With high hormone overproduction, voices deepen: "We have had a few singers who can't sing soprano anymore."

Mills cites a case study of one, Margaret, a dynamic school teacher, who had to shave daily. Her husband was happy with her high sex drive, but she found it difficult to conceive.

Eventually she succeeded in bearing a child and her hairiness regressed, but when she went back to work she became irritable and hairy all over again.

A number of contradictions are mentioned. Sometimes, the findings show a decrease in male hormone production, leading to loss of libido and depression.

Mill advocates that the main solution is for women to insist that their husbands help more in the home.

As the article implies, a link between excess stress in women and hairy chests and lust was observed. Indeed, a potential psychobiological mechanism was even implied, "strain on a woman's brain is related to hormonal changes that include the production of excess male hormones." Although this example may appear farfetched at first glance, a question one must ask when critically reviewing the stress–illness link is whether the associations that appear so plausible on the surface are actually based upon empirical research. Stress should be viewed as any other risk factor when evidence of its role in the etiology of illness is evaluated. (Chapter 3 provided a framework for evaluating the role of suspected risk factors.)

As discussed in Chapter 3, a critical consideration of any risk factor requires the review of several lines of research, including some combination of retrospective, prospective, and experimental research strategies. The first section of this chapter will review the various models used to explain the possible role of stress in the development of illness or "stress as precursor to illness." The second section of the chapter focuses on "stress as a response to illness," in an effort to address more specifically the role stress may play in the exacerbation and maintenance of illness. Research on stress and illness is growing at a rapid rate, and this chapter should help place this research in perspective.

## STRESS AS PRECURSOR TO ILLNESS

How is stress linked to illness? A number of models have been proposed to explain the potential role of stress in the etiology, exacerbation, and maintenance of physical illness (e.g., Levi, 1972; Minuchin, Baker, Rosman, Liebman, Milman, & Todd, 1975; Rahe & Arthur, 1978; Schwartz, 1977, 1978; Selye, 1956). Although the various proponents of these models have quite diverse backgrounds, a number of commonalities across models exist. This section briefly reviews these models.

One model that is frequently cited as the first serious attempt to link stress to illness is that proposed by Selye (1956). While a young medical student, Selye observed that a variety of different diseases appeared to have a number of characteristics in common. He noted that, regardless of the disorder, patients often complained of diffuse pains in joints and muscles, intestinal disturbance with loss of appetite, and loss of weight (general sense of discomfort), among others and referred to this as simply the "syndrome of just being sick." Later, in the laboratory, he was able to reproduce these clinical manifestations in rats following the injection of a variety of toxic substances. He argued that some degree of nonspecific damage to the organism is superimposed on the specific characteristics of any disease and perhaps on the specific effects of any drug. He also noted that certain nonspecific curative measures, often provided by physicians, such as suggestions to rest and take it easy, eat only very digestable foods, protect against drafts or variations in temperature, were useful to patients with a variety of diseases. In addition, the history of medicine is replete with a long list of nonspecific treatments, such as injections of substances foreign to the body, fever therapy, shock therapy, or blood letting, which were unquestionably therapeutic in certain cases. From these observations, Selye hypothesized that a general nonspecific reaction pattern of the organism in response to a threat of damage must exist and that it is this nonspecific response that permits the body to mobilize against these threats. Following a series of studies, primarily in laboratory animals, Selye proposed a general theory of stress that attempts to describe and explain this nonspecific response.

First, Selye defines stress as the nonspecific response of the body to any demand made upon it. As discussed in Chapter 5, positive as well as negative experiences can evoke the stress response. Many patients with so-called stress-related disorders report that enjoyable activities (e.g., a special social gathering) are often associated in time with the problem disorders (e.g., a migraine headache). This nonspecific pattern of exposure to stressors was referred to by Selye as the general adaptation syndrome (GAS).

The GAS evolves through three stages: (1) alarm reaction, (2) resistance, and (3) exhaustion. The alarm reaction is the most rapid component observed in response to a specific stressor. It is primarily a function of epinephrine release and is related to high levels of physiological arousal and negative affect. During the alarm reaction, the organism's susceptibility to increases in intensity of the specific eliciting stressor and to other extraneous stressors is reduced. During this stage, heightened susceptibility to illness presumably occurs. If the stress is severe and unavoidable, death occurs within hours or days of initiation of the alarm reaction. With less severe nonfatal stressors, however, prolonged exposure sets the slow components of the GAS into play through pituitary-adrenocorticotropic hormones (ACTH), so initiating the resistance stage.

In the stage of resistance, physiological arousal remains *high*, but decreases somewhat through adaptation, while the parasympathetic branch of the autonomic nervous system (ANS) attempts to counteract sympathetic discharge. During this stage, the organism is able to endure the particular stressor and to *resist* further debilitating effects. However, the threshold for eliciting the alarm reaction is lowered, so that a heightened sensitivity to stressors is apparent while the adrenal cortex is replenished.

If exposure to stress continues at intense levels, the hormonal reserves are depleted, fatigue sets in, and eventually the organism enters the final stage of GAS exhaustion, with a decreased ability to resist either the original stressor or extraneous stressors. The affective experience during this stage is often depression. This stage often persists for some time following the removal of the stressor.

Selye had good reasons for calling this three-stage sequence the *general adaptation syndrome*. It is general in that it is produced by agents that have a *general* effect on many bodily systems. It is *adaptive* because it stimulates defense and thereby assists in the acquisition and maintenance of a stage of *restoration*. It is a *syndrome* because its individual components are coordinated and interdependent. The stages of the GAS are summarized in Table 6-1. The other models to be reviewed will emphasize the psychobiological aspects of the stress–illness association to a greater degree than the GAS.

Levi (1972) and his associates have proposed a model for psychosocially mediated disease. This model is illustrated in Figure 6-1. Levi argues that any psychosocial change can act as a stressor or a stimulus, eliciting a nonspecific biological response. This stimulus acts on an individual with a preexisting "psychobiological program" or propensity to react neuroendocrinologically in accordance with a certain pattern. This propensity is a function of genetic factors and environmental influences. The response prepares the organism for some type of physical activity (e.g., fight or flight) in a variety of situations, in some of which a response of this nature is maladaptive. This nonspecific stress response then influences the precursors of disease or malfunctioning psychological or physiological systems that have not yet reached a state of disability. If stimulation persists, disease will result. Disease is defined as disability in or failure of a psychological or somatic system to perform an

## TABLE 6-1
### General Adaptation Syndrome

| | |
|---|---|
| Stage I | Alarm Reaction |
| | Enlargement of adrenal cortex |
| | Enlargement of lymphatic system |
| | Increase in hormone levels |
| | Response to specific stressor |
| | Epinephrine release associated with high levels of physiological arousal and negative affect |
| | Increased susceptibility to increased intensity of stressor |
| | Heightened susceptibility to illness |
| | If prolonged, the slower components of the general adaption syndrome are set into motion beginning with Stage II |
| Stage II[a] | Resistance |
| | Shrinkage of adrenal cortex |
| | Lymph nodes closer to normal size |
| | Hormone levels sustained |
| | Physiological arousal remains high, but parasympathetic branch of the autonomic nervous system counteracts |
| | Individual can endure the stressor and resist further debilitating effects |
| | Heightened sensitivity to stress |
| | If stress continues at intense levels, hormonal reserves are depleted, fatigue sets in, and individual enters Stage III or Exhaustion |
| Stage III[a] | Exhaustion |
| | Enlargement/dysfunction of lymphatic structures |
| | Increase in hormone levels |
| | Depletion of adaptive hormones |
| | Decreased ability to resist either original or extraneous stressors |
| | Affective experience often depression |

[a]Stages I and II are continuously repeated throughout life.

essential task. Levi also hypothesizes the existence of interacting variables, or intrinsic or extrinsic psychological or physiological variables, that modulate the action of causal factors at the mechanism (stress response), precursor, or disease stage. These interacting variables can facilitate the disease process.

Rahe and Arthur (1978) proposed the model depicted in Figure 6-2 and postulated that the significance of recent life changes or situations is influenced by an individual's perceptual set. This perceptual set is, in turn, influenced by the current level of social supports and biographical assets or liabilities. The biographical assets or liabilities are a function of the individual's past experiences (e.g., death of parents, religious upbringing, financial situation). Biographical assets are presumably the result of positive early life influences, whereas biographical liabilities are the result of negative early life experiences. The second step in the

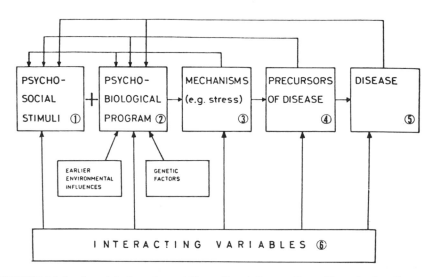

**FIGURE 6-1.** Levi model of psychosocially mediated disease. From "Introduction: Psychosocial Stimuli, Psychophysiological Reactions, and Disease by L. Levi in *Stress and Distress in Response to Psychosocial Stimuli* edited by L. Levi. Copyright 1972 by Pergamon Press. Reprinted by permission.

model involves the psychological defenses or, in psychodynamic terms, *ego defense mechanisms*. Rahe and Arthur suggest that certain psychological defenses are associated with reduced physiological arousal and therefore reduced susceptibility to illness.

The third step involves the psychophysiological response pattern to life events. Rahe and Arthur divide these responses into two categories: responses associated with awareness (e.g., sweating, pain, muscle tension) and responses not associated with awareness (e.g., elevated serum lipids, mild to moderate elevations in blood pressure, mild to moderate hypoglycemia). These responses can be immediate and/or delayed, and they are interactive. Step 4 in the model is related to the strategies the individual implements to reduce the psychophysiological response pattern. The use of these strategies is motivated by an *awareness* of the psychophysiological response complex and the perception that this response represents a health threat. The strategies include a variety of approaches, including relaxation techniques, broadly defined, physical exercise, medication, and cognitive coping techniques (e.g., minimalization, distraction, avoidance, selective awareness). If the response management is not completely successful in eliminating symptoms, step 5 occurs. At this stage, the individual directs his or her attention to persistent bodily symptoms, seeks medical care, and may develop "sick

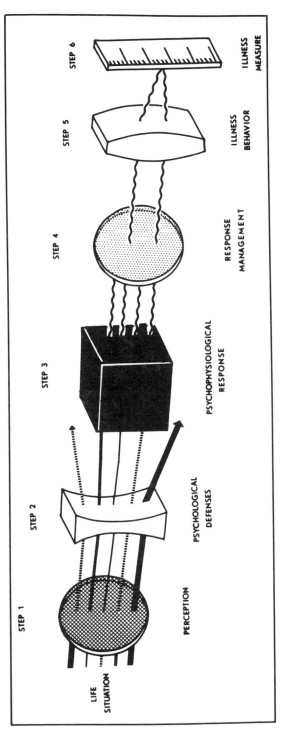

**FIGURE 6-2.** Rahe and Arthur's (1978) model of life change and illness. From "Life Changes and Illness Studies: Past History and Future Directions" by R. H. Rahe and R. J. Arthur, 1978, *Journal of Human Stress, 4*, 3–15. Copyright 1978 by Heldref Publications. Reprinted by permission.

role" behaviors, such as lost time from work, bed rest, and dependence on medical caretakers. Step 6 is the actual recorded medical diagnosis. As Rahe and Arthur emphasized, tests of the model indicate modest correlations among various steps or stages; the "further apart were any two steps in the model, the greater the scatter in their relationship."

Although both the Levi and the Rahe and Arthur models provide explanations for the influence of psychosocial factors on illness, they place considerable emphasis on "stress" as the mediating factor. Although the stress construct is often defined in these models, the psychosocial factors considered to be stressors within the models are quite general. A model proposed by Minuchin et al. (1975) is a good example of an attempt to operationalize such psychosocial constructs, particularly stress, to conflict within the family. These investigators proposed a multiple feedback model of psychosomatic illness in children, the open systems family model. This model postulates three necessary conditions for the initiation and maintenance of severe psychosomatic problems in children: (1) a certain type of family organization that encourages somatization, (2) child involvement in parental conflict, and (3) physiological vulnerability. The model hypothesizes that problematic family interaction patterns may trigger the onset or maintain the psychophysiological process associated with a given disorder. The symptoms function as a homeostatic mechanism regulating dysfunctional family transactions. The family transactions fall into four categories: enmeshment, overprotectiveness, rigidity, and lack of conflict resolution (see Table 7-10 in Chapter 7 for description of the categories). These transactional patterns reduce the ability of the family to solve conflict. The child's symptom is assumed to be primarily responsible for the avoidance of irrevocable conflict within the family.

Although the open systems family model is an attempt to operationalize stress, it is limited by its focus on the family system to the exclusion of other factors that may play a role, on the primary emphasis on childhood illness, and on classical psychosomatic illnesses. The model is, however, one of the first serious attempts to identify patterns of social interaction, rather than psychological traits, as contributing to the etiology and maintenance of physical illness.

Schwartz (1977) has proposed a biobehavioral model to account for the influence of stress, which is an application of systems theory to health and illness. The basic subsystems of the model, as depicted in Figure 6-3, include (1) environmental demands or input stimulation; (2) an information processing system; (3) output in the form of behavioral, autonomic, and glandular responses; and (4) a negative feedback loop. Specifically, Schwartz (1978) proposes the following:

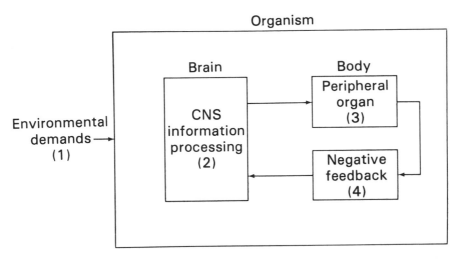

**FIGURE 6-3.** Schwartz's biobehavioral model. From "Psychosomatic Disorders and Bio-feedback: A Psychobiological Model of Disregulation" by G. E. Schwartz in *Psychopathology: Experimental Models*, edited by J. D. Maser and M. E. P. Seligman. Copyright 1977 by W. H. Freeman & Co. Reprinted by permission.

> When the environment (Stage 1) places demands on a person, the brain (Stage 2) performs the regulatory functions necessary to meet the specific demands. Depending upon the nature of the environmental demand on stress, certain bodily systems (Stage 3) will be activated, while others may be simultaneously inhibited. However, if this process is sustained to the point where the tissue suffers deterioration or injury, the negative feedback loops (Stage 4) of the homeostatic mechanism will normally come into play, forcing the brain to modify its directives to aid the afflicted organ. Often these negative feedback loops lead to the experience of pain. (p. 76)

The negative feedback loop in this model has a self-regulatory function in that it informs the brain of an existing problem, triggering it to influence the individual's behavior in an effort toward correction. It is this disruption in the health-maintaining feedback loop that can lead to a state of instability or *disregulation*. Disregulation may occur at any one stage or at multiple stages in the model. It is a condition in which the brain can no longer regulate an organ or a physiological system. Thus, the goal of the investigator and/or clinician is to identify the various stages involved in a specific disease state and then determine the complex interactions among these stages or pathways responsible for its etiology, exacerbation, and maintenance. Although there is little direct empirical evidence for the overall validity of the model, various aspects have been supported (cf. Schwartz, 1977, 1978).

Two major issues inherent in each of the models discussed require more specific attention. First, each assumes that stress contributes *directly* to the etiology and maintenance of a number of disorders. Unfortunately, with the exception of a limited number of disorders (e.g., coronary heart disease), psychological stress has not been empirically identified as contributing to physical illness. Indeed, even in those disorders in which psychological "stress" is presumed, by most investigators and clinicians, to significantly contribute to a given disorder, the relationship is largely indirect or speculative.

A case in point is illustrated in the areas of migraine headache in adults and of the recurrent abdominal pain (RAP) syndrome in children. In both cases, clinical reports and specifically, in the case of migraine, patient reports suggest that environmental stress may play a role in their etiology and/or exacerbation. However, there have been *no* longitudinal prospective studies on the impact of this factor on migraine (cf. Feuerstein & Gainer, 1982) or RAP (cf. Barr & Feuerstein, 1983). Although it is likely that such factors as environmental stress exacerbate the pain episodes, the data are either nonexistent, as in the case with RAP (Barr & Feuerstein, 1983) or scant, as with migraine (Henryk-Gutt & Rees, 1973). Finally, at the level of psychobiological mechanisms, most of the research on the psychophysiological reaction to laboratory stress in migraine and RAP is either inconclusive or indicates the *absence* of autonomic response patterns specific to these patient groups (e.g., Feuerstein, Barr, Francoeur, Houle, & Rafman, 1982; Feuerstein, Bush, & Corbisiero, 1982). A second problem with the current models is that only a general pathway linking psychological and biological factors to various forms of illness has been described.

## STRESS AND EPISODIC PAIN: AN ILLUSTRATIVE MODEL

Let us consider the role stress may play in the exacerbation of a symptom or pain episode to illustrate the potential complexities of the stress–illness link. Consider the symptom of pain. It is commonly assumed that pain episodes for which no pathogenic agent or pathophysiological process is readily apparent are frequently associated with stress. That is, various stressors trigger the symptom episode. Many symptom episodes, regardless of the presenting complaint, are episodic or irregular in nature, and patients frequently report minimal association between such episodes and the occurrence of stressors. In addition, certain patients may report an association with a stressor for one episode, but no such link for a subsequent episode. Another interesting clinical observation is the report of "good and bad periods," when patients will experience no symptom for hours, days, weeks, or months, and times where the symptom is quite frequent. These clinical observations, in conjunction with the apparent lack of stable, reliable differences in the way various patients with such symptoms respond psycho-physiologically to laboratory stressors, suggest an alternative model for investigating the stress–symptom/pain interaction.

Figure 6-4 represents the position that patients with a recurrent symptom, such as pain, actually display a stable psychobiological pattern that is fixed over time. Although the pattern illustrated is that of an oscillating wave, this wave simply represents diurnal changes. The assumption here is that patients display a characteristic psychobiological reactivity that differs from normal individuals in tonic levels, phasic response, or recovery components of the stress response. That is, these patients are operating at higher levels of autonomic arousal and they display a greater magnitude response to a stressor and/or delayed recovery from exposure to a stressor. It is this overactivity, existing as "trait," that predisposes the individual to recurrent symptom attacks. As discussed earlier, the empirical support for the hypothesis of a traitlike overreactivity is limited. What might an alternative pattern of psychobiological reactivity look like and how can such a pattern be conceptually integrated with the episodic nature of symptoms and exposure to stressors?

Figure 6-5 shows a pattern of psychobiological reactivity in which there are periods of relative stability followed by periods of increased reactivity or heightened psychobiological activity. This heightened psychobiological activity should be manifested in one or several physiological systems that are directly related to the symptom (e.g., temporal

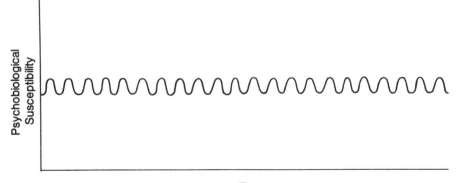

Time

**FIGURE 6-4.** Stable psychobiological pattern over time.

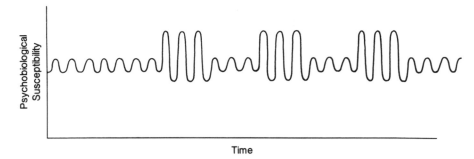

**FIGURE 6-5.** Fluctuating psychobiological pattern over time.

artery, in the case of migraine headache, or prostaglandin levels) or at a more general level (e.g., the immune system, stress hormones reflecting general sympathetic nervous system activity, and/or at a central neurochemical level reflecting central modulation of pain/discomfort (e.g., beta endorphin activity). Psychological changes may accompany these periods of heightened reactivity. Such psychological changes are a function of the individual's cognitive coping style and general level of awareness of emotional state. A major point is the concept of periods or *windows* of heightened activity. Such windows, in time, may reflect the clinical phenomenon of "good and bad" periods.

Figure 6-6 adds two additional dimensions to the model: (1) episodes of symptoms and (2) presence of stressors. The symptoms may occur alone or in clusters, whereas the stressors may precede, co-occur, or follow the symptom or may not be temporally related. With the

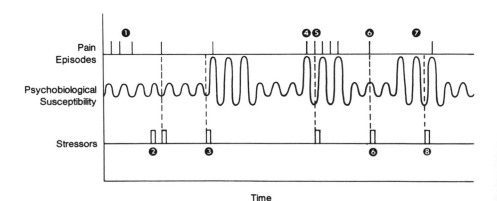

**FIGURE 6-6.** Dynamic psychobiological model of stress, psychobiological susceptibility, and episodic pain.

## TABLE 6-2
Patterns of Stressor, Psychobiological Susceptibility, and Symptom and/or
Pain Episodes

1. Pain episode or multiple pain episodes during low susceptibility
2. Stressor occurs before pain episode during low susceptibility
3. Stressor occurs before co-occurrene of pain episode and high susceptibility
4. Pain episode during high susceptibility
5. Pain episode co-occurring with stressor during high susceptibility followed by
   multiple pain episodes
6. Pain episode co-occurring with stressor during low susceptibility
7. High susceptibility with no concurrent pain episode or stressor
8. Stressor occurs before pain episode during period of high susceptibility

periods of psychobiological reactivity superimposed, the student can begin to appreciate the complexities in such a system. Table 6-2 lists the various combinations of stressor, psychobiological vulnerability, and symptom patterns that can emerge. The model in Figure 6-6 is simply a working set of hypotheses that must be validated if it is to assist in understanding stressor–symptom interactions and their treatment. Such validation could procede as follows: (1) determine whether the periods of heightened psychobiological activity exist over time within certain key physiological measures and within certain episodic disorders; (2) identify patterns of stressor–symptom interactions; and (3) identify the existence of stressor, psychobiological vulnerability, and symptom patterns. Such a model, if validated could help in the management of patients with recurrent symptoms, providing insight as to when to intervene pharmacologically and what to direct such interventions at (i.e., periods of heightened reactivity). Biobehavioral treatments could also be fine-tuned to affect the underlying symptom process to a greater degree.

## THE AIR TRAFFIC CONTROLLER HEALTH CHANGE STUDY: IN SEARCH OF THE STRESS–ILLNESS LINK

As discussed in Chapter 3, when reviewing research strategies, Rose *et al.*, (1978) conducted a five-year prospective study of job stress and health using air traffic controllers as subjects. The significance of the study was that it is the only longitudinal study of job stress that also investigated the possible psychological and psychobiological mechanisms relating job stress to health outcome while the subjects were actually working. The importance of this aspect of the research is considerable, since such a study permits the analysis of situation-specific changes in hypothesized physiological mechanisms of health and disease. Physiological, behavioral, and psychological reactivity to a structured, recurrent environmental stimulus (i.e., the well-defined work environment) and their relationship to health outcome was determined with such a design. In addition, the more common static measurement of biological, medical, psychological, and psychosocial variables was obtained.

Rose and colleagues summarized their findings in three broad categories: (1) examination of physiological activity during the day; (2) relationships among biological, psychological, and work variables; and (3) the relationship between physiological activity and physical and psychiatric morbidity. Approximately 416 air traffic controllers (male; mean age = 36.2; $SD = 5.0$) were studied.

In the first study, 20-minute integrated plasma cortisol and growth hormone measures over a 5-hour typical work period across three repeated studies (days) indicated that the controllers were secreting more cortisol and less growth hormone than the most comparable group of normal controls (there were no controls in the study; the control data come from the literature). The two measures were not related to each other and both measures were inconsistent across days in terms of average levels and episodic secretory activity. No habituation across days was evidenced for either measure (Rose, Jenkins, Hurst, Livingston, & Hall, 1982).

In the second study, 76 psychosocial variables, including 21 measuring attitude, coping resources, and social supports; three peer ratings of work performance; 11 measuring work satisfaction and job attitude; 3 measuring magnitude of life change; 34 variables from two personality inventories; and 4 measuring Type A behavior, were obtained. To quote the researchers directly, "there was very little relationship between any of these 76 variables and average endocrine responses. . . . These analyses cast doubt on the existence of *stable trait* characteristics as predictors of endocrine response, at least in this study" (Rose, Jenkins, Hurst, Herd, & Hall, 1982, p. 115). This second study did, however, show a relationship between increased behavior at work and increased average cortisol levels, yet the findings were weak and potentially unreliable. Taken as a whole, the findings suggest the insensitivity of a *normative* approach (comparisons across individuals using group data) to the analysis of such data. More interesting findings emerged when the data were examined using an *ipsative* or individual approach.

The ipsative approach indicated that those men who showed increases in cortisol response with increasing work were psychologically different from the other subjects. These men were *not* more dissatisfied or less competent, nor did they display increased levels of distress. Rather, they were more satisfied with their work; they were regarded by their peers as more competent; and they reported greater work freedom, high job satisfaction, and low life change events. These findings contradict those theories of stress that hypothesize that increased levels of strain are associated with increased distress and heightened physiological activity and illustrate the complexities involved in findings from naturalistic stress studies.

In the third study, Rose, Jenkins, Hurst, Kreger, Barrett, and Hall (1982) reported on the relationship between physical health change, psychopathology, and work responsivity or reactivity to cortisol. Those subjects with the *lowest* rates of mild to moderate physical health change showed a modest tendency toward *greater* average cortisol. Those men who displayed the workload–cortisol relationship also had higher average cortisol levels. The men who experienced greater psychiatric symptomatology, including impulse control problems, alcohol abuse, and subjective distress, had slightly higher average cortisol levels at work. Physical health change, level of psychopathology, and cortisol response to increased workload were independent predictors of average cortisol levels.

The air traffic controller study indicated the importance of an ipsative approach to research on stress and illness and their underlying physiology. And, contrary to expectations, higher cortisol reactivity to work pressure is associated with factors that indicate less distress, and perhaps reflects increased job involvement. The increased cortisol activity tends to be associated with *lower* rates of change in physical health status, but *higher* rates of psychopathology. The conclusion drawn from this research is that traditional models of stress and illness should be viewed with caution.

## WHO STAYS HEALTHY UNDER STRESS?

Is it possible to encounter stress and remain healthy? This type of question leads to an approach that differs from the one that attempts to predict and explain stress–illness associations, but it is equally important. There is only limited work in this area, represented by Kobasa, Hilker, and Maddi (1979), researchers in the field of personality. Kobasa *et al.* based their investigation on the anecdotal observation that certain individuals, regardless of exposure to stress, somehow manage not to succumb to stress disorders. Also, the stress–illness correlations are modest ($r = .30$) and the standard deviations of these associations are quite extreme suggesting considerable variability across individuals in the degree to which stress is associated with illness.

Kobasa *et al.* (1979) studied two groups of managers from a large public utility in a major metropolitan area. Two groups of subjects were identified as either high in stress but low in illness or high in stress and high in illness. High stress scores were obtained before the high or low illness scores. The two groups were homogeneous on a number of variables (income, stable family, etc.), and all subjects were males. A discriminant function analysis (multivariate statistical procedure that identifies the best *combination* of variables for explaining differences between groups) was conducted using a number of variables. These variables included measures of alienation from self, measures of perceived control, and tendency to seek novelty and challenge, all characteristics hypothesized to be associated with health. The results indicated that the high stress/high illness subjects were more alienated from self, whereas alienation from work, interpersonal relations, social institutions, and family did not discriminate between the two groups. High stress/low illness subjects were less nihilistic than high stress/high illness subjects, indicating a belief that one can control events in one's environment. High stress/low illness subjects tended to be more interested in novel experience, as well as more oriented toward achievement, and displayed greater endurance. High stress/low illness subjects perceived less threat in personal, financial, and interpersonal areas than did high stress/high illness subjects. The discriminant function explained 74% of the total variance of the difference between the groups, leaving only 26% unexplained. Although this study was not longitudinal, it represents an attempt to describe or identify differences between groups exposed to stress who do and do not report illness. The causal link remains unclear.

## STRESSORS INDIRECTLY INFLUENCING HEALTH OUTCOME

Stressors can also have an indirect effect on health outcome. That is, exposure to a major life event or events may be associated with the occurrence of some type of accident that affects health status. An interesting study suggesting such a link is one reported by Knudson-Cooper and Leuchtag (1982) on the stress of a family move on children's burn accidents. These investigators observed that children are at greater risk of being burned following a family move. The relationship among family moves, life change events, age and sex of child, and type of burn (flame, scald, other) was analyzed. Of the total 330 in the study sample, 63% (208) had experienced one or more major life change events,

(Schedule of Recent Experience) and 35% (117) had moved within the year prior to the burn accident. Those who had moved also reported more life change events, excluding the move, than those who did not move. Girls were approximately twice as likely as boys to experience three major life events. These findings were concordant with subjective reports of stress: 66% of the movers, in contrast to 34% of the non-movers, indicated that they felt the family had been under greater stress than usual over the year before the burn accidents. Children under five who were scalded were more likely to have moved than were older children who had sustained a flame burn. A period at 2 to 5 months after the move, was identified as critical, when the child is particularly vulnerable to burn accidents.

## STRESS AS RESPONSE TO ILLNESS

In addition to the effects that stress may have in the etiology or development of various physical illnesses, the illnesses themselves, and their associated treatments, also constitute stressors the individual must confront. Therefore, stress can also be studied as a set of complex responses to illness. Several health psychologists have proposed various models in an attempt to explain how individuals cope with such stress; both acute and chronic illnesses have been studied. This section will provide a detailed consideration of coping, and reviews the modern psychological theories of coping. The stress experienced following severe burn will be used to illustrate the complexities involved in coping with illness.

A discussion of coping first requires answering the question, Coping with what? Given that our discussion will focus on stressors associated with various health states, it is important to review the various stressors encountered during medical illness and treatment. Cohen and Lazarus (1979) identified a series of stressors from the literature on stress and medical illness and its treatment. Table 6-3 lists these various stressors. As the table indicates, a wide variety of potential threats characterize this list of stressors. These threats include threat to life and fear of dying, threat to body integrity and comfort, threats to one's self-concept and future plans, threat to one's emotional stability, threats to the fulfillment of customary social role and activities, and threat involving the need to adjust to a new physical or social environment. Given this diversity of stressors representing potential threats to biological integrity, as well as the social and psychological states, the study of coping in relation to medical illness and treatment provides fertile ground for research on stress and coping. One goal of such research is to

**TABLE 6-3**
Stressors Associated with Medical Illness and Treatment

- Threats to life and fears of dying
- Threats to bodily integrity and comfort (from the illness, the diagnostic procedures, or the medical treatment itself)
  — Bodily injury or disability
  — Permanent physical changes
  — Physical pain, discomfort, and other negative symptoms of illness or treatment
  — Incapacitation
- Threats to one's self-concept and future plans
  — Necessity to alter one's self-image or belief systems
  — Uncertainty about the course of the illness and about one's future
  — Endangering of life goals and values
  — Loss of autonomy and control
- Threats to one's emotional equilibrium, that is, the necessity to deal with feelings of anxiety, anger, and other emotions that come about as a result of other stressors described
- Threats to the fulfillment of customary social roles and activities
  — Separation from family, friends, and other social supports
  — Loss of important social roles
  — Necessity to depend on others
- Threats involving the need to adjust to a new physical or social environment
  — Adjustment to the hospital setting
  — Problems in understanding medical terminology and customs
  — Necessity for decision making in stressful and unfamiliar situations

*Note.* From "Coping with the Stress of Illness" by F. Cohen and R. S. Lazarus in *Health Psychology: A Handbook* (p. 229) edited by G. C. Stone, F. Cohen, and N. E. Adler. Copyright 1979 by Jossey-Bass, Inc. Reprinted by permission.

answer the question, How do the stressors effect the exacerbation and maintenance of various illnesses and their associated social and psychological consequences? The majority of research on stress as a response to illness has emphasized the cognitive factors associated with the modulation of the stress response, rather than emphasizing the stress response itself or the nature of the specific environmental stressors. Such an approach is consistent with the transactional models of stress reviewed in Chapter 5.

Our own experience with family members exposed to the stressors of medical illness or hospitalization and/or very painful or anxiety-provoking medical procedures shows that humans have the ability to buffer the effects of severe personal tragedy quite effectively. Whereas coping or adjustment to these tragedies often occurs, as we are also unfortunately well aware, certain individuals have extreme difficulty coping with such situations, and oftentimes this leads to a variety of emotional and interpersonal difficulties and the prolongation and/or exacerbation of the illness itself. Indeed, depending upon the extent and period of such maladaptive coping, a set of complicated illness behaviors, as discussed in Chapter 9, can ensue. What are the factors proposed to be involved in adaptive coping with physical illness? Models have been proposed by Moos and Davis Tsu (1977), Lazarus (1974), Cohen and Lazarus (1979), and Taylor (1983).

## PSYCHOLOGICAL THEORIES OF COPING WITH ILLNESS

Lazarus and colleagues have perhaps had the greatest impact in the study of stress and coping. Therefore, Lazarus's theory and its application to coping with the stressors of illness will be carefully reviewed. As shown in Chapter 5, cognitive factors are assumed to play a major role in emotion and adaptation. If cognitive factors influence the effects of stressful events; the choice of coping patterns; and the cognitive, physiological, and behavioral reactions to stressors, it is important to identify these key cognitive factors. Recall that, according to Lazarus, cognitive appraisal, or evaluation, of potentially stressful events mediates psychologically between the individual and the environment when the individual encounters a stressful event. It is the individual's evaluation that determines whether a stressor is harmful or potentially harmful. The evaluation is, in turn, partly a function of the resources available to the individual to neutralize or tolerate the stressor. The individual continually reevaluates judgments made about demands and constraints characteristic of various interactions with the environment and the various options and resources he or she has for meeting these demands. These cognitions determine the individual's stress reaction, the emotions experienced, and the adjustment or adaptational outcome. The extent to which an individual experiences psychological stress, then, is determined by the evaluation of both what is at stake (primary appraisal) and what coping resources are available (secondary appraisal).

*Primary appraisal* represents evaluations of whether the transaction is (1) irrelevant to the individual's well-being, (2) benign-positive, or (3) whether stress occurs as a judgment of harm or loss, threat, or challenge. Primary appraisal addresses the question, Am I OK or am I in trouble? *Secondary appraisal* refers to the individual's continuous judgments concerning coping resources, options, and constraints. Secondary appraisal processes involve evaluation of the cost of different strategies and their probability of success. Factors that influence secondary appraisals in a given stressful situation are a function of the individual's past experience with such situations, general belief patterns, and availability of coping resources at that particular time. According to this model, secondary appraisal in a specific stressful situation is a function of the individual's previous encounter with similar situations, general beliefs regarding self and environment, and the availability of certain resources, for example, personal health, level of energy, problem-solving skills, degree of social support, and material resources (Folkman, Schaeffer, & Lazarus, 1979). Therefore, with secondary appraisal, the individual asks the question What can I do about this situation? Although the distinction is made between primary and secondary appraisal processes, this distinction is to assist researchers and clinicians in identifying various factors that comprise these processes, as well as the variables affecting cognition, coping, and adaptation to stress. The two evaluative processes are interrelated and not empirically distinct in many environmental situations. Such observations question whether they are, in fact, different at all; this dichotomy, however, does appear useful when we conceptualize the coping process.

Now that we have looked at the process of cognitive appraisal involved in coping, according to Lazarus's transactional model of stress, it is important to define operationally what we mean by *coping*. Coping, according to Lazarus and colleagues, is defined as the cognitive and behavioral efforts necessary to manage environmental and internal demands and the conflicts among them. These cognitive and behavioral actions, or efforts, are directed at mastering, tolerating, reducing, and/or minimizing environmental and internal demands and conflicts that strain an individual's resources. Although coping is commonly conceptualized as occurring in reaction to stressful situations, it can also occur before a stressful confrontation. This form of coping is *anticipatory coping*. Coping can also occur in reaction to a present or past confrontation with a harmful stressor. Anticipatory coping activities have been emphasized by Lazarus and colleagues (Lazarus & Cohen, 1977; Lazarus & Launier, 1978). This emphasis on anticipatory coping argues that the portion of our time that is spent dealing with the environment involves an active regulation of emotional reactions, selecting environments that we must respond to, shaping our interaction with such environments, which includes planning, choosing, avoiding, tolerating, postponing, escaping, and manipulating (Folkman, 1984).

Coping is hypothesized to have two main functions: (1) the alteration of an ongoing person–environment relationship (problem-focused coping) and (2) the control of stressful emotions or physiological arousal (emotional regulation). Problem-focused coping involves the individual's efforts to deal with the source of stress through the modification of his or her own problem-maintaining behavior or through the modification of environmental conditions. An example of such problem-oriented coping would be learning appropriate ways of handling anger directed toward one's boss through various anger management approaches (see Chapter 7 for a discussion of anger management) or modifying the work environment whereby whatever triggers such anger is bypassed or removed. Emotional regulation involves coping efforts directed at modifying emotional distress and maintaining the moderate level of arousal or internal state that is necessary for effective information processing and action. An example of emotional regulation involves learning relaxation techniques or active involvement in aerobic exercise, with the intent of reducing heightened levels of physiological arousal associated with the stress response.

A recent study on stress and coping in middle-aged individuals revealed that both forms of coping (problem-focused coping and control of stressful emotions and physiological arousal) were used in 98% of the specific stressful episodes reported over the course of a year (Folkman & Lazarus, 1980). Problem-solving efforts to cope with the threat itself and efforts to regulate emotional distress can be mutually facilitative. An example of such mutual facilitation is the case in which the reduction of emotional distress may help the individual concentrate more effectively on work that needs to be completed, thus improving performance. As discussed in Chapter 5, the inverted U function of arousal and performance suggests that optimal performance occurs at an optimal arousal level, whereas extreme arousal affects performance adversely. It is also possible that one coping function can interfere with the effectiveness of the other coping function, as in the case in which denial that a breast lump could be anything serious leads to a delay in seeking medical care, (i.e., instrumental actions), and increases the risk of advanced stage cancer (Katz, Weiner, Gallagher, & Hellman, 1970). Coping efforts that are totally palliative or directed at reducing emotional distress can be problematic, particularly if the justification for such stress reduction is not based in reality. The interaction of these two functions of coping must be considered when the effects of such coping on adaptation are studied. That is, it is often the combination of both forms of coping that influence the outcome of stress. Let us now consider the various coping modes or forms of coping that can achieve the two functions described.

According to Cohen and Lazarus (1979), a number of coping strategies specifically relevant to the health care setting have been proposed, yet there is no widely agreed-upon system for describing such coping. Investigators who study coping in health care situations typically direct their attention to those strategies that seem to emerge from the data obtained from specific patient populations. This typically results in a listing of the various mechanisms described in these different studies. Coping strategies have been described for patients with serious illnesses (Lipowski, 1970), families of children with polio (Davis, 1963), and women facing breast biopsy (Katz et al., 1970). Lipowski (1970) does suggest two central cognitive coping styles: *minimalization* and *vigilant focusing*. Lipowski suggests that these coping styles can be expressed behaviorally in one of three ways: (1) tackling the problem, (2) capitulating, or (3) avoiding.

Within the Lazarus transactional model of stress and coping, four major modes or forms of coping have been delineated. These forms include information seeking, direct action, inhibition of action, and intrapsychic or cognitive processes. Cohen and Lazarus (1979) define information seeking as one of the more basic forms of coping in situations that are novel, and of which little is known, or under conditions of ambiguity. Here the individual attempts to determine if problems exist and what, if anything, must be done. Interestingly, in the case of certain chronic illnesses, for example, various forms of chronic pain, patients can conduct an insatiable search for information regarding their problem. In contrast, other patients with severe illness prefer to avoid such information and place themselves in the hands of some health care provider. The degree of information seeking displayed across individuals varies widely. Direct actions include behaviors directed at doing something about the problem (i.e., running away, taking medication). Inhibition of action is also considered a mode of coping. As the term suggests, here the individual simply fails to make an effort to cope with a stressor. Intrapsychic processes, or cognitive processes, include a wide variety of coping modes, such as denial, avoidance, intellectualized detachment, and use of humor in a difficult situation. Many of these approaches have traditionally been considered defenses with potential long-term negative consequences. Cohen and Lazarus (1979) added a fifth mode of coping; turning to others for assistance and support. As discussed in Chapter 5, such social support can enhance effective coping.

Illness is frequently viewed as threatening, and many patients appraise the situation as a challenge or a task to be mastered. A number of investigators have reviewed the various adaptive tasks that must be dealt with for an appropriate adjustment to illness. Consideration of these adaptive tasks allows the reader to identify goals of patients' coping efforts and provides a perspective when types of interventions that might be helpful in facilitating coping are considered. The research dealing with the adaptive tasks involved with illness, as summarized by Cohen and Lazarus (1979), include (1) reduce harmful environmental conditions and enhance prospects of recovery; (2) tolerate or adjust to negative events and realities; (3) maintain a positive self-image; (4) maintain emotional equilibrium to reduce the possible effects of depression, fear, anxiety, and anger, which are considered normal responses to such situations; and (5) continue satisfying relationships with others.

In their review of coping with the stressors of illness, Cohen and Lazarus (1979) draw a number of conclusions after considering both the basic (i.e., nonintervention) and clinical research in this area. The research as a whole is characterized by contradictory results, few replications, and the inability to compare studies because of various differences in independent and dependent measures and lack of preciseness about the potential effective components of certain psychological interventions used to enhance coping. However, a number of conclusions were drawn. Trait measures of depression (nonsurgical illnesses), state measures of depression (recovery from surgery), state measures of preoperative fear (surgery), inhibition or expression of emotion (nonsurgery), and vigilant coping modes (surgery) were found to predict (fairly) consistently negative medical outcomes in nonintervention studies. Currently, it is unclear what types of information are most helpful in facilitating coping with illness. In addition, types of information may interact with a number of other characteristics of the patient (e.g., personality), and the degree of interaction requires further investigation.

Cohen and Lazarus suggest a number of factors that could improve research in this area. These include (1) using a wider range of outcome variables when examining coping strategy naturally, or through the examination of coping strategies using intervention studies; (2) specifying which coping strategies are most effective across several illnesses and which are valuable in dealing with specific illnesses; (3) using both trait and process measures of emotion in studying outcome, since each of these measures have some significant relationship with certain medical outcomes, but not with others; (4) limiting generalization from results of nonintervention studies to interventions to aid patients coping, given that these generalizations are not consistent and do not justify clinical application at present; (5) considering the outcome measures carefully, including both short-term and long-term measurement, and (6) broadening the assessment of coping so that coping changes over time and across situations can be identified. In fact, given the transactional nature of the Lazarus model of stress and coping, it is not surprising that inconsistent findings have been observed in this area. That is, many of the assessment and measurement procedures used to date in the studies discussed by Cohen and Lazarus were based upon a more static model of stress and not on the transactional or interactional feedback model proposed by Lazarus and colleagues. Measures are needed that reflect this complex interactional process.

Taylor (1983) proposes a theory of *cognitive adaptation* to threatening events. She argues that the readjustment process involved in dealing with a threatening event includes three general themes: (1) a search for meaning in the experience; (2) an attempt to regain mastery over the event, as well as over life in general; and (3) an effort to enhance one's self-esteem through self-enhancing evaluations, that is, to feel good about one's self again, despite the personal setback.

According to the cognitive adaptation theory, the search for meaning involves a need to understand why the stress occurred and what its impact has been (causal attributions). The tendency to search for meaning is based upon *attribution theory*, which argues that, following a traumatic or threatening event, individuals tend to make attributions regarding that event so as to understand, predict, and control their environment (Wong & Weiner, 1981). In Taylor's research with cancer patients, she noted that patients attempt to understand why they developed cancer. Ninety-five percent of her respondents provided some explanation for why their cancer occurred, in contrast to spouse's rates of such attributions, which were approximately 63%. This finding suggests that the need for some explanation was apparently more cogent for the cancer patient than for her spouse or the relatively less involved individual.

In an effort to determine whether a certain type or form of attributional explanation enhances the search for meaning to a greater degree than others, Taylor evaluated the specific content of cancer patients' explanations and related these to overall psychological adjustment. The largest number, 41%, attributed their cancer either to general stress or to a particular type of stress. Interestingly, when a particular stressor was mentioned, it was either an ongoing problematic marriage or a recent divorce. Thirty-two percent of the sample reported some suspected carcinogen (birth control pills, DES, or Primarin) or an environmental situation (e.g., living near chemical dumps or nuclear testing sites). Twenty-six percent of the women attributed cancer to hereditary factors, 17% to diet, and 10% to a blow to the breast, such as one occurring in an automobile accident or a fall. Taylor points out that, with the exception of heredity, all the attributive causes represent *past* rather than ongoing events, or they are events over which one currently has some control, such as stress or diet. The issue of control is a key factor in this model. No single attribution was related to overall psychological adjustment. The finding that no specific attribution is associated with improved adjustment suggests that the causal meaning itself is the goal of the attribution. In addition to understanding why the event occurred, subjects were also concerned over its implications for quality of life. In sum, the attempt to identify meaning in the cancer experience takes at least two forms: (1) causal analysis providing an answer to the question of why it happened, and (2) a rethinking of one's attitudes and priorities to restructure life along more satisfying lines. Various quotations were provided by Taylor (1983) to illustrate these changes:

I have much more enjoyment of each day, each moment. I am not so worried about what is or isn't or what I wish I had. All those things you get entangled with don't seem to be part of my life right now. (p. 1163)

You take a long look at your life and realize that many things that you thought were important before are totally insignificant. That's probably been the major change in my life. What you do is put things into perspective. You find out that things like relationships are really the most important things you have—the people you know and your family—everything else is just way down the line. It's very strange that it takes something so serious to make your realize that. (p. 1163)

Of course, this experience is not positive for everyone, and the variation is considerable. Taylor gives the following example:

I thought I was a well-cared for, middle-class woman who chose her doctors carefully and who was doing everything right. I was rather pleased with myself. I had thought I could handle pretty much what came my way. And I was completely shattered. My confidence in myself was completely undermined. (p. 1163)

Sudden threatening events can undermine one's sense of control over one's body and life in general. The second component of the adjustment process, according to Taylor, is *gaining a sense of control* over the event, so as to manage it or to keep it from recurring. Data from Taylor suggest that cancer patients appear to handle the concern for mastery or self-control by assuming that they can personally avoid recurrence of cancer. Of the patients she interviewed, 67% reported they had at least some control over the course or recurrence of their cancer, and 37% believed they had considerable control. Some of the remaining 33% believed that although they personally had no control over the cancer, the doctor or continued treatment would help control the disease. In contrast, the significant others used as a control indicated that both the patients' and physicians' ability to control the cancer was less. This belief that one can control one's cancer or that the physician or treatments can control it are strongly associated with overall positive adjustment. Interestingly, many of the patients' efforts at control were psychological. Many patients considered that a positive attitude would keep the cancer from recurring. An example from Taylor follows: "I believe that if you are a positive person your attitude has a lot to do with it. I definitely feel I will never get it again. . . . I think that if you feel you are in control of it you can control it up to a point. I absolutely refused to have any more cancer" (p. 1163). Attempts to control the side effects of treatments represent another effort at mastery. Ninety-two percent of the patients who received chemotherapy reported doing something to control its side effects. Another form of control or mastery can be the acquisition of information. That is, certain patients obtain information regarding the illness in an effort to cope as illustrated by the following (Taylor, 1983): "I felt that I had lost control of my body somehow, and the way for me to get back some control was to find out as much as I could. It really became almost an obsession" (p. 1164).

The third component to Taylor's description of cognitive adaptation is the *process of self-enhancement*. Here, coping efforts are directed at enhancing the self and restoring self-esteem, the loss of which is frequently associated with the consequence of exposure to threatening events. In certain cases, self–esteem-enhancing cognitions can be quite direct. Taylor asked subjects to describe changes that had occurred in their lives since the cancer incident. After reporting such changes, the subjects were also asked to indicate whether these changes were positive or negative. Only 17% reported any negative changes in their lives, whereas 53% reported only positive changes, with the remainder indicating no change. When Taylor asked these women to compare how well they were doing with other women who were coping with the same crisis, only two indicated that they were doing less well. Taylor suggests that these results imply that women are making downward social comparisons, contrasting themselves with women who were less fortunate than they, which suggests that downward comparisons are a fairly effective method of self-protection against threat. Of course, as with any explanation of this type, further research is necessary to support such an assumption. Social comparison is only one method of coping and is, presumably directed at enhancing self-esteem. Other dimensions for comparison could include the severity of the disorder, the extent of surgery, or current social status (married or presence of significant other). Examples of such social comparisons are as follows (Taylor, 1983):

> I had a comparatively small amount of surgery. How awful it must be for women who have had a mastectomy. I just can't imagine, it would seem it would be so difficult. (p. 1166)

> The people I really feel sorry for are those young gals. To lose a breast when you are so young must be awful. I'm 73; what do I need a breast for? (p. 1166)

> If I hadn't married I think this thing would have really gotten me. I can't imagine dating or whatever knowing you have this thing and not knowing how to tell the man about it. (p. 1166)

The themes of meaning, mastery, and self-enhancement were observed in practically every patient as a reaction to the threat she was experiencing. However, the form through which the theme was expressed differed from patient to patient. Whereas the specific attributions made by these cancer patients varied, virtually each patient had some theory about her cancer. The same type of finding occurred for control and social comparisons, implying that the specific form of the cognitions these patients held regarding their illness may not be as important as the *functions* of the cognitions. Taylor (1983) concludes that specific cognitions may represent different things under different circumstances, that they may be functionally overlapping rather than functionally distinct, and that they may satisfy several functions simultaneously. Such a position differs from the assumptions of cognitions in laboratory psychological research, in which cognitions are conceptualized as having consistent meanings across situations rather than multiple or changing meanings.

Taylor also emphasized that an important characteristic of cognitive adaptations to threatening events is that they tend to be *illusion based.* That is, the cognitions on which meaning, mastery, and self-enhancement depend are, to some extent, founded on illusions. The causes for cancer, the belief in control over one's cancer, and the self-enhancing social comparisons may or may not have any basis in reality, yet they tend to be beneficial with regard to psychological adaptation. This contrasts considerably with past notions regarding mental functioning in which positive adaptation was assumed to be associated with reality-based appraisals. Indeed, as Lazarus (1983) points out, "everyone knew that self-deception was tantamount to mental disorder" (p. 1). Lazarus (1983) emphasized that denial is no longer viewed as a primitive, ultimately unsuccessful defense, but rather that it possesses value in protecting individuals against crisis both in the initial stages of threat and intermittently when people must come to terms with a terminal illness. Illusion has been observed in normal cognitive functioning and apparently represents a factor differentiating depressive individuals from normal individuals. Normal individuals tend to inflate others' views of them (Lewinsohn, Mischel, Chaplin, & Barton, 1980), and they are more prone to an illusion of control if the perception is that they can control objectively uncontrollable outcomes (Alloy, Abramson, & Viscusi, 1981). Greenwald (1980) suggests that these illusion-based cognitions assist in the maintenance of the "self" as a highly organized information processing system producing behavioral persistence. Taylor (1983) concludes then that the effective individual is one who allows the development of illusions, nurtures these illusions, and as a result can adaptively cope with various threats.

A potential problem with the adaptive significance of illusion is that these illusions are susceptible to disconfirmation. Beliefs that one can control cancer can be abruptly disconfirmed by a recurrence. Physicians or a knowledgeable friend can quickly disconfirm ideas regarding the cause of cancer as well. If these illusions are challenged or modified, what happens to the maintenance of such illusions? This represents an important issue in social cognition, especially relative to psychological control. Both the *reactance model* and *learned helplessness* model suggest that when lack of control exists in actuality, those who attempted to exercise such control will experience difficulties behaviorally, emotionally, cognitively, and motivationally, in contrast to those who did not believe they were in control. The cognitive adaptation theory proposed by Taylor (1983) represents an alternative to models of disconfirmation (i.e., learned helplessness and reactance).

## RESPONSE TO THE STRESS OF BURNS: CLINICAL OBSERVATIONS

Based on a sample of 35 patients (19 women, 16 men) admitted to a hospital for burn care with burns over 7% of the body surface area, and 18 years or older, Steiner and Clark (1977) present a model of the psychological reactions of the adult burn patient. This model is actually a representation of the course of psychological and physiological changes observed in patients with significant burns. The model provides a clinical example of the complex reaction to a significant stressor. The description involves three basic stages, Stage I representing the state of physiological emergency, Stage II the stage of psychological emergency, and Stage III the stage of social emergency. These stages are illustrated in Figure 6-7.

Steiner and Clark (1977) describe the first stage of physiological emergency as occurring between weeks 2 to 4 following the burn. This period represents a major physiological strain on the individual, particularly patients with large burns when reserves must be mobilized to meet this physiological stress. A number of marked physiological changes occur, including anoxia, acidosis, and carbon monoxide intoxication. The cardiovascular system is stressed by the injury and by the large volumes of fluid needed for resuscitation and the loss of eletrolytes and proteins, mostly through the burned area. The burn is susceptible to infection, which must be continuously guarded against. Endocrine changes that are indicative of severe stress (see the GAS model) occur, and wound debridement and various operative procedures must be performed. Psychologically, delirium characterized by a global, but reversible impairment in thinking, memory, and perception is characteristic. The symptoms accompanying this delirium include hallucinations, delusions, confabulations, apathy, agitation, and withdrawal. These clinicians noted that significant fluctuations in this symptomatology occurred in that patients were frequently worse at night, reporting fewer

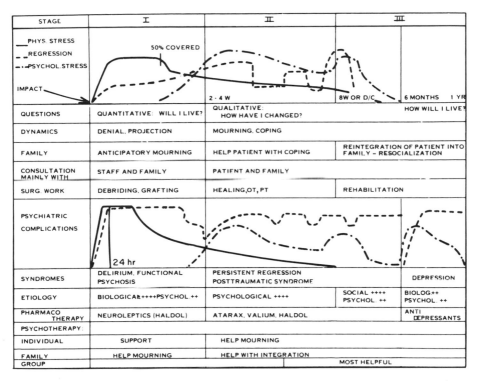

| STAGE | I | II | III | |
|---|---|---|---|---|
| ___PHYS. STRESS<br>__ _REGRESSION<br>_.._PSYCHOL.STRESS<br><br>IMPACT | 50% COVERED | 2 - 4 W | 8W OR D/C | 6 MONTHS   1 YR |
| QUESTIONS | QUANTITATIVE:   WILL I LIVE? | QUALITATIVE:<br>HOW HAVE I CHANGED? | | HOW WILL I LIVE? |
| DYNAMICS | DENIAL, PROJECTION | MOURNING, COPING | | |
| FAMILY | ANTICIPATORY MOURNING | HELP PATIENT WITH COPING | REINTEGRATION OF PATIENT INTO<br>FAMILY – RESOCIALIZATION | |
| CONSULTATION<br>MAINLY WITH | STAFF AND FAMILY | PATIENT AND FAMILY | | |
| SURG. WORK | DEBRIDING, GRAFTING | HEALING, OT, PT | REHABILITATION | |
| PSYCHIATRIC<br>COMPLICATIONS | 24 hr | | | |
| SYNDROMES | DELIRIUM, FUNCTIONAL<br>PSYCHOSIS | PERSISTENT REGRESSION<br>POSTTRAUMATIC SYNDROME | | DEPRESSION |
| ETIOLOGY | BIOLOGICAL++++PSYCHOL.++ | PSYCHOLOGICAL ++++ | SOCIAL ++++<br>PSYCHOL. ++ | BIOLOG++<br>PSYCHOL. ++ |
| PHARMACO<br>THERAPY | NEUROLEPTICS (HALDOL) | ATARAX, VALIUM, HALDOL | | ANTI<br>DEPRESSANTS |
| PSYCHOTHERAPY:<br>INDIVIDUAL | SUPPORT | HELP MOURNING | | |
| FAMILY<br>GROUP | HELP MOURNING | HELP WITH INTEGRATION | MOST HELPFUL | |

**FIGURE 6-7.** Sequence of psychological and physiological changes in burn patients. The upper half of the figure represents the material pertinent to the normal psychological reaction to burn injury: acute grief. There are three focal points in the temporal progression of this process. First, the closing of the burn wound or reduction of the size of the wound by 50%, after which there is usually a significant decrease in the physiological stress imposed on the patient. Survival is usually no longer an issue. Second, the transition into Stage II at which time the focus of patient activity changes to healing and rehabilitation, which presents qualitative issues previously denied and an increase in psychological demands. Stage III is the time of discharge which once again means an increase of psychological stress for the patient who has to face a generally familiar, but somewhat less supportive, environment while simultaneously he is forced to recognize whatever deformity or disabilities may remain. The lower half of the figure outlines the psychiatric complications that occur when the natural progression of the grieving process is arrested in a regressive state. The complications are related to the different stresses represented by the curves. Every patient in each stage has a curve generally similar to these curves. From "Psychiatric Complications of Burned Adults: A Classification" by H. Steiner and W. R. Clark, 1977, *The Journal of Trauma, 17,* 134–143. Copyright 1977 by Williams & Wilkins Co. Reprinted by permission.

of these symptoms during the day with more familiar stimulation. It was suggested that the patient's isolation from family or other support systems may contribute to the psychological problems. Steiner and Clark (1977) present a case illustrating this first phase:

> D. R., a 52-year-old woman with 60% third degree body surface area burn, was kept in a single room. During her first three weeks of hospitalization, the patient was mostly apathetic alternating with periods of agitation. She was at times able to respond to questions. However, most of the time it was an effort for her to do so. She complained of difficulties in keeping her thoughts together and of forgetting a lot. She was disoriented to time and place, and briefly even to person. In her more lucid moments she demonstrated a clear concern for her physical status, asking us whether or not we thought she would survive. Her denial assumed psychotic proportions when she told the staff to debride the sick women in bed with her while she and her husband went to have a cup of coffee in the cafeteria. (p. 137)

The stage of *psychological emergency*, or Stage II, may last from 2 to 8 weeks postburn. During this stage, the patient is usually physiologically stable. Basic survival is typically no longer a problem. Most of the burn has healed or has been covered with skin grafts, and treatment is focused on increasing patient activity, with considerable emphasis on physical and occupational therapy. Although these activities are painful, the primary problem, from a psychological perspective, is the developing awareness of certain losses. It is at this stage that the patient must confront the long-term outcomes regarding changes in work capacity, functional ability, and social adjustment. Steiner and Clark (1977) report that adjustment depends upon the effectiveness and completeness of the mourning process over these losses. If such mourning does not occur, problematic behavior may be observed in the form of hostile dependent or depressive-withdrawn attitudes, demanding behavior, temper tantrums, refusal to cooperate, various diffuse somatic complaints, emotional lability, irritability, hypersensitivity, anorexia, insomnia, and night terrors. Many of these difficulties focus around the issue of pain, and it is this pain that may represent a strategy to negotiate dependency needs rather than a physical complaint. An example of such a situation is the following (Steiner & Clark, 1977):

> M. P. a 25-year-old man with a 30% body surface area burn second and third degree had an IQ of 83, a history of a passive-dependent personality and habitual excessive drinking. In his third post-burn week he became increasingly uncooperative and demanding. He complained of pain despite adequate analgesia, to the point that he would not let anyone near him for dressing changes or debridement. The staff reacted angrily to his conduct, which in turn led to a perpetuation and increase in his complaints and demands. In a series of brief interviews the

*motivation for his conduct was elucidated. He had a very exaggerated view of the nature of his injury, expecting it would render him a cripple for life and unable to support himself or his family. He feared discharge and the subsequent demands of his family. (p. 138)*

Stage III, or the stage of *social emergency*, extends from the time of discharge through the first post-burn year. Discharge typically is associated with anxieties about some issues faced initially in Stage II. During this period, the patient must undergo a "desensitization" in which he must learn to cope with the curiosity and even hostility of those individuals he interacts with. Psychological problems during this stage usually include depression and a "posttraumatic neurosis" or a syndrome characterized by many of the same symptoms described in Stage II. The following excerpt from Steiner and Clark (1977) presents a patient in Stage III:

*A. F. a 50-year-old divorced man, returned for a follow-up visit six months after his 40% body surface area burn, which had left him with hands severely scarred and stiff. He had complaints of restlessness, insomnia, anorexia, tearfulness, preoccupation with his injury, feelings of worthlessness, and uselessness. After discharge, he had moved in with his daughter and her husband in hopes that he would be able to take care of repair work that needed doing around the house. When it became clear that he was unable to do any of these things to his satisfaction, he became increasingly depressed. His depression persisted despite the fact that his daughter and her husband remained very supportive and accepting of him and sought to alleviate his distress in many ways. The patient also developed rather poor judgment in his social interactions in that he began a one sided love affair with a nurse significantly younger than he and entertained plans to marry her in spite of the fact that she did not encourage this. On reviewing his case it turned out that he had indeed been a very "good patient, quiet and cooperative." He never asked any questions about the details or the implications of his illness and had not shown any of the symptoms associated with grieving during his hospitalization. (p. 139)*

It is important to indicate that this particular series of stages represents psychological complications of burned adults, not normal psychological coping. Steiner and Clark distinguish between an individual's adaptive response to trauma, acute grief, or mourning, on the one hand, and the individual's maladaptive response or the psychological complications, as discussed above, on the other. This work also represents a more psychodynamic conceptualization of coping and maladapative coping. Acute grief is here considered an adaptive response, given that some of the losses burn patients experience represent considerable changes in health, well-being, sense of vulnerability, and separation from family. The burn patient must also respond to the loss of attractiveness, lovability, various body parts, and an acute loss of a protective skin, which often leads to feelings of losing one's body boundaries. As argued by Steiner and Clark, these losses must be mourned.

This acute grief and mourning has a self-limited course, with a duration of 3 to 6 months and is characterized by three clinically distinct stages, according to Engel (1961). In the initial stage immediately following the injury, the patient is in a state of shock and disbelief. So-called primitive defenses, such as denial and projection, are used to avoid facing reality and losses. The questions the patient has at this stage relate to survival and physiological function. The second stage of uncomplicated grief begins with an awareness of the magnitude of the loss. There is a transition from denial to recognition, which develops in a series of approximations until a total understanding of reality is achieved. Clinically, at this stage, the patient increases his focus of attention and information-seeking behavior as a way of coping with anxiety. At this point, the mourning process proper begins and continues in spite of brief periods of "regression" and depressive symptoms. The final stage of acute grief occurs where the patient accepts his losses emotionally, comes to grip with reality, and returns to the best possible level of functioning. This three-stage coping process or grief response represents a classical psychodynamic perspective and is presented here to highlight this common view of coping. When such a grief response does not occur, as discussed earlier, multiple psychological complications are common. This position is quite different from more recent views of coping in which denial is considered a legitimate, functional, coping strategy. The reader may wish to contrast this view with more recent conceptualizations of coping as discussed in this chapter and Chapter 5.

Steiner and Clark (1977) report on 35 patients. Interestingly, 65% of these patients reported psychiatric or psychological complications significant enough to interfere with treatment and to warrant psychiatric consultation. No complications were reported in the remaining 12 patients. Psychiatric or psychological complications operationalized here as maladaptive coping were found to be associated with age, degree of body surface area burned, and premorbid psychiatric diagnosis. All these factors were associated in a positive direction. That is, older individuals, those with greater burn surface area, and those with a premorbid psychiatric diagnosis experience significant complications following burn. Clinical impressions reported by these authors suggest that the "good patient" who had not gone through the normal grief reaction during hospitalization adjusted poorly in the long run. Also, patients who had a history of difficulty handling stress (i.e., premorbid psychiatric diagnosis) repeated their maladaptive response to the burn stressor. If one looks carefully at the various stages reported, the three stages do closely approximate the three stages hypothesized in the general adaptation syndrome proposed by Selye (1956). A cognitive behavioral approach to assist in the management of burns is discussed in the next chapter.

## SEARCH FOR PSYCHOBIOLOGICAL MECHANISMS: AUTONOMIC NERVOUS SYSTEM ACTIVITY

As we consider the various models linking stress to illness, the autonomic nervous system is regularly hypothesized as playing a major role in the transduction from stressor exposure to illness. There is research that suggests that sympathetic nervous system changes are associated with both acute (infectious) and chronic diseases. Typically, the research has focused on the influence of psychosocial stressors on susceptibility to *chronic* disease, although recent research has been conducted on the *acute* infectious diseases as well. In this section, the role of the autonomic nervous system in both chronic and acute illness will be illustrated, using diabetes mellitus as the example of chronic illness and acute infectious episodes (cough, sore throat, cold, or flu) as examples of acute illness.

Diabetes mellitus is a complex metabolic illness representing a major health problem for up to 5% of the American population. The disorder is associated with premature death, blindness, kidney failure, premature cardiovascular disease, and gangrene of the lower extremities. Diabetes mellitus is characterized by *chronic* hyperglycemia (high blood glucose [sugar] concentration). Individuals with diabetes mellitus do not secrete enough insulin (the substance that regulates glucose metabolism), which allows glucose to accumulate in the blood. Unable to metabolize glucose, the cells metabolize glycogen, fat, and protein. Weight loss and dehydration occur, leading to either hyperosmolar coma or to ketoacidosis and death. Diabetes mellitus is of two types: *Insulin-dependent diabetes* (IDDM or Type I) and *Noninsulin-dependent diabetes* (NIDDM or Type II). Basically in Type I diabetes, the beta cells of the pancreatic islets of Langerhans secrete little or no insulin, and the patient must have daily insulin injections. In the Type II form, considerable beta cell function is intact, although increased resistance to insulin places an increased demand on the insulin-secretory capacity of the system in individuals who cannot release sufficient insulin to meet these demands. How does stress and sympathetic nervous activity influence these forms of diabetes?

Surwit, Feinglos, and Scovern (1983) and Surwit and Feinglos (1984) have reviewed the role of stress in diabetes. These investigators provide a simplified schematic diagram of the major effects of the sympathetic nervous system (SNS) on glucose metabolism (Figure 6-8). The specific role of the sympathetic nervous system is described in the authors' terms (Surwit & Feinglos, 1984) below:

> The autonomic nervous system is intimately involved in the regulation of carbohydrate metabolism. The effects of the autonomic nervous system on insulin action are both facilitatory and inhibitory. Branches of the right vagus nerve innervate the pancreatic islets, and stimulation of the right vagus causes increased insulin secretion. Stimulation of pancreatic islet cell beta adrenergic receptors also facilitates insulin secretion. Conversely, insulin secretion is inhibited by stimulation of the sympathetic nerves of the pan-

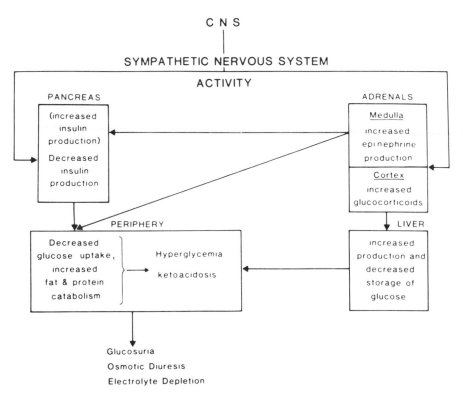

**FIGURE 6-8.** Effects of the sympathetic nervous system on glucose metabolism. The diagram oversimplifies the process involved to provide a general overview of how behavioral manipulation of the SNS can influence glucose metabolism in the normal and in the diabetic individual. Note that the important contributions of the hypothalamic-pituitary axis and the parasympathetic nervous system have been omitted for the sake of simplicity. (CNS = central nervous system.) From "Stress and Diabetes" by R. S. Surwit and M. N. Feinglos, 1984, *Behavioral Medicine Update, 6*(1), 9. Copyright 1983 by the American Psychological Association. Reprinted by permission.

creas through the activation of alpha adrenergic receptors. This sympathetic and parasympathetic innervation of the pancreas may modulate insulin secretion in the normal regulation of carbohydrate metabolism.

The autonomic nervous system has additional metabolic effects. Beta adrenergic stimulation facilitates the conversion of glycogen to glucose in the liver as well as fat to free fatty acids in adipose tissue. (Free fatty acids are further metabolized to ketoacids in the liver.) Neurogenic stimulation of the hypothalamic-pituitary axis leads to the secretion of cortisol from the adrenal cortex, which elevates blood glucose and impairs glucose tolerance. Low-dose exogenous epinephrine infusions (to levels comparable to those achieved in minor stress) can also adversely affect glucose tolerance. Thus, the autonomic nervous system, particularly the sympathetic branch, has both direct *neural* as well as indirect *hormonal* control pathways in the regulation of glucose metabolism. Yet, although the role of the sympathetic nervous system in the body's response to acute hypoglycemia has been known for years, the importance of sympathetic nervous system activity in normal glucose metabolism is only beginning to be appreciated. (p. 8)

Surwit and Feinglos (1984) review the experimental evidence regarding stress in the development or expression of diabetes in animal and human studies. The animal literature can be characterized along two dimensions: research on the effects of laboratory stressors on blood glucose and the interaction of stress and other risk factors in the development of Type II diabetes using animal models. The former type of research suggests that exposure to a repeated restraint stress results in permanent diabetes in a large percentage of pancreatectomized rats (Capponi, Kawada, Varela, & Vargas, 1980). Huang, Plout, Taylor, and Wareheim (1981), however, reported that light shock could inhibit the development of streptozotocin-induced diabetes in young mice. This latter finding is consistent with other research indicating that the administration of exogenous steroids *inhibits* the development of another streptozotocin-induced model of diabetes (Roudier, Portha, & Picon, 1980). Surwit and Feinglos (1984) suggest that these findings indicate a potential *protective* effect of shock on the development of diabetes in animals treated with a single dose of streptozotocin and that such an effect may be mediated through the adrenocorticotropic effects of stress. These studies also illustrate the complex nature of the impact of stress in the development of diabetes in susceptible animals. Animal research has also addressed the impact of stress on existent diabetes (i.e., exacerbation of diabetes).

In a series of well-designed, well-conceptualized studies, Surwit and colleagues have investigated the role of stress in the expression of diabetes in the *ob/ob* mouse, an animal model of Type II diabetes (Surwit, Feinglos, Livingston, Kuhn, & McCubbin, 1984). Essentially, 24 obese mice and their littermates were housed in cages, with 4 to 6 animals per cage. Half the animals were immobilized for 60 minutes;

during the final 30 minutes, they were shaken moderately for five minutes (stressor condition). At 60 minutes, blood was drawn. The control animals (both obese and lean) were caged until the blood samples were obtained. The stressor increased plasma glucose in both the lean and obese animals, although the increase was significantly greater in the obese animals. A similar pattern was observed for plasma insulin; insulin decreased in all animals exposed to the stressor, although the decrease was greater in the obese animals. When Surwit and his colleagues conducted a similar experiment using epinephrine in place of the environmental stress (in an effort to test the effects of drug-induced increased sympathetic arousal on serum glucose and insulin), similar results were obtained. Epinephrine increased plasma glucose in all subjects, with the obese animals showing a greater response. Plasma insulin decreased in the obese animals only. Similar effects were not observed for saline injections.

Surwit *et al.* (1984) noted that the basal (resting) blood glucose values were not consistently elevated in the obese as compared to the lean mice, although severe hyperglycemia was noted in obese mice during exposure to the environmental stressor or following the administration of exogenous epinephrine. These findings indicate that the obesity itself was not associated with tonic-heightened levels of blood glucose, but that the obesity was associated with greater glucose *reactivity* to stress.

Early investigations in humans suggested a heightened response of blood glucose and ketones to stress in diabetic patients (e.g., Hinkle, Evans, & Wolf, 1951). This early work, however, was poorly controlled and represented the anecdotal approach commonly used in psychosomatic medicine in the 1940s to 1950s. Findings in humans are contradictory at present. A controlled evaluation of the effects of induced stress on subjects, the majority with insulin-dependent diabetes, indicated a *decrease* in blood glucose (Vanderbergh, Sussman, & Titus, 1966). Although these findings were replicated (Vanderbergh, Sussman, & Vaughan, 1967), other investigators have observed a hyperglycemic response in insulin-dependent and noninsulin-dependent diabetic patients during surgery, as compared to controls (McLesky, Lewis, & Woodruff, 1978). In a study on the effects of epinephrine on blood glucose and ketone release, Baker Barcai, Kaye, and Hague (1969) observed significant elevations in both measures in diabetic children, compared to controls. Of considerable interest is the finding that acute beta-adrenergic blockade with propranolol *prevented* exogenous epinephrine and experimental stress-induced hyperglycemia in diabetic children (Baker, Minuchin, Milman *et al.*, 1975). The experimental findings, as a whole, suggest a glucose overreactivity to stress in diabetics. If these findings are reliable, the implications of such an overreactivity in the daily management of diabetes are considerable. Exposure to stressors could further offset glucose metabolism, potentially exacerbating the complications of the disorder. These findings suggest the potential importance of stress reduction techniques in the management of diabetes.

Shifting from chronic illness to acute infectious illness, Gruchow (1979) studied the relationship of catecholamine activity and reported symptomatic infectious disease episodes in a group of 47 volunteer university students (24 male, 23 female). The major question addressed in this research was whether variations in the activity of hormones associated with the stress response (catecholamine activity) could be linked with episodes of infectious disease. In this prospective analysis, urine specimens were obtained for 28 days, and diaries of daily symptoms were kept (list of 10 health status items to elicit reporting of acute respiratory symptoms). The specific measure of catecholamine activity was vanillylmandelic acid (VMA), rather than free catecholamines, because of its relative stability as a measure of catecholamine activity. The lag in excretion resulting from metabolic breakdown reduces the potential short-term increases that can occur with other measures of catecholamines. Given that the intent of the research was to identify daily dynamic fluctuations, the VMA titer was thought to be an appropriate measure despite the fact that with such VMA measurements it is impossible to differentiate sympathetic nervous system activity from adrenal medullary activity. (See Chapters 4 and 5 for further details.)

During the four-week study period, 34 respondents (17 males, 17 females) reported cold or flu symptoms at least one day (the average was 5.5 days on which symptoms were reported). An *illness episode* was operationally defined as two or more consecutive days of reported respiratory symptoms occurring at a minimum of three days following onset and preceding the cessation of the monitoring period. Seventeen subjects (10 males, 7 females) met these criteria; this represented a total of 19 illness episodes. The results indicated a characteristic *pattern* of variation in VMA values, which coincided with the onset of reported symptoms in 13 of the 19 (68%) episodes. The pattern that emerged was one in which VMA values peaked three days *before* the onset of symptoms. The question arises whether such a peak also occurred in controls. Subjects who reported illness episodes had the highest frequency of VMA spikes on days 3 and 2 before symptom onset and the lowest frequency on the day after onset. This pattern was *not* observed in the control group. Also, the extent of variation in relative frequency of VMA spikes from day to day was greater in the cases reporting illness episodes than in the controls, which illustrated greater variability in the illness group. These findings are consistent with the hypothesis that susceptibility to disease may be enhanced by fluctuating sympathetic-adrenal medullary activity.

This increased catecholamine activity, as reflected in higher VMA levels, may reduce immune response and thus increase susceptibility to infectious disease agents. The immune system, however, is quite complex. Stressors can both inhibit and facilitate various components of the immune system. Also, it is unclear whether psychosocial stressors were linked to spikes in VMA activity or whether the VMA spike preceded or followed invasion by the infectious agent. Nevertheless, this study illustrates the potential role of catecholamine activity in infectious disease episodes. The prospective nature of the study also adds to the validity of the findings. We will now shift to methods used to influence or manage the stress response, including the presumed activation of the sympathetic nervous system.

## SUMMARY

Stress is commonly assumed to play a role in the etiology, exacerbation, and maintenance of several health problems. In this chapter we have reviewed the possible relationship between stress and health. Stress as a precursor to illness was first considered in a review of the major theories of the role stress plays in the development of illness. Theories that illustrated diverse perspectives rather than one theoretical orientation were emphasized. Exacerbation of symptoms was next discussed, and a model was proposed by the authors to illustrate the complexities the health psychologist is faced with when considering a fluctuating biological system. The results from the air traffic controller health change study, discussed in Chapter 3, were presented to illustrate the point that our hypotheses regarding stress and illness and associated biological mechanisms are often not as consistently supported as one would assume. The modulating role of personality in the stress–illness association was also discussed.

Stress can indirectly influence health outcome, and such an association was illustrated using burn accidents in children following a move in residence. The response to illness also represents a variant of the stress–illness relationship. Often the illnesses and their associated treatments represent a set of stressors that the individual must cope with. The concept of coping is a major area in health psychology research and treatment. Therefore, much of this chapter dealt with the coping concept, using "coping with the stress of illness" as a model problem to highlight issues regarding adaptation to stress, transactional models of stress, cognitive coping mechanisms and cognitive appraisal processes, anticipatory coping, functions of coping, coping and development, and cognitive adaptation. Certain of these theoretical and laboratory- or research-based phenomena were then illustrated, using such clinical problems as breast cancer and severe burns.

The final section of the chapter emphasized psychobiological mechanisms hypothesized to play a role in stress-mediated illness. Diabetes mellitus and acute infectious disease were used to illustrate the potential role of autonomic nervous system activity in the transduction process. Although we emphasized that there are no simple answers to the complex relationship between stress and health/illness, research on several fronts in health psychology is providing significant knowledge toward answering some of the major questions in this important health area.

## REFERENCES

Alloy, L. B., Abramson, L. Y., & Viscusi, D. (1981). Induced mood and the elusion of control. *Journal of Personality and Social Psychology, 41*, 1129–1140.

Baker, L., Barcai, A., Kay, R., & Hague, N. (1969). Beta adrenergic blockade and juvenile diabetes: Acute studies and long-term therapeutic trial. Evidence for the role of catecholamines in mediating diabetic decompensation following emotional arousal. *Journal of Pediatrics, 75*(1), 19–29.

Baker, L., Minuchin, S., Milman, L. *et al.* (1975). Psychosomatic aspects of juvenile diabetes mellitus: A progress report. *Modern Problems in Pediatrics, 12*, 332–343.

Baker, L., Minuchin, S., Milman, L., Liebman, R., & Todd, T. (1975). Psychosomatic aspects of juvenile diabetes mellitus: A progress report. In Z. Lawon (Ed.), *Diabetes in juveniles: Medical and rehabilitation aspects: Vol. 12. Modern problems in pediatrics.* New York: Karger.

Barr, R. G., & Feuerstein, M. (1983). Recurrent abdominal pain syndrome. How appropriate are our basic clinical assumptions? In P. McGrath & P. Firestone (Eds.), *Pediatric and adolescent behavioral medicine.* New York: Springer.

Capponi, R., Kawada, M. E., Varela, C., & Vargas, L. (1980). Diabetes mellitus by repeated stress in rats bearing chemical diabetes. *Hormone Metabolism Research, 12*, 411–412.

Cohen, F., & Lazarus, R. S. (1979). Coping with the stresses of illness. In G. C. Stone, F. Cohen, & N. E. Adler (Eds.), *Health psychology.* San Francisco: Jossey-Bass.

Davis, F. (1963). *Passage through crisis.* Indianapolis, IN: Bobbs-Merrill.

Engel, G. L. (1961). Is grief a disease? *Psychosomatic Medicine, 23*, 18–22.

Feuerstein, M., & Gainer, J. (1982). Chronic headache: Mechanism and management. In D. M. Doleys, R. L. Meredith, & A. R. Ciminero (Eds.), *Behavioral medicine: Assessment and treatment strategies.* New York: Plenum Press.

Feuerstein, M., Barr, R. G., Francoeur, T. E., Houle, M. M., & Rafman, S. (1982). Potential biobehavioral mechanisms of recurrent abdominal pain in children. *Pain, 13*, 287–298.

Feuerstein, M., Bush, C., & Corbisiero, R. (1982). Stress and chronic headache: A psychophysiological analysis of mechanisms. *Journal of Psychosomatic Research, 26*(2), 167–182.

Folkman, S. (1984). Personal control and stress and coping processes: A theoretical analysis. *Journal of Personality and Social Psychology, 46*(4), 839–852.

Folkman, S., & Lazarus, R. S. (1980). An analysis of coping in a middle-aged community sample. *Journal of Health and Social Behavior, 21*, 219–239.

Folkman, S., Schaeffer, C., & Lazarus, R. S. (1979). Cognitive processes as mediators of stress and coping. In V. Hamilton & D. M. Warburton (Eds.), *Human stress and cognition: An information processing approach*. London: Wiley.

Greenwald, A. G. (1980). The totalitarian ego: Fabrication and revision of personal history. *American Psychologist, 35*, 603–618.

Gruchow, W. H. (1979). Catecholamine activity and infectious disease episodes. *Journal of Human Stress, 5*(3), 11–17.

Henryk-Gutt, R., & Rees, W. L. (1973). Psychological aspects of migraine. *Journal of Psychosomatic Research, 17*, 141–153.

Hinkle, L. E., Jr., Evans, F. M., & Wolf, S. (1951). Studies in diabetes mellitus III: Life history of three persons with labile diabetes, and the relation of significant experiences in their lives to the onset and course of their disease. *Psychosomatic Medicine, 13*, 160–202.

Huang, S. W., Plout, S. W., Taylor, G., & Wareheim, B. A. (1981). Effect of stressful stimulation on the incidence of streptozotocin-induced diabetes in mice. *Psychosomatic Medicine, 43*, 431–437.

Katz, J. L., Weiner, H., Gallagher, T. F., & Hellman, L. (1970). Stress, distress and ego defenses. Psychoendocrine response to impending breast tumor biopsy. *Archives of General Psychiatry, 23*, 131–142.

Knudson-Cooper, M. S., & Leuchtag, A. K. (1982). The stress of a family move as a precipitating factor in children's burn accidents. *Journal of Human Stress, 8*, 32–38.

Kobasa, S. C., Hilker, R. R. J., & Maddi, S. R. (1979). Who stays healthy under stress? *Journal of Occupational Medicine, 21*(9), 595–598.

Lazarus, R. S. (1974). A strategy for research of psychological and social factors in hypertension. *Journal of Human Stress, 4*, 35–40.

Lazarus, R. S. (1983). The costs and benefits of denial. In S. Breznitz (Ed.), *Denial of stress*. New York: International Universities Press.

Lazarus, R. S., & Cohen, J. (1977). Environmental stress. In I. Altman & J. Wohlwill (Eds.), *Human behavior and environment* (Vol. 2). New York: Plenum Press.

Lazarus, R. S., & Launier, R. (1978). Stress-related transactions between person and environment. In L. A. Pervin & M. Lewis (Eds.), *Perspectives in interactional psychology*. New York: Plenum Press.

Levi, L. (1972). Introduction: Psychosocial stimuli, psychophysiological reactions, and disease. In L. Levi (Ed.), *Stress and distress in response to psychosocial stimuli*. Oxford: Pergamon Press.

Lewinsohn, P. M., Mischel, W., Chaplin, W., & Barton, R. (1980). Social competence and depression: The role of illusory self-perceptions. *Journal of Abnormal Psychology, 89*(2), 203–212.

Lipowski, Z. J. (1970). Physical illness, the individual and the coping process. *Psychiatry in Medicine, 1*, 91–102.

Manchester Guardian. (1977). Excess stress in women—hairy chests and lust. London.

McLesky, C. H., Lewis, S. B., & Woodruff, R. E. (1978). Glucogen levels during anesthesia and surgery in normal and diabetic patients. *Diabetes, 27*(S2), 492.

Minuchin, S., Baker, L., Rosman, B. L., Liebman, R., Milman, L., & Todd, T. C. (1975). A conceptual model of psychosomatic illness in children: Family organization and family therapy. *Archives of General Psychiatry, 32*(8), 1031–1038.

Moos, R. H., & Tsu-Davis, V. (1977). The crisis of physical illness: An overview. In R. H. Moss (Eds.), *Coping with physical illness* (pp. 3–21). New York: Plenum Press.

Rahe, R. H., & Arthur, R. J. (1978). Life change and illness studies: Past history and future directions. *Journal of Human Stress, 4*(1), 3–15.

Rose, R. M., Jenkins, C. D., & Hurst, M. W. (1978). Health change in air traffic controllers:

A prospective study. I. Background and description. *Psychosomatic Medicine, 40*(2), 142–165.

Rose, R. M., Jenkins, C. D., Hurst, M., Herd, J. A., & Hall, R. P. (1982). Endocrine activity in air traffic controllers at work. II. Biological, psychological, and work correlates. *Psychoneuroendocrinology, 7,* 113–123.

Rose, R. M., Jenkins, C. D., Hurst, M., Kreger, B. E., Barrett, J., & Hall, R. P. (1982). Endocrine activity in air traffic controllers at work. II. Relationship to physical and psychiatric morbidity. *Psychoneuroendocrinology, 7,* 125–134.

Rose, R. M., Jenkins, C. D., Hurst, M. W., Livingston, L., & Hall, R. P. (1982). Endocrine activity in air traffic controllers at work. I. Characterization of cortisol and growth hormone levels during the day. *Psychoneuroendocrinology, 7,* 101–111.

Roudier, M., Portha, B., & Picon, L. (1980). Glucocorticoid-induced recovery from strep- tozotocin diabetes in the adult rat. *Diabetes, 29*(3), 201–205.

Schwartz, G. E. (1977). Psychosomatic disorders and biofeedback: A psychobiological model of disregulation. In J. D. Maser & M. E. P. Seligman (Eds.), *Psychopathology: Experimental models.* San Francisco: W. H. Freeman.

Schwartz, G. E. (1978). Psychobiological foundations of psychotherapy and behavior change. In S. L. Garfield & A. E. Bergin (Eds.), *Handbook of psychotherapy and behavior change: An empirical analysis* (2nd ed.). New York: Wiley.

Steiner, H., & Clark, W. R. Jr. (1977). Psychiatric complications of burned adults: A classification. *The Journal of Trauma, 17*(2), 134–143.

Surwit, R. S., & Feinglos, M. N. (1984). Relaxation induced improvement in glucose tolerance is associated with decreased plasma cortisol. *Diabetes Care, 7*(2), 203–204.

Surwit, R. S., Feinglos, M. N., Livingston, E. G., Kuhn, C. M., & McCubbin, J. A. (1984). Behavioral manipulation of the diabetic phenotype in ob/ob mice. *Diabetes, 33,* 616– 618.

Surwit, R. S., Feinglos, M. N., & Scovern, A. W. (1983). Diabetes and behavior: A para- digm for health psychology. *American Psychologist, 38*(3), 255–262.

Taylor, S. E. (1983). Adjustment to threatening events: A theory of cognitive adaptation. *American Psychologist, 38,* 1161–1173.

Vanderbergh, R., Sussman, K. E., & Titus, C. (1966). Effects of hypnotically induced acute emotional stress on carbohydrate and lipid metabolism in patients with diabetes mellitus. *Psychosomatic Medicine, 28,* 382–390.

Vanderbergh, R., Sussman, K. E., & Vaughn, G. D. (1967). Effects of combined physical– anticipatory stress on carbohydrate–lipid metabolism in patients with diabetes mellitus. *Psychosomatics, 8*(1), 16–19.

Wong, P. T. P., & Weiner, B. (1981). When people ask "why" questions, and the heuristics of attributional search. *Journal of Personality and Social Psychology, 40,* 650–663.

# STRESS MANAGEMENT

In recent years, much effort has been devoted to the application of methods in clinical psychology to reduce the impact of stress. These techniques have evolved from a diverse set of theoretical frameworks, ranging from principles of Eastern philosophy to learning principles that form the foundation of behavioral psychotherapy. In this chapter, various stress-management techniques will be reviewed. The chapter first focuses on a description of several techniques and then gives examples of their application to the prevention and treatment of stress-related health problems.

## TECHNIQUES FOR STRESS MANAGEMENT

Given the rise in incidence of stress-related disorders in our modern society, the development of strategies to reduce stress has become of primary importance to many of today's health care providers.

An individual's stress response may be viewed as his or her attempts at cognitive, behavioral, and physiological adjustment to major environmental demands, for example, life in highly overpopulated areas, job pressures, and organismic demands (e.g., physical illness). As pointed out in Chapters 5 and 6, the person's perception and interpretation of these stimuli are crucial to how he or she responds to stress. Conceptually, the reduction of stress is comprised of three basic elements: (1) physical alteration of environmental stressors, for example, relocating factories to an industrial zone; opting out of the rat race in the case of an executive promoted beyond the level of his or her competence; (2) modification of a person's cognitive attributions, for example, refocusing thought or reinterpreting situations as less problematic; and (3) alteration of behavioral and physiological responsivity, for example, the use of various relaxation techniques or pharmacological methods. The next section will describe a variety of stress-management procedures used to reduce the impact of stress.

### Progressive Relaxation Training

Historically, progressive relaxation training, as it is known today, originated in the late 1920s with the work of Edmund Jacobson who, at that time, was conducting research on the knee jerk reflex in the Department of Physiology at the University of Chicago. Jacobson discovered, while engaged in clinical practice, that the amplitude of the knee jerk reflected the degree of tension a patient was experiencing. As the patient learned to relax, the amplitude of his or her knee jerk tended to decrease.

In his attempt to find more sophisticated and sensitive methods of measuring and quantifying muscle tension levels, Jacobson invented the integrating neurovoltmeter, which could measure action potentials from muscle groups and from nerves at levels as low as a microvolt. Jacobson's research led him to the conclusion that if an individual is to experience a sense of relaxation in mind and body, he or she must relax a multiplicity of the interacting systems of the body. Jacobson suggested that by teaching a person to relax the skeletal musculature directly, a decrease in central nervous system (CNS) arousal, as well as a decrease in autonomic nervous system (ANS) arousal, would follow.

Jacobson (1978) proposed that the main mechanisms influencing relaxation effects lie with the patient's ability to perceive the differences between tension and relaxation. Each time a muscle contracts, the receptors within the muscle are activated. In turn, these activated receptors produce a series of neural impulses that are transmitted to the brain along afferent neural fibers. Tension may be viewed as the result of this generation and conductance of afferent neural impulses. When muscle contraction occurs, neural impulses are transmitted to the brain and instigate complex CNS activity. Subsequently, neural impulses return to the muscles along efferent neural fibers and produce further muscle contraction. As a result, additional neural impulses are directed to and from the brain along numerous neuromuscular circuits throughout the body. By teaching the patient to recognize excessive contraction of the skeletal muscles, one is then able to teach the patient how to relax specific muscle groups to relieve tension.

The specific physiological effects of progressive muscular relaxation training are less understood than the effects of certain other stress reduction techniques (i.e., the Benson relaxation response). The research on progressive muscular relaxation however, suggests that the technique is associated with reductions in the electromyogram (EMG), which measures muscle activity; the heart rate; the respiratory rate; and possibly, skin conductance. Unfortunately, the specificity of these changes is currently unclear, since in several studies the effects of the technique were not studied in a control group requested to sit quietly for a sufficient length of time. Also, some reviews have indicated approximately equivalent changes for relaxation technique groups and controls (Borkovec & Sides, 1979). This is surprising, given that relaxation training can be considered the "aspirin" of the clinical health psychologist. It is perhaps one of the most commonly used techniques in clinical work with patients experiencing stress-related health problems.

The lack of consistent physiological changes may relate to the types of measures used in the various studies. Very few studies, if any, employed systematic biochemical measures of the stress response. These measures, which were discussed in Chapters 4 and 5, may reflect more accurately the psychobiological mechanisms of stress reduction.

Progressive muscular relaxation involves the successive tensing and relaxing of various muscle groups. Throughout training, the patient typically sits or reclines in a comfortable chair in a quiet, dimly lit room with closed eyes. In order to enhance the relaxation effect, the therapist speaks in a slow and quiet tone of voice and usually has the patient successively tense and relax the following muscle groups: hands and forearms, upper arms (biceps), wrists, forehead, eyes, mouth, neck, shoulders, chest, stomach, buttocks, thighs, calves, and feet. Table 7-1 lists the methods of tensing particular muscle groups. The patient repeats the procedure twice for each muscle group. The therapist may explain to the patient that it is not necessary to obtain the maximum muscle tension possible. Also, it is up to the therapist to determine the rate at which the patient should relieve muscle tension, that is, suddenly "letting go" versus gradually relaxing the muscle. The progressive relaxation method should be tailored to the needs of each individual patient, with one to two practice sessions per day. Often therapists suggest the

TABLE 7-1
Brief Instructions for Progressive Muscular Relaxation

| Muscle group | Method of Tensing |
|---|---|
| 1. Dominant hand and forearm | Make a tight fist while allowing upper arm to remain relaxed. |
| 2. Dominant upper arm | Press elbow downward against chair without involving lower arm. |
| 3. Nondominant hand and forearm | Same as dominant. |
| 4. Nondominant upper arm | Same as dominant. |
| 5. Forehead | Raise eyebrows as high as possible. |
| 6. Upper cheeks and nose | Squint eyes and wrinkle nose. |
| 7. Lower face | Clench teeth and pull back corners of the mouth. |
| 8. Neck | Counterpose muscles by trying to raise and lower chin simultaneously. |
| 9. Chest, shoulders, and upper back | Take a deep breath; hold it and pull shoulder blades together. |
| 10. Abdomen | Counterpose muscles by trying to push stomach out and pull it simultaneously. |
| 11. Dominant upper leg | Counterpose large muscle on top of leg against two smaller ones underneath (specific strategy will vary considerably). |
| 12. Dominant calf | Point toes toward head. |
| 13. Dominant foot | Point toes downward, turn foot in, and curl toes gently. |
| 14. Nondominant upper leg | Same as dominant. |
| 15. Nondominant calf | Same as dominant. |
| 16. Nondominant foot | Same as dominant. |

Note. From "Progressive Relaxation: Abbreviated Methods" by D. A. Bernstein and B. A. Given in *Principles and Practice of Stress Management* (p. 51) edited by R. L. Woolfolk and P. M. Miller. Copyright 1984 by Guilford Press, Inc. Reprinted by permission.

use of audiotapes of the therapist reviewing the relaxation procedure, particularly in the initial phases of therapy.

## The Relaxation Response

Most individuals at some time in their lives have experienced or will experience a nonpharmacological, self-induced altered state of consciousness. Individuals experiencing one of these states have reported feelings of increased creativity and "inner peace." Despite the long-standing recognition of the existence of such a phenomenon in Eastern cultures, it is only in the last 30 years or so that the Western world has witnessed a growing interest in the physiological changes and possible health benefits of the relaxation-associated properties underlying these altered states of consciousness. First identified by Hess (1957) and termed the *trophotropic response*, it was later to be described by Benson (1975) as the *relaxation response*. Stimulation of anterior areas of the hypothalamus apparently elicit the relaxation response whereas its counterpart—the fight-or-flight reaction—can be elicited by stimulation of posterior areas of the hypothalamus. The relaxation response, according to Benson, is mediated by the parasympathetic nervous system and electrical stimulation of the anterior hypothalamus results in hypo- or adynamia of skeletal musculature, decreased blood pressure, decreased respiratory rate, and constricted pupils. Benson noted that these physiological changes are consistent with a generalized decrease in sympathetic activity and are distinctly different from the physiological changes recorded during quiet sitting or sleep.

Elicitation of the relaxation response requires four basic elements:

1. *Mental device*—presence of a constant stimulus such as a sound, word, or phrase repeated silently or audibly, or fixed gazing at an object. The purpose of these procedures is to reduce a person's distractibility.
2. *Passive attitude*—if distracting thoughts do occur during the above procedure, they should be disregarded and attention should be redirected to the technique. One should not worry about how well he or she is performing the technique.
3. *Decreased muscle tonus*—the individual should be in a comfortable posture so that minimal muscular work is required.
4. *Quiet environment*—a quiet environment with decreased environmental stimuli should be used. The individual is usually instructed to close his or her eyes.

The effects of the relaxation response on reducing autonomic functions and sympathetic responsivity have been well documented in the scientific literature (Bradley & McCanne, 1981; Hoffman, Benson, Arns, Stainbrook, Landsberg, Young, & Gill, 1982; Morse, Martin, Furst, & Dubin, 1977; Walrath & Hamilton, 1975). An example of such effects can be drawn from the work of Benson, Dryer, and Hartley (1978). These authors found decreased oxygen consumption (measure of metabolism) in four males and four females who had been taught to elicit the relaxation response while working at a fixed work intensity, compared to their oxygen consumption before eliciting the relaxation response under the same conditions.

## Meditation Procedures

*Yogic Therapy.* The yogic method of meditation was first developed as a self-help system of health care and spiritual development forming an integral part of an ancient Indian culture. The term *yoga* means union or oneness with life. The practice of yoga has been central to the maintenance of health in Eastern cultures for thousands of years. Although the precise origins of yoga are unclear, engraving of yoga postures dating back to 3000 B.C. have been found.

Typically, the yogic method of meditation may consist of a sequence of postures called *asanas*, whereby a person is able to gain substantial control over individual muscles and body movements resulting in a general sense of suppleness and relief from musculoskeletal symptoms. Physiologically, the principles of yoga aim at the reduction of sympathetic arousal through activating a hypometabolic response and eliciting the relaxation response. Five steps need to be taken in order to achieve this effect:

1. The patient is taught to discriminate between appropriate and inappropriate responses to specific situations in everyday life and made aware of how his or her perceptions of these situations influences the intensity of the response.
2. The patient is taught a simple rhythmic, diaphragmatic breathing exercise to induce physical and mental calmness.
3. The patient is next instructed in progressive deep-muscle relaxation to reduce the sympathetic responsiveness of the hypothalamus.
4. After several sessions of breathing exercise and deep-muscle relaxation, the patient is instructed in how to relax mentally. The main goal for the patient here is to learn how to relax mentally by passively concentrating on a visual image and eventually meditating.
5. The final step is to help the patient integrate the relaxation response into daily activities. Specific situations that evoke the stress response in a patient's life are identified and the patient is encouraged to practice the relaxation response in those situations.

## Recent Modifications of Meditation

The more recent forms of meditation have attempted to simplify this technique of stress reduction and to free it from some of its cultic associations. Transcendental meditation (TM) is the most popular of Westernized forms of meditation. However, the TM method has not been widely used in clinical settings because it still adheres to certain cultic traditions.

Currently, the two most commonly used clinically oriented meditation techniques have been "clinically standardized meditation" (CSM)

(Carrington, 1978) and "respiratory one method" (ROM) (Benson, 1975). Both these techniques are essentially noncultic and meant to be used in clinical practice. Some basic differences between the two methods need to be highlighted, however.

In learning CSM, the individual is free to select a sound from a standard list of sounds or to create one according to directions. This sound is then repeated mentally by the person in an effortless manner, without any attempt at structure and without intentionally linking the sound to the breathing pattern. On the other hand, ROM requires the individual to repeat to himself or herself mentally a word (e.g., "ore," "out") while linking this word with each exhalation. The latter technique, therefore, differs from CSM in terms of being relatively more structured and requiring more discipline.

The commonly held assumption that meditation produces a state of profound rest has produced a proliferation of research demonstrating the effects of simplified meditation techniques on physiological arousal (e.g., Wallace, Benson, & Wilson, 1971). Despite this abundance of studies, a recent review by Holmes (1984) of the research literature on the effects of meditation on somatic arousal reduction shows that there is no conclusive evidence to show that meditation is more effective in reducing somatic arousal than is simple rest. A comparison of somatic arousal of asymptomatic meditating subjects with somatic arousal of asymptomatic resting subjects did not indicate any consistent differences between meditating and resting subjects on measures of heart rate, electrodermal activity, respiration rate, systolic blood pressure, diastolic blood pressure, skin temperature, electromuscular activity, blood flow, or various biochemical factors. Similarly, Holmes (1984), in his review of the literature on the effects of meditation in controlling arousal in threatening situations, did not find any consistent differences between meditating and nonmeditating (no-treatment, antimeditation, or relaxation) subjects. The implication of these findings, based on the experimental evidence available, is that the personal or professional use of meditation as an antidote for high somatic arousal does not seem to be justified. Further controlled comparative studies are needed to validate the effectiveness of meditation as a useful stress management technique.

## Hypnosis

The use of hypnotic induction procedures in medical settings may be traced back to the modern origin of "animal magnetism" in the work of the Viennese physician Franz Anton Mesmer (1734–1815). The early use of hypnosis emphasized its possibilities as an analgesic. An English surgeon, James Endaile, for instance, while working in India during the years 1845 to 1851, reported using hypnosis as an analgesic in approximately 1,000 operations, 300 of which were major. Since that time, hypnosis has become a relatively accepted form of treatment in both medicine and clinical psychology.

Suggestibility is considered to be a critical factor in mediating the effects of hypnosis. The two have been equated by Barber (1974) and his collaborators who argue that individuals, when given direct suggestions without a hypnotic induction, display behavior similar to that of subjects given a formal induction. Another conceptualization of hypnosis has been offered by Fromm (1977) and Hilgard (1968) who view this phenomenon as an altered state of consciousness.

According to Barber (1984), hypnotic induction procedures typically consist of suggestions for deep relaxation and are intended to enhance responsiveness to subsequent suggestions. Once the preliminary hypnotic induction is completed, two additional types of suggestions are often made. These include suggestions for limb heaviness, hand numbness, age regression, and posthypnotic behavior and indirect and direct therapeutic suggestions, as in the case of losing weight or stopping smoking. A typical example of suggestions for deep relaxation or for use in modern hypnotic inductions may run as follows (Barber, 1984):

> Close your eyes and take a deep breath. As you breathe out slowly, you feel all the tensions leaving. Letting go of tensions, worries, frustrations, and becoming more and more calm, at ease, deeply relaxed. Floating on a soft, cushiony cloud (or lying on a pleasant beach, feeling the warm sand and the sun) . . . more and more comfortable, tranquil, serene, relaxed. . . . Breathing slowly and gently. Thoughts slowing down. . . . Time slowing down, lots of time, so much time. . . . Mind and body slowing down. Arms relaxing, legs relaxing, face relaxing, body and mind relaxing. Warm and comfortable. . . . At peace, calm, more and more relaxed and drowsy . . . moving slowly, calmly down (an escalator) and becoming more and more deeply relaxed. . . . Peaceful, quiet, drifting, floating, deeper and deeper relaxed.

Barber (1984) offers several reasons for the need for suggestions for deep relaxation: (1) They define the situation as "hypnosis" and may enhance the patient's positive expectancy about hypnosis. (2) The suggestions are easy, so that most subjects can "pass" them. (3) They can help reduce critical and analytical thinking so that the patient is less concerned about time, place, and person. (4) Suggestions for deep relaxation can change the situation from a formal, reality-oriented one to one in which fantasy and primary processes take over. (5) Suggestions for deep relaxation can help the patient in thinking through solutions to life problems. (6) Deep relaxation suggestions let the patient mentally rehearse the carrying out of tasks and performance, which can be accomplished most effectively when the individual is calm instead of tense. (7) Suggestions for deep relaxation can produce a high degree of tranquility, which allows the person to mentally rehearse overcoming such addictions as smoking or overeating. Finally, (8) deep relaxation suggestions enhance the state of deep relaxation, which is useful for overcoming such stress-related disorders as migraine headache, asthma, skin rashes, insomnia, and mild hypertension. No clear evidence has as yet emerged for the superiority of hypnosis over other relaxation procedures (Morse *et al.*, 1977; Shapiro, 1980).

## Biofeedback

Biofeedback represents a technological advance in the treatment of stress-related disorders. Several theoretical frameworks have been derived from a variety of experimental approaches to explain the mechanisms of biofeedback: operant conditioning (Black, Cott, & Pavoski, 1977); complex skills learning (Lang, 1977); discrimination of internal bodily responses and processes (Brener, 1977); "mediation" of physiological responses and control through somatomotor and cognitive change (Katkin & Murray, 1968); cybernetic formulations derived from electrical engineering and control systems theory (Anliker, 1977; Mulholland, 1977); and psychobiological patterning models (Schwartz, 1977).

Blanchard and Epstein (1978) have defined biofeedback as: "a process in which a person learns to reliably influence physiologial responses of two kinds; either responses which are not under voluntary control or responses which are ordinarily easily regulated but for which regulation has broken down due to trauma or disease" (p. 2).

Three basic operations are involved in the biofeedback process. First, detection and amplification of a biological response must occur. Second, some form of signal processing of the response is necessary. And third, there must be immediate feedback or information regarding the status of the response. Once the person generates a response it is detected, amplified, processed, and fedback as new input. The individual can then observe this new input and use it to modify the physiological response. Feedback is usually by visual or auditory signals, which reflect minute changes in the physiologial response. Typically, the patient attempts to influence the signals in order to change the physiological response in the desired direction. This usually involves a trial-and-error strategy with guidance by a technician. Figure 7-1 illustrates the components of the biofeedback process. As indicated, the biofeedback instrumentation converts a complex signal typically beyond the conscious awareness of the patient (weak complex signal) into a

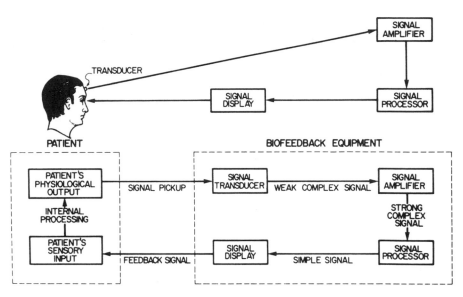

**FIGURE 7-1.** Components of a biofeedback system. From "Scientific Foundations of Bio-feedback Therapy" by K. R. Gaarder and P. S. Montgomery in *Clinical Biofeedback: A Procedural Manual* (p. 24) edited by K. R. Gaarder and P. S. Montgomery. Copyright 1977 by Williams & Wilkins Co. Reprinted by permission.

simple signal that can be more easily processed by the patient. An example of such a feedback system is the case in which a patient with a paraspinal lumbar muscle spasm and associated pain receives auditory feedback in the form of a continuously fluctuating tone that reflects the continuous change in skeletal muscle activity in the lower back region. As minute changes in muscle tension occur, the pitch of the feedback tone increases. Patients are instructed to modify the muscle tension while receiving such biological feedback. The goal is to assist the patient in learning skeletal muscle self-regulation so he or she will ultimately be able to reduce or increase skeletal muscle activity as necessary. It is frequently assumed that this regulation assists certain patients with pain reduction (i.e., those patients in which there is a link between skeletal muscle tension and pain). The goal of such training, therefore, is to increase the patient's ability to control biological systems that have been functioning maladaptively and that may have been beyond conscious control.

Budzynski (1973) lists the three stages involved in biofeedback training as (1) *awareness* of the response so that biofeedback training teaches the patient how certain thoughts as well as certain bodily events influence the particular response, (2) *control* of the response using the biofeedback signal, and (3) *transfer* of the control into everyday life situations (i.e., generalization). The major physiological response systems for which biofeedback has been employed include heart rate (HR), galvanic skin resistance (GSR), skin conductance (SC), blood pressure (BP), muscle activity (via the EMG), finger temperature (FT), and brain-wave activity (via the EEG). Table 7-2 lists the type of feedback procedures employed for specific disorders.

## Autogenic Biofeedback

"Autogenic training," developed in Germany at the turn of the century, focuses on the gradual acquisition of autonomic control (Schultz & Luthe, 1969) through a "system of psychosomatic self-regulation." Rather than utilizing active control strategies, the patient engages in a type of "passive concentration." Although the intention is to achieve certain effects, such as relaxation, the patient remains detached as to his or her actual progress. Throughout training, the patient's attention is focused on visual, auditory, and somatic imagery, which is employed to induce such specific physiological changes as hand warmth or muscle relaxation. Autogenic training in combination with biofeedback training, which relies on a conscious control of physiological parameters by the patient, comprises *autogenic biofeedback training* (Green, Green, Walters, Sargent, & Meyer, 1975) (see Figure 7-2).

Since the emphasis in autogenic biofeedback training is on self-regulation, the patient is expected to assume and/or maintain responsibility for his or her stress response, healing process, and state of wellness. This approach requires the patient to participate actively in the treatment process, and the therapist should convey all relevant information about the patient's condition (blood tests, X-ray results, etc.) to the patient, with the goal of increasing the patient's self-awareness. Only verbal feedback is typically given during the first autogenic biofeedback experience to reduce the possibility of performance anxiety induced at this stage by direct instrument feedback. At the end of the first session, the therapist and the patient discuss the experience and homework assignments, which should be practiced daily between therapy sessions.

## Cognitive-Behavioral Approaches

One of the major cognitive-behavioral approaches to stress reduction has been stress-inoculation (SI) training. Stress-inoculation training was originally developed and described by Meichenbaum and Cameron (1983) as a self-instructional method for teaching individuals to cope with stress. Stress-inoculation procedures may be conceptualized as a

**TABLE 7-2**
Biofeedback Applications

| Disorder | Biofeedback procedure |
| --- | --- |
| Anxiety | Frontal EMG biofeedback |
| Asthma | Frontal EMG biofeedback |
| Bruxism | Masseter EMG biofeedback |
| Cardiac neurosis | HR biofeedback (+ gradual hierarchy presentation) |
| Eczematous dermatitis | Hand temperature biofeedback (+ relaxation training) |
| Essential blepharospasm | Electrooculogram biofeedback (+ massed practice and contingent shock)[a] |
| Essential hypertension | Forearm & frontalis EMG biofeedback (+ autogenic training) |
| | GSR biofeedback (+ meditation-relaxation training) |
| | Diastolic BP biofeedback |
| | Systolic BP biofeedback |
| Fecal incontinence | External sphincter pressure biofeedback |
| Functional diarrhea | Bowel sounds biofeedback |
| Heart rhythm and rate disturbance | HR biofeedback |
| Insomnia | Theta EEG biofeedback[a] |
| Migraine headache | Temperature (absolute) biofeedback |
| | Temperature (differential) biofeedback |
| | Temporal artery vasomotor biofeedback |
| | Alpha EEG biofeedback |
| Muscle retraining to increase activity | EMG biofeedback (+ physical therapy) |
| Muscle retraining to decrease activity | EMG biofeedback |
| Obsessive ruminations | Alpha EEG biofeedback[a] |
| Outpatient psychiatric | Alpha EEG biofeedback[a] |
| | GSR biofeedback |
| Penile tumesescence | Erection biofeedback (+ contingent aversive sound)[a] |
| Raynaud's disease | Temperature (absolute) biofeedback (following relaxation training and autogenic imagery) |
| | Temperature (differential) biofeedback |
| | Vasomotor biofeedback |
| Seizure disorders | Alpha EEG biofeedback[a] |
| | Sensorimotor rhythm EEG biofeedback |
| Stuttering | GSR biofeedback |
| Tension headache | Alpha EEG biofeedback[a] |
| | Frontalis EMG biofeedback |
| Vaginismus | Contraction pressure biofeedback |
| Writer's cramp | EMG biofeedback |

Note. From "Biofeedback: Clinical and Research Considerations" by F. Andrasik, D. Coleman, and L. Epstein in *Behavioral Medicine: Assessment and Treatment Strategies* (p. 85) edited by D. M. Doleys, R. L. Meredith, and A. R. Ciminero. Copyright 1982 by Plenum Press. Reprinted by permission.
[a]Rarely used in common clinical practice.

Trainee's Initials _____     Date _____

Initial Temperature_____

Meter Reading (at the
start of each phrase)                        Phrases

| left | right | Phrases |
|------|-------|---------|
| | | 1. I feel quite quiet. |
| | | 2. I am beginning to feel quite relaxed. |
| | | 3. My feet feel heavy and relaxed. |
| | | 4. My ankles, my knees, and my hips feel heavy, relaxed, and comfortable. |
| | | 5. My solar plexus, and the whole central portion of my body, feel relaxed and quiet. |
| | | 6. My hands, my arms, and my shoulders feel heavy, relaxed, and comfortable. |
| | | 7. My neck, my jaws, and my forehead feel relaxed. They feel comfortable and smooth. |
| | | 8. My whole body feels quiet, heavy, comfortable, and relaxed. |
| | | 9. Continue alone for a minute. |
| | | 10. I am quite relaxed. |
| | | 11. My arms and hands are heavy and warm. |
| | | 12. I feel quite quiet. |
| | | 13. My whole body is relaxed and my hands are warm, relaxed and warm. |
| | | 14. My hands are warm. |
| | | 15. Warmth is flowing into my hands; they are warm, warm. |
| | | 16. I can feel the warmth flowing down my arms into my hands. |
| | | 17. My hands are warm, relaxed and warm. |
| | | 18. Continue alone for a minute. |
| | | 19. My whole body feels quiet, comfortable, and relaxed. |
| | | 20. My mind is quiet. |
| | | 21. I withdraw my thoughts from the surroundings, and I feel serene and still. |
| | | 22. My thoughts are turned inward, and I am at ease. |
| | | 23. Deep within my mind I can visualize and experience myself as relaxed, comfortable, and still. |
| | | 24. I am alert, but in an easy, quiet, inward-turned way. |
| | | 25. My mind is calm and quiet. |
| | | 26. I feel an inward quietness. |
| | | 27. Continue alone for a minute. |
| | | 28. The relaxation and reverie is now concluded, and the whole body is reactivated with a deep breath and the following phrases: "I feel life and energy flowing through my legs, hips, solar plexus, chest, arms and hands, neck and head . . . The energy makes me feel light and alive." Stretch. |

Final Temperature _____

FIGURE 7-2. Representative monitoring form for autogenic biofeedback training. From "Autogenic Biofeedback in Psychophysiological Therapy and Stress Management" by N. A. Norris and S. L. Fahrion in *Principles and Practices of Stress Management* (p. 236) edited by R. L. Woolfolk and P. M. Lehrer. Copyright 1984 by Guilford Press, Inc. Reprinted by permission.

form of coping-skills therapy. These procedures are basically concerned with developing the individual's competence to adapt to stressful events in such a way as to enable the individual to alleviate his or her stress and achieve personal goals. The therapeutic process involves discussing with the patient the nature of the perceived emotion and stress reaction, rehearsing coping self-statements and relaxation skills, and testing those skills under actual stress conditions. The SI approach, therefore, generally involves three basic phases: *cognitive preparation, skill acquisition,* and *application practice.* The paradigm for SI procedure may be described by means of a flowchart as presented in Table 7-3.

A number of variables play a role in the maintenance of generalization of induced changes following SI training. Dunbar (1980) has suggested that therapists may be more effective if they are seen as approachable. This means that the therapist engages in behaviors that put the patient at ease and allow for open expression of concerns. An example of behaviors that may enhance perceived approachability include the therapist's warmth, empathy, general friendliness, and spontaneity. Other variables that may affect responses to treatment include the patient's expectations. If a patient has unrealistically positive initial expectations that are disconfirmed during the course of therapy, this may be demoralizing. Helping the patient achieve small changes that build progressively toward the final objective can enhance his or her sense of progress and morale.

Finally, the inclusion of other family members in the patient's treatment has been shown by several authors to enhance patient involvement (Baekeland & Lundwill, 1975; Cobb, 1979). One can see that a variety of important factors may positively influence patient involvement in the treatment process and have an impact on treatment outcome.

An example of how SI training may be applied to a specific problem area relevant to the stress–illness link is clearly seen in the work of Novaco (1975) on anger management. Using the SI paradigm, the patient is typically taught, during the cognitive preparation phase, the functions of anger, and his or her personal anger patterns are discussed. During the skill acquisition phase, the patient is provided with cognitive and behavioral coping skills. In terms of cognitive skills, the patient is taught to view provocation events alternatively (Kelly, 1955) and to modify the importance he or she often attaches to the events (Ellis, 1973). In terms of behavioral coping skills, behavioral interventions aim at providing the patient with skills that are incompatible with anger to increase competence in interpersonal communication and to solve problems. Relaxation techniques form the basic behavioral component of the treatment procedure and are used as a counter-conditioning procedure

**TABLE 7-3**

Flowchart of Stress-Inoculation Training

Phase One: Conceptualization
(a) Data collection–integration
   • Identify determinants of problem via interview, image-based reconstruction, self-monitoring, and behavioral observance.
   • Distinguish between performance failure and skill deficit.
   • Formulate treatment plan—task analysis.
   • Introduce integrative conceptual model.
(b) Assessment skills training
   • Train clients to analyze problems independently (e.g., to conduct situational analyses and to seek disconfirmatory data).
Phase Two: Skills Acquisition and Rehearsal
(a) Skills training
   • Training instrumental coping skills (e.g., communication, assertion, problem solving, parenting, study skills).
   • Train palliative coping skills as indicated (e.g., perspective-taking, attention diversion, use of social supports, adaptive affect expression, relaxation).
   • Aim to develop an extensive repertoire of coping responses to faciliate flexible responding.
(b) Skills Rehearsal
   • Promote smooth integration and execution of coping responses via imagery and role play.
   • Self-instructional training to develop mediators to regulate coping responses.
Phase Three: Application and Follow-Through
(a) Induce application of skills
   • Prepare for application using coping imagery, using early stress cues as signals to cope.
   • Role play (a) anticipated stressful situations and (b) client coaching someone with a similar problem.
   • "Role play" attitude may be adopted in real world.
   • Exposure to in-session graded stressors.
   • Use of graded exposure and other response induction aids to foster *in vivo* responding and build self-efficacy.
(b) Maintenance and generalization
   • Build sense of coping self-efficacy in relation to situations client sees as high risk.
   • Develop strategies for recovering from failure and relapse.
   • Arrange follow-up reviews.
General Guidelines for Training
   • Attend to referral and intake process.
   • Consider training peers of clients to conduct treatment. Develop collaborative relationship and project approachability.
   • Establish realistic expectations regarding course and outcome of therapy.
   • Foster optimism and confidence by structuring incremental success experiences.
   • Respond to stalled progress with problem solving versus labeling client resistant.
   • Include family members in treatment when this is indicated.

against the physiological arousal associated with anger-eliciting situations. Anger-management self-statements rehearsed in SI training are presented in Table 7-4. Finally, during the application practice phase of treatment, the patient is allowed to practice his or her proficiency in anger-control methods through imaginal and role-playing inductions of anger.

Novaco (1975) demonstrated the usefulness of SI training on anger control in a study in which he trained 34 volunteers who had problems controlling anger to resist responding angrily to provocation. The patients were first told that anger reactions consisted of a series of states involving cognitive processes and arousal. Next, they were taught muscle-relaxation exercises and adaptive self-statements for each stage—preparing for provocation, impact, and confrontation; coping with arousal; and reflecting on outcome. Finally, the patients rehearsed coping with provocation by imagining provoking situations that were hierarchically graded from least to most provoking. The results of the study

TABLE 7-4
Self-Statements in Anger Management

Preparing for a provocation
    This could be a rough situation, but I know how to deal with it. I can work out a
    plan to handle this. Easy does it. Remember, stick to the issues and don't take it
    personally. There won't be any need for an argument. I know what to do.
Impact and confrontation
    As long as I keep my cool, I'm in control of the situation. You don't need to prove
    yourself. Don't make more out of this than you have to. There is no point in getting
    mad. Think of what you have to do. Look for the positives and don't jump to
    conclusions.
Coping with arousal
    Muscles are getting tight. Relax and slow things down. Time to take a deep breath.
    Let's take the issue point by point. My anger is a signal of what I need to do. Time
    for problem solving. He probably wants me to get angry, but I'm going to deal with
    it constructively.
Subsequent reflection
(a) Conflict unresolved
    Forget about the aggravation. Thinking about it only makes you upset. Try to shake
    it off. Don't let it interfere with your job. Remember relaxation. It's a lot better than
    anger. Don't take it personally. It's probably not so serious.
(b) Conflict resolved
    I handled that one pretty well. That's doing a good job. I could have gotten more
    upset than it was worth. My pride can get me into trouble, but I'm doing better at
    this all the time.
    I actually got through that without getting angry.

Note. From "Anger and Coping with Stress" by R. W. Novaco in Cognitive Behavior Therapy (p. 150) edited by J. P. Foreyt and D. P. Rathjen. Copyright 1978 by Plenum Press. Reprinted by permission.

indicated that the training program had a positive effect in reducing the patients' self-report of and physiological indices of anger.

An example of the application of the anger management technique is illustrated by the following case seen by the authors:

> M.C., a 44-year-old white, single female business executive, presented with multiple somatic symptoms, including chest pain, tachycardia, sleep disturbance, general restlessness and irritability. Following evaluation, it was determined that the major stressors were related to her job situation and difficulties in interaction with her mother and father who required much attention because of their deteriorating physical condition. In terms of job-related problems, M.C. indicated that although she was in a position of authority, she found it difficult to delegate responsibility because of the "incompetence" of her staff. This resulted in M.C. completing most of the jobs herself, with considerable feelings of anger toward her staff. A similar situation existed with regard to her parents; her brother took no responsibility in handling parental care problems and thus left M.C. with "excessive family demands." Both the job and the family situation triggered multiple episodes of anger outbursts, resulting in significant management problems at work and considerable distress among family members. Treatment was directed at teaching the patient more appropriate ways of dealing with these anger-provoking situations. The techniques to achieve this goal included relaxation training, self-monitoring of anger-provoking situations, and the behavioral, physiological, and cognitive reactions to such situations, and identifying and role-playing alternative ways of responding to such situations. This latter goal was partly achieved by helping the patient conceptualize the anger situation along the stages proposed by Novaco (preparing for provocation, impact, and confrontation; coping with arousal; and reflecting on outcome). The patient was able to utilize the specific strategies taught and displayed considerable ability at more direct communication in both the work and the family environments. Symptoms were successfully eliminated and treatment gains were maintained at 1-year follow-up.

## Pharmacological Treatment

Clinicians commonly agree that psychopharmacological intervention can play a useful role in the management of the stress response. Its greatest utility, perhaps, has been considered to be the way it relieves the acute symptoms of excessive stress that interfere with other forms of therapy. Table 7-5 lists the antianxiety drugs available today.

The popularity of a major group of antianxiety drugs, the benzodiazepines, is evident from the rapid rise in consumption of these drugs. Diazepam (Valium) was the most frequently prescribed drug in the United States by 1972, and chlordiarepoxide (Librium), its close analogue, was the third most often prescribed drug. Prescriptions for benzodiazepines are primarily written by nonpsychiatrists—typically family physicians, orthopedists, gynecologists, general practitioners, and pedi-

TABLE 7-5
Drugs Used in the Management of Anxiety

| Generic name | Trade name | Usual dose range (mg/day) |
| --- | --- | --- |
| Barbiturates | | |
| Phenobarbital | Luminal | 30–120 |
| Amobarbital | Amytal | 100–200 |
| Secobarbital | Seconal | 100–200 |
| Propanediols | | |
| Meprobamate | Miltown | 800–2000 |
| | Equanil | 800–2000 |
| Tybamate | Tybatran | 750–2800 |
| Antihistamines | | |
| Hydroxyzine | Vistaril | 75–400 |
| Diphenhydramine | Benadryl | 75–300 |
| Benzodiazepines | | |
| Chlordiazepoxide | Librium | 15–100 |
| Diazepam | Valium | 5–40 |
| Oxazepam | Serax | 30–120 |
| Clorazepate | Tranxene | 15–60 |
| Prazepam | Centrax | 20–60 |
| Lorazepam | Ativan | 1–60 |
| Tricyclic antidepressants | | |
| Doxepin | Sinequan | 75–225 |
| | Adapin | 75–225 |
| Amitriptyline | Elavil | 75–225 |
| β-Adrenoceptor antagonists | | |
| Propranolol | Inderal | 30–240 |

*Note.* From "Pharmacological Methods" by M. Lader in *Principles and Practice of Stress Management* (p. 311) edited by R. L. Woolfolk and P. M. Lehrer. Copyright 1984 by Guilford Press, Inc. Reprinted by permission.

atricians. In a review of benzodiazepine usage by nonpsychiatric practice, Lasagna (1977) found that tranquilization was the major desired action.

In a cross-national study of benzodiazepine usage, Balter, Levine, and Manheimer (1973) found that in the United States and the United Kingdom, approximately 14% of the adult population reported tranquilizer use at some time during the year before the survey. Belgium and France were found to have higher than average usage, whereas Holland and Spain had lower than average. Sex differences were also noted, with usage among females about twice that among males, increasing with age for females but not with males. Also, usage in females was higher in the lower social classes.

The basic mode of action of the benzodiazepines is a potentiation of the activity of the neurotransmitter γ-aminobutyric acid (GABA). This neurotransmitter is active at several types of synapses and is thought to decrease neuronal activity through an inhibitory process, both presynaptically and postsynaptically. Four main sites for the action of the benzodiazepines have been identified: (1) the spinal cord, where presynaptic and postsynaptic inhibition produce muscle relaxation; (2) the brainstem, which is thought to account for the anticonvulsant effect of most benzodiazepines; (3) the cerebellum, which may mediate the common side effects (ataxia) of high doses of benzodiazepines; and (4) the limbic and cortical areas, specifically those associated with emotional integration and response (benzodiazepines may inhibit arousal systems from the reticular formation to the limbic and cortical areas).

In contrast to barbiturates, Lader (1984) points out several advantages in the use of benzodiazepines in the symptomatic treatment of anxiety and stress-related conditions: (1) drowsiness and psychological impairment is less with benzodiazepines than with barbiturates when given in effective antianxiety doses; (2) benzodiazepines tend to be safer in overdosage than barbiturates; (3) the risk of dependence is less with benzodiazepines than with barbiturates; and finally (4) metabolic interactions with other drugs are relatively infrequent with benzodiazepines as compared to the barbiturates.

Lader (1984) also discussed the potential adverse effects of the benzodiazepines. These may include drowsiness, torpor, excessive weight gain, skin rash, impairment of sexual function, menstrual irregularities, and (rarely) blood abnormalities. Such respiratory problems as chronic bronchitis and emphysema may be exacerbated by benzodiazepines, which can cause respiratory depression. Gaind and Jacoby (1978) have also reported on the paradoxical reactions to benzodiazepine. These may include such uncharacteristic criminal activities as shop-lifting and sexual offenses (self-exposure) and excessive emotional responses, including uncontrollable giggling or weeping. Further, as with most depressant drugs, the effects of alcohol can be significantly potentiated. Prescribing such antianxiety agents as benzodiazepines, therefore, requires that the clinician and the patient ultimately must decide as to whether the benefits of antianxiety medication outweigh the risks of dependence or the creation of a medical issue out of a basically interpersonal or environmental problem.

Another group of drugs with secondary sedative properties are the tricylic antidepressants amitriptyline, doxepin, and mianserin. These drugs are primarily prescribed for depressed patients who show secondary signs of anxiety and agitation, and they are not appropriate for the treatment of primary anxiety states. The monoamine oxidase inhibitors, used to treat atypical depressives, are generally felt to be of little value in the management of stress response, although some patients with phobic anxiety have been found to respond well to full doses of phenelzine or tranylcypromine.

There has been recent interest in another major class of antianxiety agents, the β-adrenoceptor antagonists (beta-blockers). Their central mode of action is to block overactivity of the β-adrenergic sympathetic neurons. The palpitations, tremor, and gastrointestinal problems (e.g., diarrhea) often associated with anxiety states may be viewed as a consequence of the overactivity of these neurons. Some physicians have found it helpful to use such beta-blockers as propranolol in the treatment of those patients whose anxiety and psychophysiological arousal are primarily manifested by these peripheral autonomic symptoms. Since the primary operative mechanism of beta-blockers is assumed to be peripheral rather than central, symptoms associated with anxiety and stress arousal will be reduced without alteration of consciousness. A good example of the type of patients who may benefit from beta-blocker intervention are stage performers who need to maintain clarity of mental functioning while alleviating the primary symptoms (e.g., diarrhea, palpitations) resulting from transient stress reactions. The use of beta-blockers is contraindicated in patients with a history of asthma or heart disease.

The effects of beta-blockers on the stress response have been studied using a variety of naturally occurring stressors. Some examples include race car driving, ski jumping, dental surgery, venipuncture, civil unrest, exam stress, public speaking, stress interviews, and stage fright. In general, these studies indicated that beta-blockers reduced tachycardia during exposure to the stressor without associated sedative effects (Frishman, Razin, Swencionis, & Sonnenblick, 1981). An oral dose of oxprenolol given to race car drivers one-hour before a race was associated with reduction of tachycardia and a lowering of plasma-free fatty acid and blood glucose levels, which were elevated in the same drivers when beta-blockers were not used (Frishman et al., 1981). This finding illustrates the effect of the beta-blockers on the phasic component of the stress response. In addition, it suggests that the effect is quite general in that it influences multiple biochemical components of the stress response. It is of interest that beta-blockade has also been observed to enhance performance on a verbal learning task in males over 60 years old (Eisdorfer, Nowlin, & Wilkes, 1970). This latter finding suggests that reducing autonomic arousal by beta-blockade affects the behavioral component of the stress response. In light of the curvilinear relationship between arousal and performance, as discussed in Chapter 4, intervention by beta-blockade may represent a useful technique for reducing sympathetic arousal and improving performance.

The therapist, in prescribing antianxiety medication, must consider the choice of drug, dosage schedules, duration of therapy, drug discontinuation, response to treatment, and finally, predictors of response.

## Exercise

Ryan (1974) has noted that the earliest use of exercise in a therapeutic capacity was in the fifth century B.C., when gymnastics were prescribed for various diseases by the Greek physician Herodicus. Three centuries later, Anchepiades prescribed walking and running in conjunction with diet and massage for diseases as well as for the ills of an "opulent" society. Following World War I, therapeutic exercise increased in the United States and it is currently practiced by millions of people.

Although exercise, in some ways, represents an intense form of the stress reaction, it differs significantly from the stress response implicated in the onset of chronic disease. Three therapeutic mechanisms of action may be identified in the clinical effectiveness of exercise: (1) mechanisms that are active during exercise; (2) mechanisms that are active in the short term following exercise; and (3) mechanisms that are active over the long term.

In the acute process of exercising, serum triglycerides (a fat implicated in the development of arteriosclerosis and coronary heart disease) (Haskall & Fox, 1974), which are released into the bloodstream during the stress response, have been found to decline. Further, resistance to blood flow to the skin and other peripheral areas increases during the stress response. However, in the context of stress from physical activity, resistance to blood flow in the skin actually decreases, cooling the body and lowering blood pressure (Bar-Or & Buskirk, 1974).

Exercise also activates short-term mechanisms that are beneficial in counteracting the stress response. DeVries (1966) speculated that since the gamma motor neural discharge may be inhibited during recovery from physical activity and since the gamma motor system is the major neural connection from the cerebral cortex to the striate musculature, the result of such inhibition is, therefore, striate-muscle relaxation.

A sustained exercise program has been found to produce desirable long-term physiological alterations, which, in turn, increase the fitness level across those systems of the body that usually experience most strain during the stress response. Wilmore (1977) has summarized these alterations as (1) increased efficiency of the heart; (2) improved pulmonary function; (3) improved utilization of blood glucose; (4) reduced body fat; and (5) reduced resting blood pressure.

Physiologically, the most beneficial type of exercise is aerobic. Exercise that increases the endurance of the pulmonary and cardiovascular systems is typically referred to as *aerobic*. Exercise that elevates the heart rate to at least 70% of maximum (about 140 beats per minute) for a minimum of five minutes increases aerobic capacity (i.e., the maximum amount of oxygen the body can process within a given time). Several forms of physical activity that have been found useful in increasing aerobic capacity include jogging, swimming, cycling, rowing, playing handball, and cross-country skiing.

Evidence for the beneficial effects of aerobic exercise and fitness is gradually accumulating in the research literature. Aerobically trained individuals, for instance, may be distinguished from their untrained counterparts on a number of cardiovascular and biochemical indices of adaptation, both at rest and during physical activity. Trained subjects, for example, have lower heart rate and greater stroke volume (Shepard, 1977), lower plasma glucose and insulin levels (Leblanc, Boulay, Dulac, Jobin, LaBrie, & Rousseau-Mogneron, 1977), and higher testosterone levels (Young & Ismail, 1978) at rest. When worked to the point of exhaustion, trained individuals also appear to have higher oxygen up-take values. When aerobically trained individuals were compared to untrained individuals on responses to a standard work load, the trained individuals had less of an increase in heart rate, coupled with a more rapid return to baseline following work termination (Clausen, 1977); less of an increase of norepinephrine (Peronnet, Cleroux, Perrault, Cousineau, de Champlain, & Nadeau, 1981) and cortisol (White, Ismail, & Bottoms, 1976); and finally, less accumulation and faster elimination of lactic acid from the bloodstream (Winder, Hickson, Hagberg, Ehsani, & McLane, 1979). These findings, as a whole, indicate that aerobic exercise influences resting levels, phasic response, and recovery from physical stress.

There is evidence of a differential reactivity to psychosocial stress among aerobically trained versus untrained asymptomatic individuals (Sinyor, Schwartz, Peronnet, Brisson, & Seraganian, 1983). Sinyor *et al.* monitored the cardiovascular, biochemical, and subjective indices of subjects who were highly trained aerobically or untrained. On exposure to a series of psychosocial stressors the heart rate and subjective measures of arousal increased indistinguishably in both groups. However, following termination of exposure to the stressors, *recovery* was more rapid in the trained group. Additionally, blood samples taken before, during, and after stressor exposure revealed that the trained subjects had *higher* levels of prolactin and attained peak levels of norepinephrine more rapidly.

Aerobic exercise has further been shown to have certain beneficial effects in alleviating anxiety and depression (Doyne, Chambless, & Beutler, 1983; Folkins & Sime, 1981; Ledwidge, 1980). Ledwidge (1980), for example, provides both a psychological and physiological rationale for the role of exercise in the treatment of depression. According to Ledwedge, fitness training may benefit the depressed individual, because the sense of accomplishment that is derived from improving one's body may generalize to a feeling that one is not helpless and that what one does indeed makes a difference. Physiologically, Ledwidge argues, exercise increases norepinephrine production, assumed to be low in certain depressed patients. Chronic fatigue, a common complaint of depressed patients, may be relieved through exercise. However, a review by Hughes (1984) of controlled studies on the effects of habitual aerobic exercise on mood, personality, and cognitive ability indicates a positive effect for self-concept, but little evidence for anxiety and depression reduction. There was only minimal support for enhanced body image, change in personality factors, and improved cognitive abilities (e.g., memory, confusion). These conclusions should be placed in perspective, given the limited number of controlled studies completed at present ($N = 12$). A number of questions regarding the effects of aerobic exercise remain unanswered. For example, What types of clinical problems are more responsive to aerobic intervention? What individual difference factors predict positive response to exercise? What psychobiological changes underlie the beneficial effects of exercise? and If regular aerobic exercise is a helpful stress reduction approach, how can this behavior be incorporated into the individual's life-style?

## GENERAL CONSIDERATIONS IN STRESS MANAGEMENT

In this section, we will discuss the proposed treatment effects of the various stress-management strategies along with the hypothesized mediators of these effects. A framework for evaluating the various stress-management approaches is also provided to help the reader appraise this significant area of clinical and research activity in health psychology. Various clinical issues regarding the use of stress management techniques will also be discussed.

Borkovec *et al.* (1984) identified a number of potential effects of various stress-management strategies. These effects include (1) reduced tension during the day and creation of a pleasant affective state; (2)

reduced anxiety response in anticipation of stressors; (3) reduced anxiety response during stressor exposure; and (4) more rapid recovery from stress events. As discussed in Chapter 5, each of these possible effects is related to various components of the stress response (i.e., cognitive, behavioral, and physiological). In addition to modifying the general stress response, the stress-management procedures should also have an effect on the presenting symptom. For example, in the case of asthma, a reduction in the frequency and severity of asthmatic attacks, in addition to changes in respiratory function, should be expected to follow stress-managment training if indeed stress is associated with the disorder.

A variety of potential mediators of the effects of stress-management procedures have been proposed (Borkovec *et al.*, 1984). These potential mediators include the ability to (1) increase parasympathetic and decrease sympathetic activity; (2) increase awareness of muscle tension and autonomic activity; (3) increase awareness of cognitive activity and stream of consciousness; (4) increase control of autonomic and cognitive activity; (5) increase control of and attention to internal biological activity; (6) increase concentration (attention focusing) on thoughts, images, physiological activity, affect, and environmental stimuli, with an implied decrease in distractibility; and (7) increase the capacity to shut off internal dialogue. Other investigators have concluded that a common pathway for the effects of various stress-management procedures is the increase in relaxation, which is associated with the decrease in sympathetic activity (Silver & Blanchard, 1978). In a review of various biofeedback and relaxation training approaches, Silver and Blanchard argue that relaxation represents a final common pathway for the treatment of several stress-related disorders. Other investigators (Stoyva & Budzynski, 1974) proposed a similar concept, *cultivated low arousal*. The basis for this hypothesized mechanism is the assumption that various stress-related disorders result from heightened sympathetic arousal and, therefore, reductions in such arousal can reduce symptoms. Gelhorn and Kiely (1972) reported that meditation, progressive relaxation, and autogenic training tend to produce a shift toward decreased sympathetic arousal. Reduction in such measures as heart rate, blood pressure, and muscle activity are often associated with this decreased sympathetic arousal, as discussed in Chapter 5. Certain forms of biofeedback have also been associated with reductions in sympathetic arousal (Silver & Blanchard, 1978). Although the decreased sympathetic arousal hypothesis generally explains the effects of various stress-management procedures in the treatment of certain somatic problems, future research in health psychology may identify more specific psychobiological mechanisms to provide a more sophisticated explanation of the effects of these procedures.

A more critical view of the effects of stress-management procedures on both resting levels of physiological activity and phasic response to stress is provided by Holmes (1984). Specifically, Holmes focused on the effects of one stress-management approach, meditation, and attempted to address the question Do subjects who meditate acutally show lower physiological arousal when they are meditating than do subjects who are simply resting? An additional question addressed by this review was Do subjects who meditate have less of a physiological response to threat or stressors than have subjects who do not? This review addressed questions regarding the effects of one stress-management procedure, meditation, and therefore the reader should be cautioned as to the generalizability of these findings to other stress reduction procedures. In addition, the Holmes' review only focused on research using asymptomatic subjects, that is, subjects not presenting with clinical problems. Lastly, as illustrated in a previously discussed case, clinical intervention typically includes a combination of approaches rather than one technique. The review itself is discussed here to illustrate the complexity of the effects of various stress-management procedures on resting levels of physiological activity and the stress response itself.

As in most studies dealing with the effects of various stress-management procedures on the stress response, Holmes identified such measures of somatic or physiological arousal as including indices of heart rate, electrodermal activity, respiration rate, blood pressure, muscle activity, skin temperature, oxygen consumption, and blood flow. Various biochemical measures of the stress response were also discussed. In a review of approximately 20 experiments, Holmes concluded that there was no measure of arousal on which the meditating subjects were consistently found to have reliably lower arousal than were resting subjects. Interestingly, there were approximately as many studies in which the meditating subjects displayed reliably higher arousal as there were studies in which they displayed reliably lower arousal than their resting counterparts. In addition, within any one experiment, there were no consistent findings to indicate that meditating subjects display reliably lower arousal across physiological measures than resting subjects. Another factor influencing the results of these studies is the sophistication of methodology used. Holmes noted that the level of sophistication in research design varies considerably across studies. The issue of research design in stress management will be discussed in a later section.

Shifting to the effects of meditation of physiological arousal in threatening situations or the effects of meditation on the stress response itself, Holmes concludes, from only four experiments, that there is no evidence to support the hypothesis that experienced meditators can produce or maintain lower levels of physiological arousal in threatening situations, in contrast to nonmeditators. In fact, the experienced meditators were observed to display *higher* levels of various physiological measures in response to stressors than nonmeditating subjects. Although this review illustrates the problems with the decreased sympathetic arousal hypothesis discussed earlier, it should be emphasized that the data reviewed were based upon one technique only, meditation, and its effects on "normal" subjects. Perhaps, more importantly, this review, with its conclusion that peripheral physiological indices, both in terms of levels as well as reactivity, do not change, suggests the need to look at more central mechanisms of change, for example, CNS biochemical markers of stress and stress reduction. Clearly, other reviews specifically looking at the effects of stress-reduction techniques on both peripheral and central physiological mechanisms involved in various physical disturbances would be most helpful in furthering our understanding of the role stress management procedures play in the treatment of somatic disturbance. A number of issues regarding methodology need to be addressed when considering such research.

In a discussion of the evaluation of experimental designs in relaxation research, Borkovec *et al.* (1984) address a number of key factors that should be considered when the relaxation literature is critically viewed. Although their focus was on relaxation research, the present authors believe that such considerations apply to all stress-management procedures. As was discussed in Chapter 3 (Research Methods), many factors can influence the outcome of intervention studies and threats to both internal and external validity must be considered. These threats to internal validity include the past history of the patient, maturation in terms of passage of time, repeated testing and the effect of such testing, measurement error, statistical regression, selection, attrition, interactions with selection, and such possible problems as non-random assignment of subjects.

Of particular concern in clinical stress research is identifying an appropriate measure of outcome or change. Does one record changes in stress response, and if so, should the focus be on behavioral, cognitive, or physiological changes? What is an appropriate way to measure the actual symptoms of clinical patients? And finally, How can a study be designed to address such questions as to whether the treatment has an effect across several different types of patient populations and over long periods of time? All these factors are commonly referred to as the *outcome criterion problem*, which is often more complicated than identifying a single outcome measure. Kazdin and Wilson (1978) have specified a number of aspects of outcome that should be considered in any comprehensive evaluation of a treatment procedure. These aspects include (1) the clinical significance of the change as opposed to the simple statistical significance; (2) the proportion of patients who change rather than the

TABLE 7-6

Checklist for Evaluating Relaxation Strategies

Internal validity and degree of specification of independent variables
—Includes no-treatment condition?
—Uses random assignment?
—Differential attrition?
—Analyses for relevant pretest differences?
—Includes placebo group?
—Credible placebo group?
—Alternative methods controlling for client expectancy?
—Uses component control design?
—Uses parametric design?
—Uses constructive design?
—Uses comparative design?
—More than one therapist?
—Controls for therapist bias?
—Taped or "live" training?
—Sufficient description of technique to judge its faithfulness?
External validity and specification of dependent variables
—Subject sample defined and specified in detail?
—Heterogeneous characteristics (e.g., age, sex, education) sampled?
—Is pretest sensitization a possibility?
—"Clinic"-like or "experiment"-like atmosphere?
—Sequential treatments?
—Multidimensional measurement of problem behavior?
—Variety of aspects of outcome measured?
—Uses auxillary outcome measures?
—Include levels of a relevant subject characteristic?
—Assesses improvement in natural setting?
—Uses detailed practice and application instructions?
—Follow-up data collected?
—Process measures obtained?
Statistical validity
—Stringent statistical tests?
—Sufficiently large sample?
—Equal $n$ per condition or homogeneous variance?
—Limited number of statistical tests or use of multivariate analyses?
—Information reported or demonstrated on stability and reliability of measures?

Note. From "Evaluating Experimental Designs in Relaxation Research" by T. D. Borkovec, M. C. Johnson, and D. L. Block in *Principles and Practice of Stress Management* (pp. 400–401) edited by R. L. Woolfolk and P. M. Lehrer. Copyright 1984 by Guilford Press. Adapted with permission.

group mean comparisons; (3) the breadth of change or the impact of the change on the patient's social, marital, and occupational adjustment; (4) the durability of change; (5) the efficiency, in terms of how therapy is administered and duration of treatment; (6) the cost, in terms of professional expertise of the therapists; (7) the cost to the patient (financial and emotional); (8) the cost-effectiveness of the therapy; and (9) the acceptability of the therapy to the population served.

Borkovec *et al.* (1984) provide a checklist for evaluating relaxation studies, which is presented in modified form in Table 7-6. Again, although Borkovec *et al.* refer to relaxation studies, the present authors assume that these factors can be used to evaluate all forms of stress-management techniques. As Table 7-6 indicates, the checklist is divided into internal validity and the degree of specification of independent variables and external validity and specification of dependent variables. This checklist allows the reader to critically evaluate various forms of stress management.

As indicated in an earlier section of this chapter, stress may be viewed as a precursor to illness as well as a response to or a consequence of illness. The following section will review the various stress-management procedures employed in preventing the potential effects of stress on illness in asymptomatic individuals (stress as precursor), as well as various applications of stress management in reducing stress as a response to illness.

## PREPARATION FOR STRESS AS PRECURSOR TO ILLNESS

Any review of procedures employed in *preparing* generally healthy individuals for coping with potentially stressful events or *preventing* exacerbations in the stress response must be prefaced by a brief discussion of the nature of positive versus excessive stress. In reality, people are seldom free of stress or without some degree of objective anxiety. Freud (1917), for instance, differentiated between neurotic anxiety and objective anxiety. He defined *objective anxiety* as an adaptative stress response if the reaction was within controllable limits, stating that the individual was responding to a real danger and was taking protective measures. Other anxiety theorists have similarly regarded anxiety as serving a positive signal function (Kutash, 1980). According to Selye (1978), an individual should not strive to avoid all stress, but rather should learn how to recognize his or her typical response to stress and then try to moderate his or her life accordingly. Prevention, therefore, would not be directed at this positive stress or *eustress* (Selye's term) experienced by an individual.

In his discussion of eustress, Selye (1978) emphasized the importance of individual differences in determining the amount of optimal stress acceptable to the person before he or she becomes incapacitated and dysfunctional as a consequence. For example, what may serve as a signal for person A in terms of his or her level of eustress, may render person B paralyzed, since this level may exceed his or her controllable limits. Bearing in mind the importance of individual differences regarding the cognitive, physiological, and behavioral components of the stress response, the reader is encouraged to view with caution the empirical evidence for the efficacy of stress-management procedures employed in the prevention of and preparation for stress.

## Preparation for Stressful Medical Procedures

The importance of psychological interventions in alleviating stress in individuals about to undergo invasive medical procedures has been underestimated for many years. It is possible that a recognition of potentially stressful situations may prevent more serious disturbances if patients are instructed in the use of adaptive coping responses. The patient is often faced with the need to undergo medical procedures, such as endoscopy or catherization, which are important for maintaining physical health. This threat of the unknown often brings about feelings of discomfort and tension, worry, and anxiety. Auerbach and Kilmann (1977) conceptualized situations in which the patient considers invasive medical procedures as *crises*. Stress-management techniques provided by health psychologists, for instance, can help make a patient's hospital experience positive, facilitate emotional well-being, improve adjustment during the actual medical procedure, and finally, influence the rate of recovery.

Psychological intervention to reduce stress during medical procedures is a recent development (Frank, 1979). A variety of strategies have been analyzed, including psychological support, provision of information, skills training, relaxation training, filmed modeling, and cognitive-behavioral interventions. Examples of each of these interventions follow.

In a study by Schmitt and Wooldbridge (1973) examining the efficacy of psychological support in conjunction with information provision and a behavioral intervention, patients were asked to attend a group (two to five patients) discussion for one hour on the evening before surgery. The discussion centered on patients sharing feelings about the forthcoming procedure, mutual reassurance that their feelings and anxieties were normal, and exhange of information about the procedure. Additional procedural and behavioral information (e.g., proper breathing and coughing techniques, leg exercises, and ways to turn and get out of bed) was provided by the group leader. On the morning of surgery, most of the treated patients also underwent a one-to-one intervention, lasting from fifteen minutes to one hour, in which they were encouraged to verbalize any anxiety they might be feeling. The therapist then provided them with support, reassurance, and some additional information. The control patients received "routine hospital care," typically consisting of some behavioral information about coughing and breathing deeply, and how to turn. Schmitt and Wooldbridge generally found that treated patients, compared to controls, showed more adaptive health behaviors, such as sleeping better, experiencing less difficulty with voiding urine and urinary retention, requiring less medication on the second and third postoperative days, resuming an oral diet sooner, and spending fewer days in the hospital. Further, no differences were found between the groups in state anxiety on the evening before surgery; however, the treated patients reported less anxiety on the morning of surgery (e.g., anticipatory anxiety).

Surman, Hackett, Silverberg, and Behrendt (1974) utilized a psychological support strategy with adult patients undergoing cardiac surgery. All patients in both the experimental and control groups were exposed to a standard educational program on heart surgery given by the nursing staff. In addition, the experimental group participated in a 60- to 90-minute interview, the goals of which were to (1) reinforce the preoperative teaching of the staff; (2) provide psychological support and a means by which the patients could express their concerns about the impending surgery; and (3) hypnotize patients and teach them self-hypnosis for their own use in the postsurgery period. Findings did not support the efficacy of the intervention, and no differences were found between the two groups on any of the dependent measures—postoperative delirium, pain, anxiety, depression, or use of medication. The authors concluded that a single preoperative visit does not appear to be an effective intervention for this medical problem.

In a review of studies on psychological preparation for stressful medical procedures, Kendall and Watson (1981) were unable to find unequivocal evidence to demonstrate the effectiveness of psychological support intervention for adult medical patients. Similarly, in the case of psychological support studies with children, they found that certain studies have produced some evidence for effectiveness but that such findings are equivocal. They suggest that psychological support is probably most effective when used in conjunction with other methods of established efficacy in the reduction of hospitalization-related stress.

A relationship between preoperative anxiety levels and postoperative recovery was first proposed by Janis (1958). On the basis of results from interviews of surgery patients experiencing moderate fear levels, Janis suggested the existence of a curvilinear relationship between preoperative anxiety levels and postoperative recovery, with best adjustment associated with moderate fear levels. According to Janis's theory, moderate levels of arousal elicit certain thoughts and fantasies about the upcoming surgery and, in experiencing these surgery-related images, the patient is able to develop a more realistic view of the stressors to be faced. By constructively engaging in the "work of worrying," the patient is thought to learn the coping skills necessary to deal with the stress. Despite the numerous studies generated by this theory, few have produced conclusive findings.

Several authors have attempted to assess the benefits of providing patients with *procedural* type information. This type of information, for example, is concerned with the medical procedure itself, where and when it will take place, and what the mortality rate is. A study conducted by Vernon and Bigelow (1974) examined the effectiveness of preoperative procedural information in reducing the anxiety among adult male hernia-repair patients. Detailed information regarding the forthcoming procedure was shared two days before surgery with the treatment patients, whereas the control patients did not receive this information. Measures of anxiety, as determined by the Multiple Affect Adjective Checklist, adjustment, and amount of information were recorded for half the treatment patients on the evening before surgery; a similar assessment was made for the other half of the treatment patients on the fourth or fifth postoperative day. No evidence was found that procedural information produced any significant differences between the treated and the control groups. The results of this study directly challenge Janis's assumptions and cast doubt on the utility of providing patients with additional information.

In contrast, however, a study by Egbert, Battit, Welch, and Bartlett (1964), using adult patients hospitalized for intraabdominal operations, investigated the utility of establishing physician–patient rapport and provided patients with *sensory* information as a component of this intervention. In addition to receiving brief procedural information preoperatively (e.g., preparation for anesthesia, time and approximate duration of the operation), the treated patients were given *sensory* information regarding what to expect postoperatively in terms of the location of pain, its severity, and its duration. Also, the treated patients were trained in such behavioral coping skills as muscle relaxation and ways to facilitate mobility. Egbert *et al.* (1964) found that, postoperatively, patients in the treated group had significantly lower levels of pain medication usage on the five successive days postsurgery, compared to the control patients, and were also released from the hospital sooner.

Despite the evidence in favor of the efficacy of this intervention procedure, this study confounds the relative effects of providing sensory information, behavioral skills training, and amount of staff attention to the treated patients.

Other studies examining the utility of providing sensory information preoperatively to reduce distress in patients undergoing gastrointestinal endoscopy examinations (Johnson, Morrisey, & Leventhal, 1973) only weakly supported the effectiveness of any of the information provision interventions.

As discussed earlier in this section, individual differences among patients play a major role in determining the type and effectiveness of preoperative information. Sime (1976) found a wide variation in the extent of information that patients desired preoperatively. The interaction between individual differences in preferred mode of dealing with stress and the influence of preoperative information on recovery in surgical patients has been demonstrated in studies of hernia-repair patients (Andrew, 1970). In the Andrew study, patients were classified as "copers" (preferred vigilant or sensitive defenses), "avoiders" (preferred to distance themselves from negative feelings), or "neutrals" (no preferred mode of coping). In the hernia-repair group of patients, copers showed the best recovery from surgery and avoiders the poorest, particularly if they received specific information about the risks of surgery before their operations. This example illustrates the importance of an *idiographic* or individual approach when implementing intervention strategies for individuals who differ in their typical modes of dealing with stress.

Melamed, Dearborn, and Hermecz (1983) raised certain important issues related to the provision of information to patients preparing for surgery and questioned whether such a procedure is uniformly beneficial. Melamed *et al*. (1983) compared the effects of presenting hospital-relevant and -irrelevant information on information acquisition, physiological reponsivity (heart rate, skin conductance), self-report of medical concern, and observed anxiety in a group of 58 children between the ages of 4 and 17 scheduled for elective surgery. Age and experience were the factors under consideration in this study. The children were shown either a hospital-relevant slide tape information package or an unrelated film the night before surgery. The results of the study supported the effectiveness of hospital-relevant information as improving the children's experience of and recovery from hospitalization for surgery. Additionally, age and experience were found to affect the amount of information acquired differentially, with older children having more information. It was also found that children under the age of 8, who had had at least one previous surgery experience, reported *increased* medical concerns if they saw the hospital-relevant presentation. In view of these findings, Melamed and her co-workers suggested that the provision of information can be helpful, but that it is contraindicated for young, experienced children who might be better prepared by alternative strategies.

In a further study examining the retention of preparatory information as influenced by time of preparation, arousal levels, and other subject characteristics, Faust and Melamed (1984) exposed two groups of children undergoing either same day or in-hospital surgery to hospital-relevant and -irrelevant information. These two groups, same day of surgery and in-hospital, retained more hospital-relevant information following preparation than did control children seeing an unrelated film. Older children were found to retain more information than younger children, regardless of population. Significantly greater decreases in skin conductance levels were noted in those in-hospital patients who saw the relevant experimental film, as compared with children seeing the same film on the day of surgery. The authors suggest that the film may have a greater impact given the context in which the children found themselves. Additionally, the nonrelevant control film seemed to serve as a distraction for these children having surgery immediately on admission and this was reflected in a reduction of their hospital fears. Also, children with previous experience who saw other relevant films showed significantly greater increases in sweat gland activity than did those children without previous experience, regardless of time of film presentation. The authors concluded that in preparing a child for surgery, it is difficult to predict his or her response to the stressful situation by preparation alone or by the amount of information the child may have acquired from preparation. Caution should be exercised in this respect, since information may only sensitize the child as the result of previous surgical experience and the temporal setting the child finds himself or herself in.

*Skills training* is another technique employed in teaching patients specific behaviors to facilitate their recovery process, reduce the distress of pain, and shorten the length of their hospital stay. An example of this approach may be seen in the work of Lindeman and Van Aernam (1971), who conducted an investigation of what they termed *structured* and *unstructured* patient teaching. Patients in the structured group were instructed in diaphragmatic breathing, leg and foot exercises, and special techniques for coughing and turning, whereas the patients in the unstructured group received routine preparative teaching provided by the nursing staff. The results of the study showed that although there were no differences between the two groups in the amount of analgesics needed postoperatively, the structured group spent significantly fewer days in the hospital (6.5 versus 8.4). The findings of this study suggest that intensive behavioral skills training may reduce length of hospitalization. Given the recent emphasis on reducing medical care costs, techniques that facilitate reduction in length of hospitalization are of considerable importance and require further study.

A later study by Johnson and Leventhal (1974) designed to examine the efficacy of skills training in preparation for an unpleasant medical examination failed to support the effectiveness of the skills training approach. No reduction in gagging, tension-related arm movements, time required for tube passage, medication needed, or heart rate increase was reported following training. On the whole, behavioral skills training does not appear to be as effective as other techniques in reducing patient anxiety and subjective distress.

Much work has recently been devoted to the study of distress often observed in patients undergoing dental procedures. Visits to the dentist's office are for many individuals highly stressful events. Imagine, for instance, that you are sitting in the waiting area of your dentist's office about to go in to have a tooth filled. Your heart begins to race, your palms become clammy, and you may begin to squirm as you recall the sound of the drill grinding against your teeth and the subsequent pain.

The dental setting itself provides a well-controlled environment with a naturally occurring time-limited stressor that is conducive to systematic empirical investigation of stress mechanisms and treatment. Such a setting further facilitates the measurement of the different components of the stress response. The patients tend to be fairly immobile throughout the dental procedure, thus allowing for a more reliable measure of physiological responding, with minimal distortion from such artifacts as movement. Observation may also be reliably made of the patient's behavioral responses to the stressor (i.e., facial grimaces, sighing, not going to the dentist). Finally, the dental setting allows the clinician to observe the variety of environmental factors, such as the dentist's reactions, and the mother's reactions in the case of a child, which may play an important role in mediating the dental patient's phobic avoidance behavior. This area, therefore, serves as a research model of the study of naturally occurring stress.

Systematic desensitization has been found to be effective in the treatment of dental fears. In a study by Gale and Ayer (1969), systematic desensitization was chosen as treatment of choice for a patient who had previously been traumatized during extractions and had avoided dentists for several years. The patient participated in constructing an anxiety hierarchy ranging from low-anxiety items ("thinking about going to the dentist," "getting in your car to go to the dentist"), to higher level anxiety situations ("having a tooth pulled," "getting two injections," "hearing the crunching sounds as your tooth is being pulled"). The patient was then trained in deep muscle relaxation. Next, the patient was exposed in imagination to these fears while in a relaxed state, beginning with the item lowest on the hierarchy, until they no longer evoked anxiety. On completion of eight sessions, the patient was able to schedule and keep appointments with the dentist and complete all necessary treatment. Relaxation training in combination with other stress management procedures appears, therefore, to have beneficial effects on reducing stress in patients fearful of dental procedures.

The earliest therapeutic effects of modeling (vicarious learning) in the reduction of fear and avoidance have been documented by Bandura and Menlove (1968). The basic clinical goals behind modeling procedures, which may involve exposure to either an actual or a filmed restorative session in which another patient is observed, include (1) allowing the patient to find out what will happen, (2) allowing the patient to see a prototype for how the patient can cope with stress, and (3) allowing the patient to experience vicariously what it feels like.

In a study with dental phobic adults, Shaw and Thoresen (1974) demonstrated that patients who had avoided treatment for a mean of 3.7 years were successfully treated using videotape modeling (including relaxation training and imagery), which produced results equivalent to systematic desensitization in less time (6.1 hours vs. 8.3 hours). Another report by Kleinknecht and Bernstein (1979) described the use of a combination of symbolic modeling (watching another patient overcome fear), graduated exposure (sequential videotape exposure to dental situations), and self-paced *in vivo* practice (sitting in the dental chair without receiving treatment) in the treatment of two patients who had avoided treatment for 13 and 6 years, respectively. After only 3½ hours of therapist contact time, the patients were able to visit their dentist and endodontist. Again, it would appear that this strategy has proven to be quite successful in the treatment of dental fears. Further research should evaluate the effect of modeling procedures, for example, on such medical procedures as heart surgery.

Cognitive-behavioral interventions as described in the previous section are strategies that seek to affect a patient's cognitive functioning and behavioral adjustment by addressing the cognitive and behavioral components of the stress response. Meichenbaum (1975), for instance, recommends that adults undergoing dental procedures should instruct themselves in coping verbalizations to reduce their level of distress. Other coping mechanisms may include humming, counting, visualizing oneself in a confident role, apathy, humor, and imagining oneself in a more pleasant environment.

In a study comparing relaxation tapes, perceived control, a distraction video game, and a control session as to the stress reaction of adult dental patients during the restorative session, Corah, Gale and Illig (1979) found that both relaxation and distraction were effective in reducing self-reported discomfort during operative dental procedures. Another study by Horan, Layng, and Pursell (1976) evaluated the use of emotive imagery in reducing self-reported discomfort in adults undergoing dental prophylaxis. When instructed to engage in pleasant emotive imagery, patients tended to report less discomfort as compared to a silent period of being instructed to imagine neutral letters. None of the conditions produced a significant difference in heart rate, however.

## STRESS MANAGEMENT IN PATIENT POPULATIONS

In this section, we will give examples of different approaches to the management of stress in those individuals experiencing a variety of health problems. More specifically, reduction of stress in diabetic patients, burn patients, and asthmatic patients will be discussed as model problems illustrating current applications of stress management. Stress management in diabetes is presented as an example of an application based upon the hypothesized link between stress-sympathetic arousal and diabetes, reviewed in Chapter 6. The focus on the burn patient and the stress inoculation approach developed by Wernick (1983) is intended to provide the reader with an example of a modern psychological management strategy for the significant set of stressors, including pain, experienced by the burn patient. Discussion of asthma provides an opportunity to critically examine specific behavior therapy procedures and to illustrate a family systems approach to the complex set of interpersonal problems that are hypothesized to characterize the families of certain asthmatic patients.

### Diabetic Patients

Although relatively little empirical evidence is available regarding stress reduction in diabetic patients, this application of stress management is quite promising. This is particularly the case given the potential role of stress in diabetes (see Chapter 6). Daniels (1939) first summarized the result of a clinical trial by Bouch (1935–1936) who used relaxation techniques to control diabetic symptoms. Patients with severe diabetes received daily muscle relaxation training, together with hypnotic suggestion, following which Bouch observed reductions in patient requirements of exogenous insulin from 10 to 60 units. More recent studies have indicated the potential role of relaxation techniques in the management of both insulin-dependent and non–insulin-dependent diabetes mellitus. In a case report of a 20-year-old, female, insulin-dependent diabetic experiencing recurrent episodes of hyperglycemia as a reaction to physical and emotional stress, Fowler, Budzynski, and Vanderbergh (1976) found that the patient's insulin requirements were halved following a six-month EMG biofeedback-assisted relaxation training program. A later study by Seeburg and DeBoer (1980) further supported the results of Fowler *et al.* (1976), utilizing a similar procedure in the treatment of a 24-year-old patient with insulin-dependent diabetes mellitus. Again, a significant reduction in the patient's insulin requirement was observed following treatment.

The effects of EMG feedback-assisted relaxation training on glucose tolerance, glucose stimulated insulin secretion, and insulin sensitivity have been studied by Surwit and Feinglos (1983). They evaluated glucose tolerance and insulin sensitivity in a sample of 12 patients before and after a 9-day hospitalization. All patients had presented with non–insulin-dependent diabetes mellitus and had previously demonstrated poor control with diets and sulfonylurea therapy. At the time of hospital admission, each patient was hyperglycemic. During the study, adjustments were made in each patient's caloric intake to maintain constant body weight, and medication was kept constant. Half of the patients received one EMG feedback session daily and practiced progressive muscle relaxation exercises with taped instruction twice a day during hospitalization. The other half of the patients were hospitalized under similar conditions, but did not practice relaxation training. Compared to the control group whose glucose tolerance deteriorated, the treated patients showed significant improvement in glucose tolerance following relaxation training. Relaxation training did not affect insulin sensitivity and glucose-stimulated insulin secretory activity, however, although plasma cortisol levels were reduced in patients trained in relaxation compared to controls (Surwit & Feinglos, 1984).

Despite the limited experimental literature dealing with the effectiveness of stress-reduction techniques in the management of diabetes mellitus, it would appear that relaxation techniques may be beneficial in the treatment of this health problem. More research is needed to evaluate the relative effectiveness of other stress-reduction procedures in this area.

## Burn Patients

Interest in the psychological problems of burn victims was initially stimulated by the anecdotal reports of Adler (1943) and Cobb and Lindeman (1943), who observed that more than 50% of their subjects who had survived the 1942 Coconut Grove fire disaster in Boston had psychological problems. Although the pain and distress experienced by burn victims has long been recognized as a major problem, little has been done in the way of systematic pain and stress management in these patients.

Three phases may be identified when considering management of the burn patient: (1) emergency phase, (2) acute phase, and (3) rehabilitation phase. These phases approximate the three stages of physiological, psychological, and social emergency discussed in Chapter 6. During the *emergency phase* (the first few days, post-burn), the patient is thoroughly examined to determine the percentage of body burned and the seriousness of the burn. Stabilization of fluids and electrolytes, maintenance of adequate respiration and circulation, and the prevention of infection are the major concerns of the burn team at this point. The invasive procedures employed (connection of tubes, lines to the patient's body), and the constant activity of the intensive care setting can be quite stressful to the patient.

The time taken before the patient is covered with new skin is considered the *acute phase,* which may last from several days to several months depending on the severity of the burn. The second-degree burn patient may typically experience severe primary pain from the burn itself, and Fagerhaugh (1974) notes that *intensity* and *long duration* are the outstanding features of such burn pain. Patients have been observed to suffer most from the pain experience of "tankings," wherein the patient is lowered on a stretcher into a large tank, the old dressings are removed, and the patient is gently scrubbed to remove encrusted medication. Severe pain in donor sites has also been reported by patients who require skin grafts (Andreasen, Noxes, Hartford, Bradland, & Proctor, 1972).

Finally, in the *rehabilitation* phase, which begins once all wounds are covered, the main concerns are the prevention of contractives, the minimization of scarring, and the return to society.

Wernick (1983) has reported the successful use of stress-inoculation (SI) training in the clinical pain experience of burn patients. Wernick randomly assigned 16 patients to either SI or no treatment control group, so that 8 patients were in each group. Selection criteria for participation in this study excluded patients with burns to less than 15% of the body, intellectually impaired patients, and patients in intensive care. Staff of the burn unit were instructed to record daily reports on pain medication requests, patient self-ratings of how they were feeling physically and emotionally, patient's rating of pain and staff's rating of patient's tolerance, six compliance behaviors considered central to patient's optimal recovery (eating, drinking, wearing splints, physical therapy or exercise, dressing changes, and tankings), nurses' global ratings (0–100) of their patients at each shift on how well the individual coped with stress (pain) during that time interval. Patients in the SI group had a 30- to 40-minute treatment session for five consecutive days. Patients in the no-treatment control group had no specific SI treatment, but the routine services provided to burn patients, such as psychiatric consultation and pain medication, were made available to them.

The SI procedure used in this study was structured over a 5-day period. In session one, the patient was told the rationale behind the treatment, the goals of therapy, and a contract was set up. Wernick (1983) calls this the educational phase in which the therapist makes the patient aware of the mechanisms of the stress cycle and how pain—the stressor in this particular case—affects the cognitive, physiological, and behavioral responsiveness of the patient. The therapist then explains how treatment aims at modifying the patient's stress response to break the stress cycle.

In session two, which Wernick calls the skills consolidation and acquisition phase, the therapist first attempts to generate a list of coping strategies based on the patient's past experience. The therapist then presents the possible treatment strategies to the patient.

In session three, the patient is instructed in the use of cognitive strategies to be used in his or her response to the appraisal of pain. Mental distraction strategies may include, for instance, watching television, daydreaming, mental arithmetic, humming, or reciting poems. Other techniques may include ignoring the pain by engaging in mental imagery or goal-directed fantasy that is incompatible with the pain experience. The patient may also try to imagine the pain experience in fantasy, but transform the sensations associated with it so that he or she imagines that a limb is made of rubber or is numb, and thus unable to feel the pain. Similarly, the patient may try to include the pain experience in fantasy, but transform the context or situation. For example, the patient might imagine himself or herself being tortured by aliens from outer space, rather than being a burn victim in the tank. In session four, patients may be taught to view the pain reaction in terms of four phases (Meichenbaum, 1977), rather than as one, overwhelming panic reaction. The phases involve assisting patients (1) to prepare for the pain, (2) to confront it, (3) to handle it, and (4) to reinforce their handling of the reaction. Table 7-7 illustrates the type of self-statements used at each phase.

Session five involves teaching the patient to look at the positive aspects of painful situations in response to the negative self-statements generated by the patients (e.g., tanking even though it is painful is necessary to remove encrusted medication and will speed the healing

TABLE 7-7
Sample of Self-Statements for Pain Control

Preparing for the painful stressor
  What is it you have to do?
  You can develop a plan to deal with it.
  Just think about what you have to do.
  Just think about what you can do about it.
  Don't worry; worrying won't help anything.
  You have lots of different strategies you can call upon.
Confronting and handling the pain
  You can meet the challenge.
  One step at a time, you can handle the situation.
  Just relax; breathe deeply, and use one of the strategies.
  Don't think about the pain, just what you have to do.
  This tenseness can be an ally, a cue to cope.
  Relax. You're in control; take a slow deep breath. Ah, good.
  This anxiety is what the trainer said you might feel.
  That's right; it's the reminder to use your coping skills.
Coping with feelings at critical moments
  When pain comes just pause; keep focusing on what you have to do.
  What is it you have to do?
  Don't try to eliminate the pain totally; just keep it under control.
  Just remember, there are different strategies; they'll help you stay in control.
  When the pain mounts you can switch to a different strategy; you're in command.
Reinforcing self-statements
  Good, you did it.
  You handled it pretty well.
  You knew you could do it.
  Wait until you tell the trainer about what procedures worked best.

Note. From *Cognitive Behavior Modification* (p. 177) by D. Meichenbaum. Copyright 1977 by Plenum Press. Reprinted by permission.

process by preventing infection); this is called cognitive restructuring. The technique requires (1) identification of the negative self-statements used by the patient in response to pain, (2) development of specific and realistic positive coping statements to counteract each of the negative self-statements, and (3) cognitively rehearsing a painful scene (e.g., having dressings changed) while at the same time imagining making the negative self-statement and, finally, replacing it with the positive coping statements.

At this point, the patient should possess a wide repertoire of techniques and should be instructed to use these interchangeably, depending on how effective they are in different situations. Throughout this part of the training, the nurse may act as a coach while the patient rehearses for the stressful event. The fifth and final session should begin before the patient's tanking, and here again the nurse may act as a coach as in session four. As tanking begins, the patient is encouraged to relax and view the tanking procedure in terms of the four phases. At the same time, the patient is instructed on how to use his or her coping strategies interchangeably. Following the tanking, the therapist should positively reinforce the patient for his or her ability to cope.

Wernick found no overall pretest differences in either demographic composition or baseline levels on dependent measures between the SI and control groups. However, patients in the SI group were found to change significantly from pretreatment to posttreatment on each measure, whereas in the control group only physical and emotional self-ratings were observed to improve significantly.

Further comparisons between the SI and control groups revealed a significant posttreatment decrease in pain medication requests for the SI group and a doubling of medication requests for the control group. Pain ratings of tankings by both patient and staff significantly improved for the SI group, compared to the controls. Additional findings regarding patient compliance to essential aspects of treatment in the burn unit showed a significant increase in this measure in the SI group, compared to the control group. Finally, individual ratings by nurses of adaptive and maladaptive behavior of each patient showed significant increases in adaptive behavior pre- to posttreatment in the SI group, with no observable change for the controls. The results of this study provide an example of the potential benefits to be derived from the application of SI training to the treatment of burn patients.

Although this program represents an innovative approach to reducing the experience of pain and distress in burn patients, Wernick has indicated that such an intervention, although well received by nursing staff, was not readily implemented. This appears to be the result of the relatively time-consuming procedures involved. Nursing staff, already burdened by multiple demands, felt that it was not feasible to continue such an approach. This problem highlights the importance of considering not only effectiveness, but also the time required for implementation of a specific program. Given that many of the interventions in health psychology will be implemented by health professionals other than psychologists, clinicians developing these programs must consider the constraints on these health providers. Programs must be efficient as well as effective.

## Asthmatic Patients

Asthma, meaning *parting* in Greek, is a symptom complex or syndrome characterized by intermittent, variable, and reversible airways constriction resulting in the impairment of air exchange and primary expiration, inducing wheezing. Asthma attacks may occur intermittently and vary as to severity. Many asthmatics will have sporadic attacks characterized by mild wheezing and will respond rapidly to medical intervention. Symptoms in such cases have been found to occur after physical exertion or seasonally in reaction to a particular allergen. Asthmatics with more severe attacks, however, can experience an acute attack so overwhelming that it may develop into a condition known as status asthmaticus, which is resistant to medical treatment, and death may occur. In order to avoid status asthmaticus, because of the difficulty in treating this condition, medical intervention has focused primarily on *managing* the symptoms of asthma.

Prevalence rates for asthma have been estimated from 2% to 20% with approximately 60% of asthmatics being less than 17 years old. Boys appear to be affected almost twice as often as girls. According to the genetic data available (Edforg-Lubs, 1971), hereditary factors may play less of a role than previously thought. Monozygotic twins produced a concordance rate of only 19% of asthma and 25% for all allergic disorders.

In a recent review of the literature of psychological influences, Alexander (1981) concluded that psychosocial variables (placebo, removing children from parents, classical conditioning, relaxation) can exert some control over lung function and the clinical course of the disorder in some individuals; however, the effects are *modest*. It is more likely that the respiratory system of some asthmatics is hypersensitive to psychological stimuli. Methods designed to identify these individuals and to further understand the basis for such hypersensitivity might result in significant health benefits.

Although the role of psychological factors in the etiology of asthma is unclear, psychological intervention has been useful in dealing with the emotional stress and adjustment consequences of asthma or asthma-related behaviors (Creer, 1982). Two major psychological approaches have been employed in reducing the asthmatic patient's distress—behavioral and family therapy.

Behavioral intervention for reducing stress responses associated with asthma has been directed at two areas: (1) *alteration of the abnormal pulmonary functioning* via relaxation training, biofeedback, and operant conditioning and (2) *alteration of maladaptive emotional concomitants,* frightening life-threatening episodes, and phobic reactions. Researchers at the National Asthma Center have attempted to evaluate the effect of relaxation training on asthma. Tal and Miklich (1976), in a study of 60 asthmatic patients, used "quasi-hypnotic" relaxation tapes in three training sessions. They found small, but statistically significant changes in forced expiratory volume in one second ($FEV_1$). In a later study, Alexander,

Cropp and Chai (1979) compared relaxation training and resting quietly while evaluating a complete battery of lung function pre- and postsessions. Results from this study again demonstrated a small, but statistically significant change in $FEV_1$.

Several questions were raised by these studies in terms of assumptions regarding the effectiveness of relaxation techniques in the treatment of asthma. Peak expiratory flow rate ($PEFR$), the dependent physiological measure used in several of the studies, is an effort-dependent measure that varies greatly, depending on the patient's cooperation. Also, the physiological changes that were observed in these studies were not clinically significant, meaning that patients' lung functioning was not in the normal range predicted for their sex, age, height, and weight after treatment. On the basis of these and findings from similar studies on asthmatics, Alexander (1981) concluded that relaxation procedures are not *clinically* beneficial in the treatment of childhood or adult asthma.

The second category of behavioral intervention included those designed to effect changes in the emotional concomitants of asthma, clear examples of which are fear and anxiety associated with asthma ("asthma panic"). Despite the paucity of controlled outcome studies, research on the deconditioning of fear associated with asthma and such behavior therapies as systematic densensitization or implosion have shown some promise in the treatment of *asthma panic*. For over a decade, numerous cases of child and adult asthma panic have been successfully treated at the National Asthma Center with either systematic desensitization or implosion. No attempt at altering lung function was made in any of the cases, anxiety or stress reduction being the measure of treatment success. Moreover, the criteria employed in evaluating success of treatment were based solely on subjective reports of improvement by the patient and observations by nurses, physicians, and other staff involved in the patient's treatment.

As mentioned earlier, Alexander (1981), in a review of behavioral approaches to the treatment of asthma, concluded that although none of the techniques (airways biofeedback, systematic desensitization, and relaxation training) have proven therapeutically effective in altering pulmonary dynamics, behavioral strategies show promise in alleviating such asthma-related difficulties as asthma panic and adjustment problems.

The behavioral approach to the management of asthma represents an individual approach, that is, one directed at the individual patient, an alternative approach, one that focuses on the family and family system, has been proposed by Minuchin, Baker, Rosman, Liebman, Milman, and Todd (1975). This family therapy approach to asthma management is based upon the family systems model discussed in Chapter 6. To review, rather than viewing illness within a linear model in which the individual's life situations or stressors and bodily illness interact in a causal chain, the alternative model shifts emphasis from the individual to the individual in his or her social context. This model also emphasizes the feedback processes between the individual and this social context. The model shifts from a focus on the "sick patient" to the "sick patient within the family" and redefines the nature of certain stress-related disorders and the scope of therapeutic change. The open systems model postulates (1) that certain types of family organization are closely related to the development and maintenance of various psychosomatic or stress-related symptoms and (2) these symptoms play a major role in *maintaining* family homeostasis. In the open systems model, illness consists of two phases: (1) the "turn-on" phase, in which the family conflict situation induces emotional arousal in the patient, and (2) the "turn-off" phase, which represents a return to baseline levels of arousal. This turn-off phase can be interrupted by the nature of family members' involvements with each other around the conflict. This latter point is the major focus of the open systems model. It is argued that since family interactions affect the psychophysiology of the patient in psychosomatic crisis, the disorder is seen in reference to the feedback processes of the patient and family. Therapeutic efforts, therefore, can be directed toward the patient, the family, and the feedback processes of the family transactional patterns in whatever combinations seem most appropriate.

In this model, which forms the basis for a type of family therapy, *structured family therapy*, three factors are necessary for the development of severe stress-related, or in this case, psychosomatic illness. It should be emphasized that this model focuses on psychosomatic illness as classically conceptualized and emphasizes illness in children. The three factors necessary for the development of severe illness include (1) that the child or adult patient is physiologically vulnerable, that is, a specific organic dysfunction is present, and (2) that the child's family has the following four transactional characteristics—enmeshment, overprotectiveness, rigidity, and lack of conflict resolution. Table 7-8 describes the characteristics of these four transactional patterns. The third component necessary for the development of illness is that the sick child plays an important role in the family's patterns of conflict avoidance. It is this role that is an important source of reinforcement for his or her symptoms. That is, the child's sickness helps the family *avoid conflict*.

Minuchin *et al.* (1975) have developed the structural family therapy approach based upon this model and have applied this technique to families with children who present with severe forms of psychosomatic disorders, including anorexia, diabetes, and asthma. The goal of this

**TABLE 7-8**
Transactional Characteristics of "Psychosomatic Families"

Enmeshment
   A high degree of responsiveness and involvement
   Intrusions on personal boundaries
   Poorly differentiated perception of self and of other members
   Various family subsystems have poor boundaries
   Executive hierarchies are confused (e.g., parent and child against parent)

Overprotectiveness
   Family members show a high degree of concern for each other's welfare
   Nurturing and protective responses are consistantly elicited and supplied
   Signs of distress can cue family members to engage in some behavior to reduce
      tension—mother weeping as she anticipates father's criticism may trigger child into
      distracting behavior

Rigidity
   Heavily committed to maintaining the *status quo*
   In periods when change and growth are necessary, emphasis on maintaining old
      patterns of relating (e.g., when child reaches adolescence—need for increased
      autonomy is squelched—because it influences the homeostasis of the family)

Lack of Conflict Resolution
   Rigidity and overprotectiveness of the family system along with consistant mutual
      interference make the threshold for conflict very low
   Some families avoid conflict—one member brings up a problem, another avoids it
   Other families simply *deny* the existence of problems

therapy is to (1) bring the faulty patterns of interaction to the family's awareness; (2) teach new patterns of interacting, and (3) teach more appropriate problem solving so the family does not avoid conflict. It is important to mention that these patterns of interaction may occur in effectively functioning families as well; however, families in the "normal range" can shift into other modes of conflict confrontation and negotiation, thus effectively adapting or coping with various forms of stress. The rigid families or the families with patients with psychosomatic illnesses are more likely to enact maladaptive sequences recurrently. The breaking of these patterns of maladaptive interactions is the goal of family therapy. In regard to specific outcome with intractable asthma in patients 6 to 16 years old, Minuchin *et al.* (1975) reported that following nine months of structural family therapy, the 10 patients experienced a "very good response." This clinical response included no absences from school, only mild attacks, and only an occasional need for the use of a bronchodilator. However, it is important to note the absence of appropriate control groups in this clinical report, as well as the small number of patients involved. This clinical approach represents a viable alternative or adjunct to behavioral therapies for the management of asthma.

## Conclusions

As can be seen in the discussion of the various stress-reduction techniques as they apply to the prevention of potential stress-related health problems and in treatment of stress-related health disorders, the stress concept has generated considerable activity both within psychology and across the various biological and behavioral sciences. Clearly, however, stress and its management continue to represent a major challenge to health psychology. Much remains to be learned regarding the actual transduction process by which exposure to stressors results in illness. In addition, more sophisticated approaches to the study of the transactional process relating stressors, coping appraisals, and stress response are required. At the intervention level, effective theraputic approaches based upon conprehensive and empirically validated models of stress-related illness must still be identified. The issue of placebo and other nonspecific effects should be investigated more carefully. Indeed, the psychobiological mechanism of potential placebo effects on stress disorders represents an important research problem. A more thorough delineation of the specific psychobiological effects of various stress management or relaxation therapies is needed. In particular, the effects of specific techniques on both resting levels of physiological activity and phasic stress responses need to be evaluated. The effects of such procedures on physiological recovery from stress is also an area to be investigated. And finally, a further identification of the interaction of individual coping strategies, personality characteristics, and type of interventions applied requires more careful delineation.

## SUMMARY

The rise in incidence of stress-related disorders in our technological society has led to the development of numerous methods aimed at reducing the impact of stress. This chapter was specifically organized to review the various stress-management techniques currently used, ranging from relaxation-based therapies to pharmacological intervention and exercise. In each case, the rationale for the use of the techniques was presented and illustrative examples were given to demonstrate their applicability to health problems. Since relaxation-based approaches continue to pervade the area of stress management, the chapter included a guide for the critical evaluation of the methodology utilized in relaxation research.

Although stress-management techniques are readily used in the alleviation of stress, the *preparation* of generally healthy individuals for coping with potentially stressful events or *preventing* exacerbations in the stress response has gained increased attention only in recent years. The chapter reviewed some of the current concepts in the preparation of individuals for stressful medical procedures, for example, hernia repair operations, and focused on dental procedures as an illustrative example of a well-controlled environment for conducting research to evaluate the efficacy of stress-management approaches. Finally, the chapter critically evaluated the applicability of stress-management procedures to individuals experiencing a variety of health problems, namely, diabetes, severe burns, and asthma.

## REFERENCES

Adler, A. (1943). Neuropsychiatric complications of victims of Boston's Coconut Grove disaster. *Journal of the American Medical Association, 123,* 1098–1100.

Alexander, A. B. (1981). Behavioral approaches in the treatment of bronchial asthma. In C. K. Prokop & L. A. Bradley (Eds.), *Medical Psychology: Contributions to behavioral medicine.* New York: Academic Press.

Alexander, A. B., Cropp, G. J., & Chai, H. (1979). Effects of relaxation training on pulmonary mechanics in children with asthma. *Journal of Applied Behavior Analysis, 12*(1), 27–35.

Andrasik, F., Coleman, D., & Epstein, L. (1982). Biofeedback: Clinical and research considerations. In D. M. Doleys, R. L. Meredith, & A. R. Ciminero (Eds.), *Behavioral medicine: Assessment and treatment strategies.* New York: Plenum Press.

Andreasen, N. J., Noxes, R. Jr., Hartford, C. E., Bradland, G., & Proctor, S. (1972). Management of emotional reactions in seriously burned adults. *New England Journal of Medicine, 286,* 65–69.

Andrew, J. (1970). Recovery from surgery with and without preparatory instruction for three coping styles. *Journal of Personality and Social Psychology, 15,* 223–226.

Anliker, J. (1977). Biofeedback from the perspectives of cybernetics and systems science. In J. Beatty & H. Legewie (Eds.), *Biofeedback and behavior.* New York: Plenum Press.

Auerbach, S. M., & Kilmann, P. R. (1977). Crisis intervention: A review of outcome research. *Psychological Bulletin, 84,* 1189–1217.

Baekeland, F., & Lunwill, L. (1975). Dropping out of treatment: A critical review. *Psychological Bulletin, 82,* 738–753.

Balter, M. B., Levine, J., & Manheimer, D. I. (1973). Cross-national study of the extent of anti-anxiety/sedative drug use. *New England Journal of Medicine, 290,* 769–774.

Bandura, A., & Menlove, F. L. (1968). Factors determining vicarious extinction of avoidance behavior through symbolic modeling. *Journal of Personality and Social Psychology, 8,* 99–108.

Barber, T. X. (1984). Hypnosis, deep relaxation, and active relaxation: Data, theory, and clinical applications. In R. L. Woolfolk & P. M. Lehrer (Eds.), *Principles and practice of stress management*. New York: Guilford Press.

Bar-Or, O., & Buskirk, E. (1974). The cardiovascular system and exercise. In W. Johnson & E. Buskirk (Eds.), *Science and medicine of exercise and sport*. New York: Harper & Row.

Benson, H. (1975). *The relaxation response*. New York: William Morrow.

Benson, H., Dryer, T., & Hartley, H. (1978). Decreased $VO_2$ consumption during exercise with elicitation of the relaxation response. *Journal of Human Stress, 44*, 38–42.

Bernstein, D. A., & Given, B. A. (1984). Progressive relaxation: Abbreviated methods. In R. L. Woolfolk & P. M. Lehrer (Eds.), *Principles and practice of stress management* (pp. 43–69). New York: Guilford Press.

Black, A. H., Cott, A., & Pavloski, R. (1977). The operant learning theory approach to biofeedback training. In G. E. Schwartz & J. Beatty (Eds.), *Biofeedback: Theory and research*. New York: Academic Press.

Blanchard, E. B., & Epstein, L. H. (1978). *A biofeedback primer*. Reading, MA: Addison-Wesley.

Borkovec, T. D., & Sides, J. (1979). Critical procedural variables related to the physiological effects of progressive relaxation: A review. *Behaviour Research and Therapy, 17*(2), 119–125.

Borkovec, T. D., Johnson, M. C., & Block, D. L. (1984). Evaluating experimental designs in relaxation training. In R. L. Woolfolk & P. M. Lehrer (Eds.), *Principles and practice of stress management*. New York: Guilford Press.

Bradley, B. W., & McCanne, T. R. (1981). Autonomic responses to stress: The effects of progressive relaxation, the relaxation response, and expectancy of relief. *Biofeedback and Self-Regulation, 6*(2), 235–251.

Budzynski, T. (1973). Biofeedback procedures in the clinic. *Seminars in Psychiatry, 5*, 537–547.

Carrington, P. (1978). *Clinically standardized meditation (CSM) instructors kit*. Kendall Park, NJ: Pace Educational Systems.

Clausen, J. P. (1977). Effect of physical training on cardiovascular adjustments to exercise in man. *Physiology Review, 57*, 779–815.

Cobb, S. (1979). Social support and health through the life course. In M. Riley (Ed.), *Aging from birth to death: Interdisciplinary perspective*. Boulder, CO: Westview Press.

Cobb, S., & Lindeman, E. (1943). Coconut Grove burns: Neuropsychiatric observations. *Annals of Surgery, 117*, 814–824.

Corah, N. L., Gale, E. N., & Illig, S. J. (1979). Psychological stress reduction during dental procedures. *Journal of Dental Research, 58*(4), 1347–1351.

Creer, T. L. (1982). Asthma. *Journal of Consulting and Clinical Psychology, 50*(b), 916–921.

Daniels, G. E. (1939). Present trends in the evaluation of psychic factors in diabetes mellitus: A critical review of the experimental, general medical, and psychiatric literature of the last five years. *Psychosomatic Medicine, 1*, 527–552.

DeVries, H. (1966). *Physiology of exercise*. Dubuque, IA: William C. Brown.

Doyne, E. J., Chambless, D. L., & Beutler, L. E. (1983). Aerobic exercise as a treatment for depression in women. *Behavior Therapy, 14*(3), 434–440.

Dunbar, J. (1980). Adhering to medical advice: A review. *International Journal of Mental Health, 9*, 70–87.

Edforg-Lubs, M. L. (1971). Allergy in 7,000 twin pairs. *Acta Allergolica, 26*, 249–285.

Egbert, L. D., Battit, G. W., Welch, C. E., & Bartlett, M. R. (1964). Reduction of post-operation pain by encouragement and instruction of patients. *New England Journal of Medicine, 270*, 825–827.

Eisdorfer, C., Nowlin, J., & Wilkie, F. (1970). Improvement of learning in the aged by modification of autonomic nervous system activity. *Science, 170*, 1327.

Ellis, A. (1973). *Humanistic psychology: The rational-emotive approach.* New York: Julian Press.

Fagerhaugh, S. Y. (1974). Pain expression and control on a burn care unit. *Nursing Outlook, 22,* 645–650.

Faust, J., & Melamed, B. G. (1984). Influence of arousal, previous experience, and age on surgery preparation of same day of surgery and in-hospital pediatric patients. *Journal of Consulting and Clinical Psychology, 52,*(3), 359–371.

Folkins, C. H., & Sime, W. E. (1981). Physical fitness training and mental health. *American Psychologist, 36*(4), 373–389.

Fowler, J. E., Budzynski, T. H., & Vanderbergh, R. L. (1976). Effects of an EMG biofeedback relaxation program on the control of diabetes. *Biofeedback and Self-Regulation, 1,* 105–112.

Frank, J. D. (1979). Psychotherapy of bodily disease: An overview. In C. A. Garfield (Ed.), *Stress and survival: The emotional realities of life threatening illness.* St. Louis: C. V. Mosby.

Freud, S. (1963). Introductory lectures on psychoanalysis. In *Standard Edition* (Volo. 15 & 16). London: Hogarth Press.

Frishman, W., Razin, A., Swencionis, E., & Sonnenblick, E. H. (1981). Beta-adrenoceptor blockade in anxiety states: A new approach to therapy. *Cardiovascular Reviews and Reports, 2,* 447–459.

Fromm, E. (1977). Altered state of consciousness and hypnosis: A discussion. *International Journal of Clinical and Experimental Hypnosis, 25*(4), 325–334.

Gaind, R. N., & Jacoby, R. (1978). Benzodiazepines causing aggression. In R. N. Gaind & B. L. Hudson (Eds.), *Current themes in psychiatry.* London: Macmillan.

Gale, F. N., & Ayer, W. A. (1969). Treatment of dental phobias. *Journal of the American Dental Association, 78,* 1304–1307.

Gellhorn, E., & Kiely, W. F. (1972). Mystical states of consciousness: Neurophysiological and clinical aspects. *Journal of Nervous and Mental Disease, 154,* 399–405.

Green, E. E., & Green, A. M. (1977). *Beyond biofeedback.* New York: Delacorte Press.

Green, E. E., Green, A. M., Walters, E. D., Sargent, J. D., & Meyer, R. G. (1975). Autogenic feedback training. *Psychotherapy and Psychosomatics, 25,* 88–98.

Haskall, W., & Fox, S. (1974). Physical activity in the prevention and therapy of cardiovascular disease. In W. Johnson & E. Burskirk (Eds.), *Science and medicine of exercise and sport.* New York: Harper & Row.

Hess, W. R. (1957). *Functional organization of the diencephalon.* New York: Grune & Stratton.

Hilgard, E. R. (1968). *The exercise of hypnosis.* New York: Harcourt, Brace, and World.

Hoffman, J. W., Benson, H., Arns, P. A., Stainbrook, G. L., Landsberg, G. L., Young, J. B., & Gill, A. (1982). Reduced sympathetic nervous system responsivity associated with the relaxation response. *Science, 215*(4529), 190–192.

Holmes, D. S. (1984). Meditation and somatic arousal reduction: A review of the experimental evidence. *American Psychologist, 39*(1), 1–10.

Horan, J. J., Layng, F. C., & Pursell, C. H. (1976). Preliminary study of effects of "in vivo" emotive imagery on dental discomfort. *Perceptual and Motor Skills, 42*(1), 105–106.

Hughes, J. R. (1984). Psychological effects of habitual aerobic exercise: A critical review. *Preventive Medicine, 13*(1), 66–78.

Jacobson, E. (1978). *You must relax.* New York: McGraw-Hill.

Janis, I. L. (1958). *Psychological stress.* New York: Wiley.

Johnson, J. E., & Leventhal, H. (1974). Effects of accurate expectations and behavioral instructions on reactions during a noxious medical examination. *Journal of Personality and Social Psychology, 29*(8), 710–718.

Johnson, J. E., Morrisey, J. F., & Leventhal, H. (1973). Psychological preparation for an endoscopic examination. *Gastrointestinal Endoscopy, 19,* 180–182.

Katkin, E. S., & Murray, E. N. (1968). Instrumental conditioning of autonomically mediated behavior: Theoretical and methodological issues. *Psychological Bulletin, 70,* 52–68.

Kazdin, A., & Wilson, G. T. (1978). *Evaluation of behavior therapy.* Cambridge, MA: Ballinger.

Kelly, G. (1955). *The psychology of personal constructs* (Vols. 1 & 2). New York: Norton.

Kendall, P. C., & Watson, D. (1981). Psychological preparation for stressful medical procedures. In C. K. Prokop & L. A. Bradley (Eds.), *Medical psychology: Contributions to behavioral medicine.* New York: Academic Press.

Kleinknecht, R., & Bernstein, D. (1979). Short term treatment of dental avoidance. *Journal of Behavior Therapy and Experimental Psychiatry, 10*(4), 311–315.

Kutash, I. L. (1980). Prevention and equilibrium–disequilibrium theory. In I. L. Kutash and L. B. Schlesinger (Eds.), *Handbook on stress and anxiety.* San Francisco: Josey-Bass.

Lader, M. (1984). Pharmacological methods. In R. L. Woolfolk & P. M. Lehrer (Eds.), *Principles and practice of stress management.* New York: Guilford Press.

Lang, P. J. (1977). Research on the specificity of feedback training: Implications for the use of biofeedback in the treatment of anxiety and fever. In J. Beatty & H. Legewie (Eds.), *Biofeedback and behavior.* New York: Plenum Press.

Lasagna, L. (1977). The role of benzodiazepines in nonpsychiatric medical practice. *American Journal of Psychiatry, 134*(6), 656–658.

LeBlanc, J., Boulay, M., Dulac, S., Jobin, M., LaBrie, A., & Rousseau-Mogneron, S. (1977). Metabolic and cardiovascular responses to norepinephrine in trained and nontrained human subjects. *Journal of Applied Physiology: Respiratory Environmental Exercise Physiology, 42,* 166–173.

Ledwidge, B. (1980). Run for your mind: Aerobic exercise as a means for alleviating anxiety and depression. *Canadian Journal of Behavioral Science/Revue Canadienne de Science de Comportement 12*(2), 126–140.

Lindeman, C. A., & Van Aernam, B. (1971). Nursing intervention with the presurgical patient—the effect of structured and unstructured preoperative training. *Nursing Research, 20,* 319–331.

Meichenbaum, D. (1975). Self-instructional methods. In F. Kanfer & A. Goldstein (Eds.), *Helping people change.* New York: Pergamon Press.

Meichenbaum, D. (1977). *Cognitive-behavior modification: An integrative approach.* New York: Plenum Press.

Meichenbaum, D., & Cameron, R. (1983). Stress-inoculation training: Toward a general paradigm for training coping skills. In D. Meichenbaum & M. E. Jaremko (Eds.), *Stress reduction and prevention.* New York: Plenum Press.

Melamed, B. G., Dearborn, M. I., & Hermecz, D. A. (1983). Necessary considerations for surgery preparation: Age and previous experience. *Psychosomatic Medicine, 45,* 517–525.

Minuchin, S., Baker, L., Rosman, B. L., Liebman, R., Milman, L., & Todd, T. C. (1975). A conceptual model of psychosomatic illness in children: Family organization and family therapy. *Archives of General Psychiatry, 32*(8), 1031–1038.

Morse, D. R., Martin, J. S., Furst, M. L., & Dubin, L. L. (1977). A physiological and subjective evaluation of meditation, hypnosis, and relaxation. *Psychosomatic Medicine, 39*(5), 304–324.

Mulholland, T. B. (1977). Biofeedback method for locating the most controlled responses of EEG alpha to visual stimulation. In J. Beatty & H. Legewie (Eds.), *Biofeedback and behavior.* New York: Plenum Press.

Novaco, R. W. (1975). *Anger control: The development and evaluation of an experimental treatment.* Lexington, MA: Heath, Lexington Books.

Novaco, R. W. (1978). Anger and coping with stress: Cognitive behavioral interventions. In J. P. Foreyt & D. P. Rathjen (Eds.), *Cognitive behavior therapy: Research and application.* New York: Plenum Press.

Peronnet, F., Cleroux, J., Perrault, H., Cousineau, D., de Champlain, J., & Nadeau, R. (1981). Plasma norepinephrine response to exercise before and after training in humans. *Journal of Applied Physiology: Respiratory Environmental Exercise Physiology, 51,* 812–815.

Ryan, A. (1974). History of sports medicine. In A. Ryan & F. Allman (Eds.), *Sports medicine.* New York: Academic Press.

Schmitt, F. E., & Wooldridge, P. J. (1973). Psychological preparation of surgical patients. *Nursing Research, 22,* 108–116.

Schultz, J. H., & Luthe, W. (1969). *Autogenic therapy: Vol. 1. Autogenic methods.* New York: Grune & Stratton.

Schwartz, G. E. (1977). Psychosomatic disorders and biofeedback: A psychobiological model of disregulation. In J. D. Maser & M. E. P. Seligman (Eds.), *Psychopathology: Experimental models.* San Francisco: W. H. Freeman.

Seeburg, K. N., & DeBoer, K. F. (1980). Effects of EMG biofeedback on diabetes. *Biofeedback and Self-Regulation, 5*(2), 289–293.

Selye, H. (1978). On the real benefits of eustress. *Psychology Today, 12*(10), 60–64.

Shapiro, D. H., Jr. (1980). *Meditation: Self-regulation strategy and altered state of consciousness.* New York: Aldine.

Shaw, D., & Thoresen, C. (1974). Effects of modeling and desensitization in reducing dental phobia. *Journal of Counseling Psychology, 21,* 415–420.

Shepard, R. J. (1977). *Endurance fitness.* Toronto: University of Toronto Press.

Silver, B. V., & Blanchard, E. G. (1978). Biofeedback and relaxation training in the treatment of psychophysiological disorders: Or are the machines really necessary? *Journal of Behavioral Medicine, 1,* 217–239.

Sime, A. M. (1976). Relationship of preoperative fear, type of coping, and information received about surgery to recovery from surgery. *Journal of Personality and Social Psychology, 34,* 716–724.

Sinyor, D. S., Schwartz, S. G., Peronnet, F., Brisson, G., & Seraganian, P. (1983). Aerobic fitness level and reactivity to psychosocial stress: Physiological, biochemical, and subjective measures. *Psychosomatic Medicine, 45*(3), 205–217.

Stoyva, J. M., & Budzynski, T. H. (1974). Cultivated low arousal—an antistress response. In L. V. DiCara (Ed.), *Recent advances in limbic and autonomic nervous systems research.* New York: Plenum Press.

Surman, O. S., Hackett, T. P., Silverberg, E. L., & Behrendt, D. M. (1974). Usefulness of psychiatric intervention in patients undergoing cardiac surgery. *Archives of General Psychiatry, 30,* 830–835.

Surwit, R. S., & Feinglos, M. N. (1983). The effects of relaxation on glucose tolerance in non-insulin-dependent diabetes. *Diabetes Care, 6*(2), 176–179.

Surwit, R. S., & Feinglos, M. N. (1984). Relaxation induced improvement in glucose tolerance is associated with decreased plasma cortisol. *Diabetes Care, 7*(2), 203–204.

Tal, A., & Miklich, D. R. (1976). Emotionally induced decreases in pulmonary flow rates in asthmatic children. *Psychosomatic Medicine, 38*(3), 190–200.

Vernon, D. T., & Bigelow, D. A. (1974). Effect of information about a potentially stressful situation on responses to stress impact. *Journal of Personality and Social Psychology, 29,* 50–59.

Wallace, R. K., Benson, H., & Wilson, A. F. (1971). A wakeful hypometabolic physiologic state. *American Journal of Physiology, 221,* 795–799.

Walrath, L. C., & Hamilton, D. W. (1975). Autonomic correlates of meditation and hypnosis. *American Journal of Clinical Hypnosis, 17*(3), 190–197.

Wernick, R. L. (1983). Stress inoculation in the management of clinical pain. In D. Meichenbaum & M. E. Jaremko (Eds.), *Stress reduction and prevention.* New York: Plenum Press.

White, J. A., Ismail, A. H., & Bottoms, G. D. (1976). Effect of physical fitness on the adrenocortical response to exercise stress. *Medical Scientific Sports, 8*(2), 113–118.

Wilmore, J. (1977). Individualized exercise prescription. In *Exercise in cardiovascular health and disease.* New York: Yorke Medical Books.

Young, R. J., & Ismail, A. H. (1978). Ability of biochemical and personality variables in discriminating between high and low physical fitness levels. *Journal of Psychosomatic Research, 22,* 193–199.

# HEALTH BEHAVIOR

## DEFINITIONS

The rising interest in health behavior today reflects a recent focus on the prevention of illness. Seven of the ten leading causes of death in the United States apppear to be associated with the *absence* of various health behaviors. Table 8-1 identifies the 10 leading causes of death in 1977 and related risk factors. Most of these causal agents are behavioral in nature or involve some behavioral response on the part of the individual. Matarazzo (1983) points out that whereas contagious and infectious diseases contribute minimally to illness and death, other illnesses have become more frequent and are of a different nature. As discussed in Chapter 2, biomedical research suggests that major breakthroughs in science have contributed significantly toward reducing the prevalence of infectious diseases. Such diseases as influenza, rubella, whooping cough, and polio are no longer a major concern of health care professionals. More deaths are now caused by heart disease (37.8% of all deaths), cancer (20%), and stroke (9.6%). Recent epidemiological studies suggest that these illnesses are the by-products of changes in twentieth-century industrial practices and personal life-styles. Health care professionals are beginning to recognize and are providing empirical evidence demonstrating that the major causes of death are ones in which behavioral pathogens are the single most important factor. *Behavioral pathogens* are the personal habits and life-style behaviors of the individual, in

**TABLE 8-1**

Leading Causes of Death in 1977

| Age groups / Problem | Infants (under 1) Rank | Rate[a] | Children (1–14) Rank | Rate[b] | Adolescents/young adults (15–24) Rank | Rate[b] | Adults (25–44) Rank | Rate[b] | Adults (45–64) Rank | Rate[b] | Older adults (over 65) Rank | Rate[b] | Total population (all ages) Rank | Rate[b] |
|---|---|---|---|---|---|---|---|---|---|---|---|---|---|---|
| **Chronic diseases** | | | | | | | | | | | | | | |
| Heart disease | | | 7 | 1.1 | 6 | 2.5 | 2 | 25.5 | 1 | 351.0 | 1 | 2334.1 | 1 | 332.3 |
| Stroke | | | 8 | .6 | 9 | 1.2 | 8 | 6.1 | 3 | 52.4 | 3 | 658.2 | 3 | 84.1 |
| Arteriosclerosis | | | | | | | | | | | 5 | 116.5 | 9 | 13.3 |
| Bronchitis, emphysema, and asthma | | | | | | | | | 10 | 12.2 | 8 | 69.3 | | |
| Cancer | | | 3 | 4.9 | 5 | 6.5 | 1 | 29.7 | 2 | 302.7 | 2 | 988.5 | 2 | 178.7 |
| Diabetes mellitus | | | | | 10 | .4 | 10 | 2.4 | 8 | 17.8 | 6 | 100.5 | 7 | 15.2 |
| Cirrhosis of the liver | | | | | | | 7 | 8.6 | 4 | 39.2 | 9 | 36.7 | 8 | 14.3 |
| **Infectious diseases** | | | | | | | | | | | | | | |
| Influenza and pneumonia | 5 | 50.6 | 6 | 1.5 | 8 | 1.3 | 9 | 3.0 | 9 | 15.3 | 4 | 169.7 | 5 | 23.7 |
| Meningitis | | | 8 | .6 | | | | | | | | | | |
| Septicemia | 6 | 32.7 | | | | | | | | | | | | |
| **Trauma** | | | | | | | | | | | | | | |
| **Accidents** | | | | | | | | | | | | | | |
| Motor vehical accidents | | | 2 | 9.0 | 1 | 44.1 | 3 | 23.1 | 7 | 18.3 | 10 | 24.5 | 6 | 22.9 |
| All other accidents | 7 | 27.7 | 1 | 10.8 | 2 | 18.4 | 4 | 18.5 | 5 | 25.5 | 7 | 78.1 | 4 | 24.8 |
| Suicide | | | 10 | .4 | 3 | 13.6 | 5 | 17.3 | 6 | 19.1 | | | 9 | 13.3 |
| Homicide | | | 5 | 1.6 | 4 | 12.7 | 6 | 15.6 | | | | | | |
| **Developmental problems** | | | | | | | | | | | | | | |
| Immaturity associated | 1 | 407.7 | | | | | | | | | | | | |
| Birth-associated | 2 | 294.4 | | | | | | | | | | | | |
| Congenital birth defects | 3 | 253.1 | 4 | 3.6 | 7 | 1.6 | | | | | | | | |
| Sudden infant deaths | 4 | 142.8 | | | | | | | | | | | | |
| All causes | | 1412.1 | | 43.1 | | 117.1 | | 182.5 | | 1000.0 | | 5288.1 | | 878.1 |

*Note.* From *Healthy People: Surgeon General's Report on Health Promotion and Disease Prevention* (p. 15) by J. A. Califano, Jr., 1979. Adapted by permission of the U.S. Government Printing Office.
[a]Rate per 100,000 live births.

contrast to the *external pathogens* (infectious agents, nutritional deficits) of earlier times.

A notion that has long been espoused by clinicians and various religious and community groups, and thought to be "common sense," is that a relationship exists between good health and such personal habits as regulation of meals and sleep, moderation in food and alcohol consumption, regular physical activity, and moderate exercise. An interesting investigation of the relationship between physical health and actual daily health practices was conducted by Belloc and Breslow (1972). They examined the relationship between several common health practices, including hours of sleep, regularity of meals, physical activity, smoking, drinking alcohol, and the subject's physical health status. A probability sample of adult residents, aged 20 and over, in Alameda County, California in 1965 were asked to complete questions on health condition and health behaviors. Usable questionnaires were received from 6,928 adults, 86% of the sample. Figure 8-1 shows that those persons who engaged in all recommended health practices had lower phys-

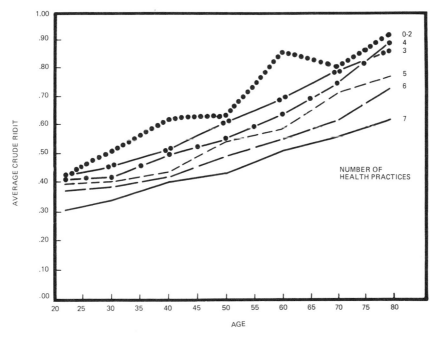

**FIGURE 8-1.** Average physical health ridit by age group by number of health practices. From "Relationships of Physical Health Studies and Health Practices" by M. B. Belloc and L. Breslow, 1972, *Preventive Medicine, 1,* 419. Copyright 1972 by Academic Press, Inc. Reprinted by permission.

ical health *ridits* (relative to an identified distribution), meaning better health, than people who did not. Health condition scores varying from severely disabled to a condition with disability, impairments, chronic condition or chronic symptoms, and great vigor converted into a scale in which the average values for a population or subpopulation are expressed in ridits. The ridit value .50 is the mean for a given population. The results of the investigation indicate that individuals who practice health behaviors tend to have positive health and that the effects were cumulative. In other words, those who practiced more or all good health behaviors were in better health, even though older, than those who failed to do so. Since this representative study, other investigations have supported the conclusion that certain behaviors are associated with better health.

An important document, *Healthy People: The Surgeon General's Report on Health Promotion and Disease Prevention* (Califano, 1979), provides further data that indicate a strong relationship between personal habits and 7 of the 10 leading causes of deaths. As additional evidence accumulates on the importance of behavior to health, attempts are being made to define just what is health and health behavior. Over the past decade, researchers have devised working models in order to understand the basis for such health behavior, with the ultimate goal of identifying factors that initiate, increase, and maintain these behaviors. The remainder of this section will discuss the several approaches used to define and understand health and health behavior.

Most research on health behavior incorporates the formulation of Kasl and Cobb (1966a,b) in their now-classic papers as a point of departure. *Health behavior,* as defined by Kasl and Cobb (1966), includes "any activity undertaken by a person believing himself to be healthy for the purpose of preventing disease or detecting it in an asymptomatic stage" (p. 531). This is distinguished from *illness behavior,* which is "any activity undertaken by a person who feels ill, to define the state of his health and to discover a suitable remedy" (p. 531), and *sick-role behavior,* which is "activity undertaken for the purpose of getting well, by those who consider themselves ill. It includes receiving treatment from appropriate therapists, generally involves a whole range of dependent behaviors and leads to some degree to neglect of one's usual duties" (p. 531).

Kasl and Cobb were interested in describing the behavioral changes that could accompany a hypothetical model of the progress of most diseases. They proposed six stages including (1) health; (2) asymptomatic disease susceptible to detection; (3) symptomatic disease not yet diagnosed; (4) manifest disease at the time of diagnosis; (5) course of disease as influenced by treatment; and (6) disease after therapy (i.e., cure, chronic state, or death). The focus was on describing and validating the behavioral roles adopted by an ill person. These included not being held responsible for incapacity, exemptions from normal social obligations, and expectations that one will try to get better. Using "role" as a central concept, four behavioral stages of health and illness were described: (1) adequate performance in usual roles; (2) diminished capacity for such performance and preparing to enter the sick role; (3) adopting the sick role; and (4) leaving the sick role.

Although Kasl and Cobb were interested in what health behaviors and preventive measures individuals engage in, until recently, most of the research has focused on preventive health behavior as defined by health care professionals. The study of the relationship between a given set of variables, for example, race, socioeconomic status, and locus of control and the performance of such health behaviors represented much of the early research in the area. The most common health prevention behaviors studied were those in which direct contact with health care professionals occurred; these included physical and dental examinations, immunization, and prenatal care. Most recently, other aspects of health behavior have been studied; these included compliance with prescribed medical regimens, which we shall discuss in more detail in a later section, and beliefs about health, and actual health behaviors of individuals not in contact with health care professionals. For instance, Berg (1976) stressed that most people are aware of what preventive health behaviors "should" be engaged in and often indicate that they would like to engage in such behaviors as exercise and sound nutrition. However, for various reasons, individuals continue their harmful habits. Berg notes that perception of illness and appropriate action may be different for different individuals and may represent important factors in understanding health behavior.

An alternate approach that does not focus on medically approved health behavior has been proposed by Harris and Guten (1979). Here it is assumed that all individuals engage in some behaviors intended to protect their health, medically sanctioned or not or objectively effective or not. Harris and Guten identified these behaviors, their dimensions, and their relation to actual health status. Essentially, the question their research addressed was What do people actually do in the belief that these behaviors facilitate health? These activities were termed *health protective behavior* (HPB) and defined as "any behavior performed by a person, regardless of his or her perceived or actual health status, in order to protect, promote, or maintain his or her health, whether or not such behavior is objectively effective toward that end." In an attempt to clarify this construct, Harris and Guten set out to identify activities an individual performs in the belief that they protect his or her health. Second, they asked "Are there patterns of relations among these activities?" "How can one determine empirically the dimensions of HPB?" Third, since the performance of HPB is not limited to asymptomatic persons (as is Kasl and Cobb's health behavior), they asked whether the nature and dimensions of HPB vary by health condition. Finally, they attempted to determine whether the health belief model, which will be described in a subsequent section, relates to HPB. Since HPB implies that individuals engage in this behavior to protect health, variables in the health belief model, which emphasizes the role of perceptions on health behavior, should be related systematically to HPB.

Harris and Guten conducted an exploratory study using 1,250 randomly chosen residents in the Greater Cleveland area. Of the 1,250 chosen respondents, 842 provided usable interview data; thus, there was a 67% completion rate. Thirty-three percent of the respondents were between the ages of 18 and 34, 35% between 35 and 54, and 32% were 55 or older; 46% were male and 25% were non-white.

The three sets of variables assessed included HPB, health condition, and health belief model variables. Health protective behavior was operationalized using two different approaches. First, respondents were asked "What are the three most important things you do to protect your health?" Responses to this question were coded by general categories determined after reviewing a sample of the replies. Table 8-2 lists the categories.

The second approach utilized a 30-item card-sort developed for the study. Each card had written on it "In order to protect my health, I (various health behaviors)." The respondent was asked to first sort through the cards and discard the ones that did not apply. Only items sorted as "almost always" engaged in were scored as part of the respondent's HPB repertoire. Health condition measures were elicited through self-report. Measures of health belief model variables consisted of questions intended to assess the respondent's concern over health matters in general; perceived vulnerability to sickness; perceived effects of illness; perceived probability that action will reduce threat of illness; and questions on sex, race, age, income, and education. The results of the study indicated that almost all the respondents practiced some type of HPB. Table 8-3 shows the percent distribution of the various behaviors. Over 70% reported HPBs related to general nutrition (specific foods eaten; how and when they ate). This is the only activity reported by the majority. The next most frequent (46%) were reports on behaviors concerning how, when, how long, or how frequently the respondents slept, rested, and relaxed. Thirty-six percent reported behavior related to exercise or physical activity and recreation. These three most frequently reported health behaviors involved everyday health habits rather than contact with health care professionals. However, one out of five re-

**TABLE 8-2**
Categories of Activities Performed to Protect Health

| Activity category | Percentage |
|---|---|
| Nutrition; foods; eating conditions | 71.3 |
| Sleep; rest; relaxation | 46.1 |
| Exercising; physical activity; physical recreation | 35.5 |
| Contact with health system | 18.8 |
| Personal hygiene or dress | 14.5 |
| Psychological, mental, or emotional well-being | 12.6 |
| Watching one's weight | 9.7 |
| Avoiding or limiting tobacco use | 8.8 |
| Use of medication | 7.8 |
| Alcohol use | 6.8 |
| Other physical activity | 5.6 |
| General environment | 5.1 |
| Home, work, or neighborhood environment | 3.1 |
| Intake of substance other than food, medicine, or alcohol | 2.4 |
| Other | 0.5 |

Note. From "Health-Protective Behavior: An Exploratory Study" by D. M. Harris and S. Guten, 1979, *Journal of Health and Social Behavior*, 20, 19. Copyright 1979 by the American Sociological Association. Adapted by permission.

spondents (18%) reported behaviors in which contact or compliance with the health care system occurred.

In order to identify the dimensions of HPB as measured by the card-sort, cluster analysis was performed. The cluster analysis indicated five clusters of HPB named by these investigators as (1) *health practices—* sleeping enough, relaxing, eating sensibly, exercising in moderation, avoiding overwork, avoiding chills, limiting certain food, and watching weight; (2) *safety practices—*repairing things, checking the condition of things, having a first-aid kit, and posting emergency phone numbers; (3) *preventive health care—*physical and dental checkups; (4) *environmental hazard avoidance—*avoiding areas of crime and pollution; and (5) *harmful substance avoidance—*no smoking or drinking. In terms of good versus poor health, the results suggest that HPB does not vary substantially by health condition. In general, those individuals classified as being in good, moderate, or poor health did *not* display considerable differences in HPB.

Finally, the results of the study indicate that the health belief model variables are only moderately predictive of selected HPB scales, and, in general, correlations were quite weak. *Preventive health care* behaviors were affected by sex, race, income, education, satisfaction with health, perceived vulnerability, and health condition. *Health practices* were af-

**TABLE 8-3**

Distribution of Behaviors to Protect Health

| Behavior | Percentage |
|---|---|
| Eat sensibly | 66.0 |
| Get enough sleep | 66.0 |
| Keep emergency phone numbers near the phone | 65.9 |
| Get enough relaxation | 56.4 |
| Have a first aid kit in home | 53.1 |
| Destroy old or unused medicines | 52.3 |
| See a doctor for a regular checkup | 51.1 |
| Pray or live by the principles of religion | 47.5 |
| Avoid getting chilled | 47.4 |
| Watch one's weight | 47.0 |
| Do things in moderation | 46.4 |
| Get enough exercise | 46.0 |
| Avoid parts of the city with a lot of crime | 41.2 |
| Don't smoke | 41.1 |
| Check the condition of electrical appliances, the car, etc. | 40.0 |
| Don't let things "get me down" | 39.3 |
| Fix broken things around home right away | 39.2 |
| See a dentist for a regular checkup | 36.6 |
| Avoid contact with doctors when feeling okay | 35.3 |
| Spend free time out of doors | 33.7 |
| Avoid overworking | 33.0 |
| Limit foods like sugar, coffee, fats | 31.9 |
| Avoid over-the-counter (OTC) medicines | 30.2 |
| Ignore health advice from lay friends, neighbors, relatives | 29.0 |
| Take vitamins | 24.1 |
| Don't drink | 24.0 |
| Wear a seat belt when in a car | 22.8 |
| Avoids parts of the city with a lot of pollution | 21.5 |
| Discuss health with lay friends, neighbors, relatives | 17.1 |
| Use dental floss | 15.9 |

Mean = 40.0; Median = 39.7

Note. From "Health-Protective Behavior: An Exploratory Study" by D. M. Harris and S. Guten, 1979, *Journal of Health and Social Behavior, 20*, 20. Copyright 1979 by the American Sociological Society. Adapted by permission.

fected by age, income, education, perceived vulnerability, health condition, and perceived control over a cold. *Safety practices* were affected by race, health satisfaction, and, to a lesser extent, age. In general then, health belief model variables influence the number of various kinds of health practice, safety practice, and preventive care behaviors performed. Also, no one variable is predictive of behavior in all three areas.

This study shows what individuals rather than professionals consider health behaviors. It was exploratory in nature and limited by the lack of a clear definition of what respondents mean or actually *do* when they report engaging in particular HPBs (e.g., what foods do they eat or avoid when they say they eat sensibly). Also, the need for a finer analysis of HPB and health status would appear warranted. Although it appears that this work calls into question the validity of *health behavior* in affecting ultimate health status (subjects classified as in good, moderate, or poor health did *not* display considerable differences in HPB), it must be emphasized that this study was not a prospective study. Also, there is a need for greater specificity with regard to type of health behaviors and their relationship to various illnesses. When this specificity approach is considered, health behavior factors (e.g., exercise, diet, no smoking) and physical illness (e.g., coronary heart disease) are significantly related. We will discuss the relationships for such disorders as coronary heart disease in later chapters.

Another approach to understanding health and risk behaviors is the one taken by Hunt, Matarazzo, Weiss, and Gentry (1979), on learning and habit. *Habit* is defined as a stable pattern of behavior marked by associative learning as well as reinforcement. Several examples are provided to demonstrate how the above definition of habit applies to issues of health acquisition and maintenance. Relapse rates of groups of individuals abstinent following treatment for certain addictive behaviors, including tobacco, alcohol, and heroin addiction, indicate that 75% of the subjects backslide by the end of three months, with a sharp leveling off between the third and sixth months; 25% remain abstinent. Hunt *et al.* (1979) hypothesizes that the relatively sharp bend in the curve depicted in Figure 8-2 as it approaches asymptote suggests that the curve might actually be the composite of two overlapping but different functions. One function is represented by the rapidly declining portion of the curve, the other by the asymptote portion. Assuming that two functions are present, Hunt *et al.* suggest that two kinds of individuals exist (those who can quit versus those who cannot) or that two levels of learning occurs. These authors argue that two types of learning—reinforcement and associative—are involved in the acquisition and maintenance of health behavior.

Hunt *et al.* (1979) cite a study that indicated the reason people give for smoking, in retrospect, often contradicts their daily diary reports at the actual time of smoking. For instance, individuals who state they smoke because of the tension-relieving properties of smoking actually reported in their diaries few instances of smoking in response to externally caused tension (Mausner & Platt, 1971). Also, Schachter (1973) noted Nesbit's paradox—in which subjects claiming to smoke to relieve tension actually showed physiological responses indicative of arousal. A

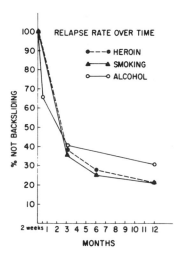

**FIGURE 8-2.** Relapse rate for addictive behaviors following treatment. From "Associative Learning, Habit and Health Behavior" by W. A. Hunt, J. D. Matarazzo, S. M. Weiss, and W. D. Gentry, 1979 *Journal of Behavioral Medicine, 2*(2), 113. Copyright 1979 by Plenum Publishing Corporation. Reprinted by permission.

final source of evidence comes from the alcohol literature, in which increased levels of alcohol ingestion led to *increased* levels of anxiety and depression in diagnosed alcoholics (McNamee, Mello, & Mendelson, 1968), as well as in non-alcoholic drinkers (Logue, Gentry, Linnoila, & Erwin, 1978), although such findings depend on a number of factors (Pohorecky, 1981). These findings have been interpreted as supporting the idea that some behaviors are determined by a cognitive or an attitudinal set, rather than by the reinforcing properties of the response itself. An alcoholic may "reach for the bottle" when upset with his wife, believing that a drink will relax him, when the effects are actually punishing. Such an effect is not in accordance with reinforcement principles. Furthermore, they propose that the reinforcement process may be short-circuited when habits become automatic and are maintained at a simple, immediate stimulus–response level. An example of this theory as applied to a specific habit is one in which a smoker, working at his desk, with a severe head cold, may respond to an open package of cigarettes by automatically reaching out, taking one, lighting it, and beginning to smoke. However, if his nose becomes irritated from the smoke, he then becomes aware of his behavior and will put the cigarette out, disengaging the pattern of smoking behavior. These automatic behaviors are commonly viewed as independent of their consequences, making them difficult, if not impossible, to extinguish, and respond to an appropriate signal or cue (Kimble & Perlmutter, 1970).

In summary, Hunt *et al.* (1979) define habit as "a pattern of behavior that is characterized by automaticity, diminished awareness, and potential independence of reinforcement." A habit is involuntary and gives the individual speed, stability, and economy in responding to his or her environment. A habit can be "good" or "bad," depending on its end result. Thus, in defining health behaviors, a habit is healthful if it contributes directly to the overall physical health of the person. Examples of health behaviors that can become "good habits" are the relaxation response, physical exercise, and proper nutrition.

We have now discussed several definitions of health behaviors. Hunt *et al.* explain health behaviors in terms of associative and reinforcement theories. The explanation acknowledges the complexity of habits, yet generates testable hypotheses. Harris and Guten's (1979) definition of health behavior emphasizes the importance of what most people consider health activities rather than what health care professionals recommend. Keeping these definitions in mind, let us now examine variables that influence the occurrence of health behavior.

## FACTORS INFLUENCING HEALTH BEHAVIOR

Although most of us are familiar with the need to engage in preventive health behaviors as discussed earlier, few of us actually do (Berg, 1976). Consider, as an example, the following description of a day in the life of an average North American male:

*After rising from a night's sleep, assisted by over-the-counter sleeping pills because of difficulty sleeping as a result of increased caffeine consumption while watching the World Series on TV, Mr. Jones sat down to a breakfast of bacon, eggs, and coffee, entered his car, lit a cigarette, and drove to work along with hundreds of others (it took him 40 minutes to travel 20 miles). While driving to work, he experienced chest pains and a slight lightheadedness. He drove to his underground parking space (polluted with carbon monoxide), then took the escalator to the main elevator of his large office building into which he had to squeeze along with 15 others, five of whom were smoking, despite the no smoking sign. He finally arrived in his office, lit a third cigarette, picked up a cup of coffee, and began to work. After sitting all morning, he decided to go out for lunch. Lunch consisted of a corned beef sandwich, french fries, and cheese cake. He returned to work and sat in his office the remainder of the day. In mid-afternoon, he again experienced pains in his chest, which he ignored. After work, he took the elevator and escalator down to his car, drove home in rush-hour traffic, and entered a house full of screaming children. He ate a large dinner and sat down in front of the TV with a cup of coffee and a piece of chocolate cake. His day was over at 12:30 A.M., and he again experienced difficulty falling asleep. The next day was no different, although he may not have experienced chest pains. Despite recurrent chest pain, Mr. Jones refuses to visit a doctor for an evaluation. Why?*

How can these behaviors, including the failure to seek diagnosis for an unexplained symptom, be accounted for? Particularly, how can one explain the absence of health behavior? Is Mr. Jones prevented from engaging in health-related behavior because of cost, time, etc.? Is there something about Mr. Jones' sociocultural background that reduces the probability of him seeking health care? What are Mr. Jones' perceptions of his symptoms and how do these perceptions motivate health behavior? These are the issues we will address in this section: What factors influence health behavior?

A number of studies have demonstrated that, despite removing what may be considered general barriers to treatment, such as providing free service, transportation, babysitting facilities, convenient location, and convenient hours, individuals continue *not* to use the health care services they need. Early explanations for this lack of compliance had focused on such *demographic* variables as age, race, socioeconomic status, and ethnicity. This research simply resulted in descriptions of populations that did and did not comply with medical regimens. The findings have been contradictory, and knowing who did not comply did not lead to an explanation of health behavior. In addition, from a practical perspective, these demographic variables are static; one cannot modify race, sex, or age, and therefore these descriptions do not easily translate into intervention. Consequently, the research focus shifted to *structural* variables, especially the characteristics of the therapy or medical regimen recommended. These structural variables include (1) economic costs of following the regimen, (2) whether the regimen requires short-term or long-term action, (3) complexity of the regimen, and (4) whether what was required is prescribed (practicing new behaviors) or proscribed (avoiding certain behaviors or consequences). Not surprisingly, it was found that compliance is lowest where the required behavior has high economic cost (absence from work), must be maintained for long periods of time, involves a complex medical regimen, and necessitates proscribed (avoidance) behaviors, such as avoiding enjoyable foods or alcohol. Unfortunately, prevention and treatment of chronic disease tends to involve all these barriers; therefore, it is not surprising that low rates of adherence are associated with treatment of such diseases. Nevertheless, certain individuals do comply with these treatment procedures. What are the factors that appear to be related to complying with or engaging in health behavior?

## The Health Belief Model

Initially proposed by Rosenstock (1966) and revised by Becker and Maiman (1975), the health belief model is one of the few models available that attempts to explain health behavior and/or compliance. It must be emphasized that this so-called sociobehavioral compliance model is simply a working system for generating and testing hypotheses regarding health behavior. See Figure 8-3 for a diagram of the health belief model.

Most of the research supporting the relationship between the various components of the model is correlational, not causative. The model proposes that the individual's subjective state of readiness to take action and engage in health-related behaviors, relative to a particular health condition, is a function of several factors. An individual's beliefs or perceptions of his or her likelihood of susceptibility to an illness and the perception of the probable severity of the consequences of having the illness represent major aspects of the model. Consequences can be both social and physical. A second factor is the perceived benefit of the action, in contrast to the perceived barrier to acting. Thus, a person's evaluation of the health behavior, both in terms of its gains or potential benefits in reducing the possible susceptibility and/or severity, as well as possible costs or barriers in terms of physical, psychological, or financial distress, are important in determining whether a person will engage in a given health behavior. A third factor involves access to cues for action. Cues to action are stimuli that trigger appropriate health behaviors. Cues can be either internal, that is, perception of bodily states, or external, that is, stimuli from the environment, such as interpersonal interactions or the mass media. Becker and Maiman also emphasize that the three factors listed above can be influenced by demographic and psychosocial factors. Thus, diverse demographic, ethnic, and social factors, as well as personality, can, in any given instance, influence health motivations and perceptions, and thereby indirectly influence the occurrence of health behaviors.

The health belief model has been useful in predicting both health behavior before illness, such as screening for cancer, and health behavior during an illness, such as compliance to medical regimens or prescribed therapies. Therefore, both preventive and sick-role behaviors can be predicted. It has been argued by Becker and others that this model also provides a useful framework for intervention. Becker suggests that by assessing which components are below a level presumed necessary for compliance for a given patient, the health care professional may be able to individualize an intervention to suit the particular needs of the patient. For example, if the individual perceives himself as susceptible, and the disease he has is quite serious, but if he simply lacks cues to action by family members, perhaps the physician can stimulate the family to motivate the patient to act. In this case, the family may need to remind the patient to keep on a diet or continue an exercise program.

A detailed review of the evidence in support of the various compo-

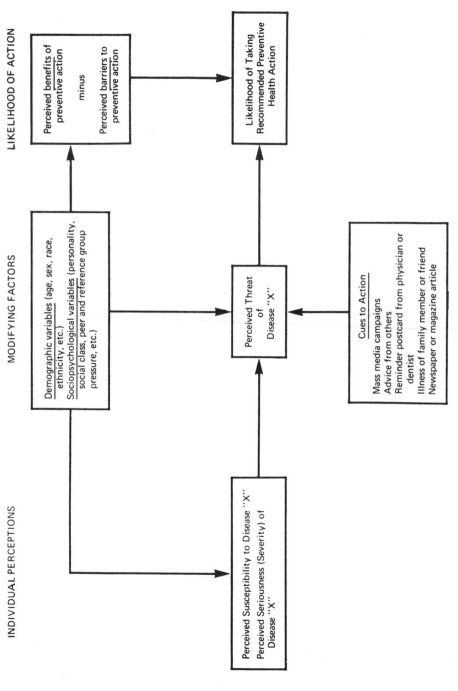

**FIGURE 8-3.** Health belief model. From "Sociobehavioral Determinants of Compliance with Health and Medical Care Recommendations" by M. H. Becker and L. A. Maiman, 1973, *Medical Care, 13,* 12. Copyright 1973 by J. B. Lippincott, Co. Reprinted by permission.

nents of the health belief model can be found in two papers by Becker and Maiman (1975) and Becker, Haefner, Kasl, Kirscht, Maiman, and Rosenstock (1977). A brief summary of supporting evidence for the various components is presented here.

*Perceived Susceptibility.* A number of retrospective and prospective studies of health behavior have reported positive correlations between relatively higher levels of subjective vulnerability and compliance to various health-related behaviors. These include medical screening for cervical, breast, and other cancers and tuberculosis, heart disease, and Tay Sachs disease; obtaining immunizations; and following an accident-preventive measure. These findings, however, are not consistent across all types of health behavior. For instance, high susceptibiles were not more likely than low susceptibiles to make preventive dental visits (Suchman, 1967). If we consider compliance to a medical regimen, there is some evidence that higher rates of compliance to treatment are associated with perceptions of recurrent susceptibility. For example, mothers who felt their child was "susceptible to a disease" because the child had previously had it or was often ill had higher rates of compliance (Elling, Whittemore, & Green, 1960).

*Perceived Severity.* Even if a person recognizes a susceptibility to a given illness, the person may not engage in health-related behavior unless there is also the perception that serious organic and/or social problems will occur. The health belief model emphasizes the individual's perceptions, rather than the medical or some other objective estimate of severity of illness. The research literature indicates that there is no association, or even a negative association, between medical opinion of severity and patient compliance. Thus, the model focuses on the predictive power of the patient's *perception* of severity of illness. There is some evidence to support the conclusion that individuals who perceive that incurring an illness will have serious effects will comply with recommended health behaviors involving dental care, preventing accidents, and seeking care in response to symptoms. However, no significant relationship has been found between perceived severity and participation in several types of screening (genetic screening) and immunization programs. Results related to perceived severity are more mixed than are those for susceptibility. For the individual without symptoms, very low levels of perceived severity are not sufficient to motivate the person to act, whereas very high levels of perceived severity and fear are *inhibiting*. In terms of clinical implications, then, threat is generally not effective. In summary, although the results of studies on perceived severity and acceptance of preventive health recommendations are mixed, the patient's estimates of the seriousness or severity of the illness in question are consistently predictive of compliance with medical recommendations. The actual presence of symptoms will probably produce a different situation, as experience of symptoms may elicit a more realistic appraisal of illness severity. It is often reported that once the patient begins to feel better or experiences fewer or less intense symptoms, he or she will discontinue compliance with the medical regimen prescribed.

*Perceived Benefits and Costs.* The relative benefits and costs of engaging in behaviors to reduce health threats is another factor that must be considered. Even if an individual perceives a high degree of susceptibility and severity of an illness for himself, a perceived payoff will need to be present in order to motivate the person to act. For example, Kegeles (1969), in a field experiment on a cervical cancer screening program, indicated that women who complied were more likely to believe that a physician or test could detect cervical cancer, that a test could reveal illness before the appearance of symptoms, and that early detection would lead to a more favorable prognosis. Other studies showed that the perceived efficacy of treatment led to subsequent compliance with preventive behaviors, such as immunization, as well as accepting treatment. In regard to barriers, fear of pain and monetary expense appear to be associated with noncompliance to preventive dental care. Other negative effects or barriers that have been studied and appear to be important in compliance include cost, extent to which new behaviors must be adopted (particularly if the patient is experiencing interpersonal or employment problems), complexity, duration, and other side effects.

*Modifying Factors.* Demographic, structural, attitudinal, interactional, and enabling factors are examples of modifying variables included in the health belief model. These represent factors that may indirectly promote or discourage health behavior. Some specific examples that have been studied and appear to be related in a positive direction to compliance are a patient–practitioner relationship in which there is good communication; a regular physician; social pressure and social group conformity; and influence of friends and family. Such factors appear to influence obtaining immunizations, undertaking fitness-exercise programs, and continued abstinence from cigarette smoking. Compliance is not consistently related to the demographic variables of sex, intelligence, education, or marital status. Noncompliance and medication errors are more likely in age extremes. The very young are less likely to ingest bad-tasting pills, whereas the very old may forget to take medication on schedule or forget that they have already taken medication.

Although no single study has provided (or could provide) definitive evidence for the health belief model, several studies of the various components of the model have produced internally consistent results in the predicted direction. When taken together, the results support this model in understanding factors influencing health-related behaviors. In a revision of the health belief model (Becker *et al.*, 1977), "motivation" was emphasized, as depicted in Figure 8-4. Motivation, or the desire or intention, to comply has been examined in several studies. Also, positive health motivation may exist and account for positive action. For example, mothers with high social mobility desires for their child and who were concerned about being "good" mothers gave their children special food and vitamins, owned a fever thermometer, and were more likely to follow a medical regimen for their child than were other mothers (Becker, Drechman, & Kirscht, 1972).

Additional research is required to validate the health belief model. Suggestions include (1) research in different settings (clinic versus physician's office), with different population groups, and with such long-term therapies as diet, smoking, exercise, and rehabilitation programs; (2) studies examining the stability of the predictive effects of psychosocial variables over time; and (3) studies on the origins of health and illness beliefs or the conditions under which they are acquired. If this information were available, it might be possible to mitigate or modify the health beliefs of children and thus minimize later psychological barriers to potentially beneficial services and behaviors. Last, there is a need for additional research directed at enhancing health behavior by modifying elements in the proposed model.

## The Conflict Theory Model

The conflict theory model, which will now be described, is another model that attempts to explain health behavior and/or compliance. It may be seen, in some ways, as an alternative to the health belief model although several similarities exist between the two models. A dramatic change has occurred in recent years in the perception of the patient's role as that of a passive recipient of health care, humbly following the doctor's orders. The patient is now seen as becoming an ever-increasingly active decision maker, influencing the type and course of treatment through a process of crucial decision making. The conflict theory model of personal decision making, unlike the health belief model, attempts to specify the conditions under which individuals "will

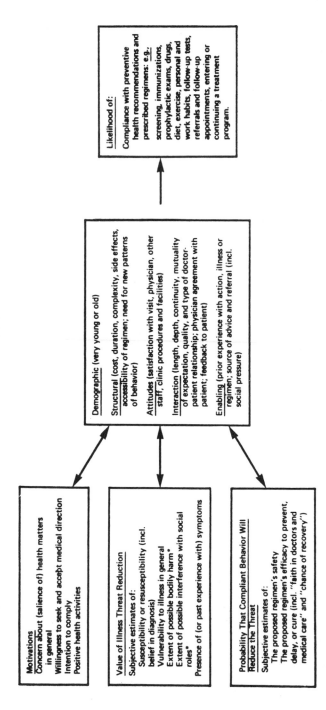

**FIGURE 8-4.** Role of motivation in the health belief model. From "Selected Psychosocial Models and Correlates of Individual Health-Related Behaviors" by M. H. Becker, D. P. Haefner, S. V. Kasl, J. P. Kirscht, L. A. Maiman, and I. M. Rosenstock, 1977, *Medical Care, 15* (Suppl. 5), 39. Copyright 1977 by J. B. Lippincott. Reprinted by permission.

give priority to avoiding subjective discomfort at the cost of endangering their lives, and under what conditions they will make a more rational decision by seeking out and taking into account the available medical information about the real consequences of alternative courses of action so as to maximize their chances of survival" (Janis, 1984, p. 332). Janis and Mann (1977) have delineated five stages that individuals go through in order to arrive at a stable decision. These five stages (Table 8-4) were identified through observing individuals who made health decisions that they subsequently carried out successfully; these included giving up smoking, losing weight on a low-calorie diet, or contemplating a series of recommended medical treatments.

As indicated in Table 8-4, Stage 1 represents the beginning of the decision-making process. The individual's current course of action is challenged. A challenge may take the form of an event or communication that conveys a threat or an opportunity. The individual now faces the task of making an active decision about it—either to ignore or reject the challenge, which would result in the continuation of the status quo, or to accept the challenge, and progress to the next stage of active decision making.

Once the present course of action is challenged, an effective decision maker will initiate Stage 2 wherein he or she will carefully consider the goals relevant to the decision and look for available alternatives that are viable in accomplishing these goals. Thoughout Stage 3, the person will evaluate the pros and cons of each alternative and may seek out

### TABLE 8-4
Stages in Stable Decision Making

| Stage | Key questions |
| --- | --- |
| 1. Appraising the challenge | Are the risks serious if I don't change? |
| 2. Surveying alternatives | Is this (salient) alternative an acceptable means for dealing with the challenge?<br>Have I sufficiently surveyed the available alternatives? |
| 3. Weighing alternatives | Which alternative is best?<br>Could the best alternative meet the essential requirements? |
| 4. Deliberating about commitment | Shall I implement the best alternative and allow others to know? |
| 5. Adhering despite negative feedback | Are the risks serious if I *don't* change?<br>Are the risks serious if I *do* change? |

*Note.* From *Decision Making: A Psychological Analysis of Conflict, Choice, and Commitment* (p. 333) by I. L. Janis and L. Mann. Copyright 1977 by The Free Press, a Division of Macmillan, Inc. Adapted by permission.

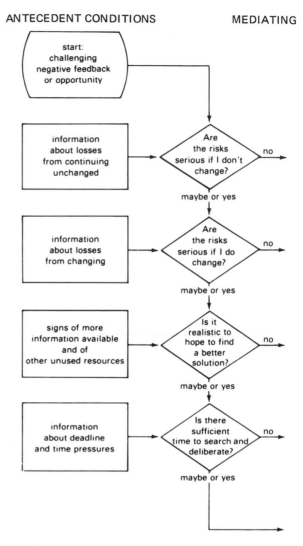

ANTECEDENT CONDITIONS                    MEDIATING

**FIGURE 8-5.** Conflict theory model of coping patterns. From *Decision Making: A Psychological Analysis of Conflict, Choice, and Commitment* by I. L. Janis and L. Mann. Copyright 1977 by The Free Press, a Division of Macmillan, Inc. Adapted by permission.

information regarding all the possible consequences of the alternatives under consideration. Based on all the information gathered, the individual will then reach a tentative decision as to which course of action to follow. Stage 4 sees the decision maker becoming increasingly committed to the new course of action as he or she informs interested parties of

PROCESSES                          CONSEQUENCES

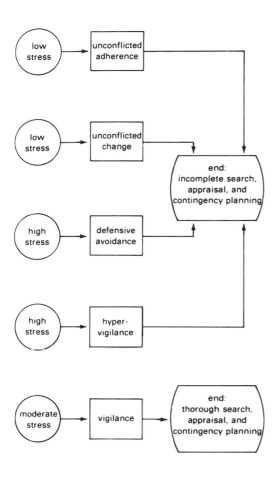

their decision. At this stage, the individual re-examines all the information gathered, works out the best way to implement the decision, and
makes contingency plans in case he or she incurs any losses. Finally, at
Stage 5, the decision maker discounts any potential new challenge, such
as threats or opportunities, remains only temporarily shaken, and continues with the task of implementing the decision.

According to the assumptions of the conflict theory model, the determinants of effective decision making can be seen as those that influence the type of coping style adopted by the decision maker to deal with decisional conflict. In this framework, the coping style used by the decision maker is determined by either the presence or absence of the following conditions: (1) arousal of conflict as the result of an awareness of serious risks for whichever alternative is chosen, (2) hope of finding a better alternative, and (3) a belief that there is time to seek out alternatives and to evaluate them before a decision is required. Figure 8-5 illustrates the determinants of the five coping patterns for an individual confronting a realistic challenge.

Janis and Mann (1977) postulate that only when the individual's coping pattern is *vigilance* will he or she be able to make a rational choice based on weighing the benefits of a recommended course of action against the perceived costs of or barriers to taking that action. The remaining four coping patterns (unconflicted adherence, unconflicted change, defensive avoidance, hypervigilance) are considered defective and are characterized by behaviors that are maladaptive when the challenge consists of symptoms of a serious disease or a warning by a physician that the illness may worsen if the decision maker procrastinates in seeking out medical treatment. If only one of these four maladaptive coping patterns is dominant, the decision maker will be unsuccessful in going through the required tasks of the four stages to reach a decision. An advantage of the conflict theory model is that it has testable implications regarding the effects of environmental circumstances and interventions that could counteract the beliefs responsible for maladaptive coping styles.

## COMPLIANCE: A CASE IN POINT

Patient noncompliance, or the lack of adherence to medical therapies, is a significant problem in health care. Compliance is a problem that is clearly behavioral; thus, health care professionals are beginning to realize the importance of the social sciences in the detection and alleviation of compliance problems. The magnitude of the problem is considerable, with at least one-third of the patients in most studies failing to comply with doctor's orders. Estimates of noncompliance range from 4% to 92%, and average from 30% to 35%.

From a biomedical perspective, the label "noncompliance" for patients usually implies that they are ignorant, lazy, or willfully neglectful. The label "noncompliant" permits differentiation of the noncompliant person from the compliant person. The health care provider may be unaware of the antecedent environmental conditions for a patient's symptoms, his or her decision to seek treatment, and also the failure to comply with treatment. Thus, the physician may not realize that symptoms may be as prevalent in those patients not seeking help as in those who seek help. Also, he or she may not perceive the purpose of the patient's visit correctly. Such a misperception may then result in inaccurate judgments regarding the likelihood and the determinants of noncompliance.

*Theoretical Considerations.* The *behavioral* approach to the problem of compliance avoids attributing the role of personality characteristics to noncompliant individuals; rather, it focuses on the environmental conditions promoting *adherence* to a structured treatment program (Stunkard, 1979). For example, in the case of evaluating adherence to a weight reduction program for obese individuals, the questions of interest to the therapist may be frequency, quantity, and type of food eaten; stimuli preceding eating; nature of eating response (slow versus rapid); the consequence of eating (how the individual feels after eating). Despite the contribution of the behavioral approach to dealing with problems of compliance, the difficulty in achieving *long-term adherence* has resulted in the need for new components to behavioral programs. Such components have included providing patients with booster sessions (Levine, Green, Deeds, Chwalow, Russell, & Finley, 1979) and social support systems (Levy, 1980). Until now, however, most behavioral attempts to resolve the problem of long-term compliance have mainly concerned themselves with the addition of cues, increasing environmental restrictions or improving the match between subjects and particular therapies (Leventhal & Cleary, 1980), rather than with examining the most effective way to integrate behavioral change into an individual's long-term life-style.

A more recent approach views the problem of adherence to behavioral medical regimens in terms of *control* or *systems* concepts (Carver & Scheier, 1982; Nerenz & Leventhal, 1983). Control theory, as applied to health or illness behavior, emphasizes that the individual creates his or her own representation of health threats and subsequently decides on a course of action relative to such a representation (Leventhal, Meyer, & Nerenz, 1980). Several factors may affect the individual's representation of a current illness episode or a future illness threat and may include information from the media, friends, health professionals, and family members and feedback from symptoms and bodily sensations. The course of action undertaken depends on both the nature of the representation and at least three other factors: (1) self-esteem or sense of self-efficacy, (2) ability to relate to problem situations and to test the effectiveness of response alternatives, and (3) fund of specific coping responses and belief in the effectiveness of these responses (Becker & Maiman, 1975; Mischel, 1973).

Whether individuals view the situation or problem as manageable is determined to a large extent by their sense of self-efficacy and self-esteem. This means that they believe that they can manage the environment and their own behaviors, as well as their own emotional reactions. Such a belief in the ability to view the problem as manageable elicits a specific coping response that is appraised for its effectiveness in meeting specified goals (Folkman & Lazarus, 1980; Leventhal & Nerenz, 1983). If such a response is, in fact, effective in achieving these goals, the behavior can be stopped or maintained at the same level of output. If, however, the coping response is ineffective, the individual will engage in a new behavior or modify the old behavior. Last, the third component of a self-regulative or self-control system is outcome appraisal. The strategy an individual uses to appraise the response, the representation of the problem, or the sense of self-efficacy is seen as either effective or ineffective (Marlatt & Gordon, 1980). Based on the principles of control theory, therefore, predictions may be made regarding a long-term self-regulative action. A behavioral treatment would need to provide the patient with an opportunity to learn the components of a self-regulation system (representation, coping, and appraisal of outcomes), as well as allowing the patient to see it as his or her own. Such self-regulation would have to make sense in the individual's total life context (Antonovsky, 1979).

Several studies have indicated that physicians underestimate the rates of noncompliance in their practice and are inaccurate in identifying noncompliant individuals. Even when noncompliance is recognized, the traditional response has been ineffective. In one study, 67% of senior physicians attributed noncompliance to the patient's "uncooperative personality," 26% thought the doctor himself could be responsible, and 40% blamed the patient's inability to understand the recommendations. Some physicians faced with noncompliance take the following steps, usually in the order indicated: (1) complete explanation of the regimen, such as "All you have to do is take this red pill three times a day and this white one four times per day"; (2) persuasion by rational argument, for example, "You'll die if you don't . . ."; (3) threat tactics, "You better or else . . ."; and (4) withdrawal from the case or referral. However, a number of studies have indicated that (1) either acquisition of knowledge or change in attitudes or both does not ensure health behavior change; (2) arousal of fear in a patient can evoke behavior that is opposite to that desired; and (3) withdrawal from a case will set negative expectations for the next physician. Because of the significance of the problem, research has been directed at two major goals. The two major areas of interest are identification of factors that predict compliance behavior and development of approaches or techniques to facilitate compliance.

*Factors Affecting Compliance.* Studies on the identification of factors that predict compliance behavior have focused on psychological characteristics of the person, such as attitudes and perception of illness and health behavior; environmental factors, such as family instability or living alone; the therapeutic regimen itself, such as complexity of the treatment or the types of behavior one must engage in (giving oneself injections of insulin); and, finally, physician–patient interaction. Some of these factors have been discussed in earlier sections; for instance, the physician–patient interaction appears sometimes to be important, although some studies show no relationship to therapeutic compliance (Davis, 1968; Kasl, 1975). In terms of the therapeutic regimen, it seems that the more complex or lengthy, the less likely the person will engage in the recommended behaviors. In terms of family instability and environmental factors, there is no clear picture of what factors are important to patient compliance. Davidson (1982) cites several studies that indicate no relationship between therapeutic compliance and the following factors: education, socioeconomic status, family interactions, distance to site of treatment, or diagnosis.

What seems to provide some initial information on factors predicting compliance behavior is the research examining attitude and perceptions of the patient, particularly within the context of the health belief model described in the previous section. For example, one study investigated the usefulness of the health belief model in predicting non-compliance with a prescribed regimen for chronic hemodialysis patients (Hartman & Becker, 1978). Fifty patients with end-stage renal disease had to follow a complex medical regimen of diet and fluid restriction, medication, and time-in dialysis. Measures of compliance were obtained for six observations, three before an interview and three after, using weight gain between dialysis treatments, serum phosphorus levels, and serum potassium levels as indices of compliance. "Compliance" was defined as whether the patient, across all six observations, was compliant more often than not. With an equal number of compliant and noncompliant scores, the patient was rated "intermediate." Information on the patient's attitudes and perceptions were obtained in a personal interview. The interview was designed to gather patients' perceptions of their state of health and other factors designed to operationalize belief dimensions of the model. A seven-point scale was generally used to rate attitude. Hartman and Becker's findings are summarized in Table 8-5. The results indicate that the health belief model appears to be useful in

TABLE 8-5

Summary of Variables Significantly Related to Compliance Behavior in End-stage Renal Disease and its Treatment.[a]

| Concern | Barriers |
|---|---|
| • General health concern (E) | • Medications |
| • Worry about kidney disease (P/W/E) | P-binder side-effects (P) |
| • Worry about sequelae of non-compliance (All) | Complexity of instructions (P/W) |
| • Worry about ability to comply (P/E) | Difficulty in following (W/K/E) |
| Susceptibility | • Difficulty in following *all* instructions (E) |
| • Likelihood of incurring sequelae of non-compliance (All) | • Satisfaction with instructions (W/K/E) |
| • Estimates of future health (P/W/K) | Self-evaluations |
| Severity | • Locus of control |
| • Seriousness if non-compliance sequelae occurred (P/W) | General (P/K) |
| Benefits | Health-specific (P/K/E) |
| • Medications | • Willingness to adopt sick role (E) |
| Phosphate binder (P/W/K) | • Frustration (K/E) |
| All medications (P/E) | • Social support |
| How close to "do OK" (P/E) | Family problems (W/E) |
| • Diet | Assistance from spouse (P/W/E) |
| Benefit (All) | • Self-report of compliance |
| How close to "do OK" (P/K/E) | Medication (All) |
| • Fluid limit | Diet (W/K/E) |
| Benefit (W/K/E) | Fluid (All) |
| How close to "do OK" (All) | All instructions (All) |
| • How close to *all* instructions to "do OK" (P/K/E) | Wears medic alert tag (All) |
|  | Sociodemographic variables |
|  | • Age (P/K/E) |
|  | • Sex (P/E) |
|  | • Marital status (W/E) |
|  | • Length of time on dialysis (All) |

*Note.* From "Non-Compliance with Prescribed Regimen among Chronic Hemodialysis Patients" by P. E. Hartman and M. H. Becker, 1978, *Dialysis and Tranplantation, 7*(10). Copyright 1978 by Creative Age Publications. Adapted by permission.
[a]Each variable is evaluated as a predictor of compliance with respect to the phosphate-binding medication (P), weight gain between treatments (W), potassium level (K), the subjective overall evaluation (E), and across all measures (All).

predicting compliant behavior in end-stage renal disease and its treatment. Measures of each of the major dimensions of the model (susceptibility, severity, benefits/barriers, self-evaluation, and socioeconomic variables) were shown to be useful predictors of therapeutic compliance. Hartman and Becker (1978) described the type of patient *less* likely to comply as follows:

> This patient is less worried about personal health matters in general and about his kidney disease in particular. Although concerned about being able to carry out all of the instructions and about potential vulnerability to the

consequences (including poorer health in the future), he still maintains that it would not be very serious if he were to experience the sequel of non-compliance during the next week. The poor complier also exhibits less faith in the value of every aspect of the therapy, feels that one can "do okay" and still not follow the medication, diet and fluid regimen closely, and sees a variety of barriers (difficulty, complexity, side effects) to compliance with the dialysis staff's instructions (with which he is relatively less satisfied) . . . self-perception . . . include tendencies toward adopting an external (fatalistic) orientation concerning ability to control life events, toward becoming easily frustrated, and toward willingness to derive secondary gain from being sick . . . more likely to be young, female, unmarried, to have relatively less social support, and to have been under dialysis treatment for a shorter period. (pp. 982–983)

Although many studies of psychological predictors of compliance focus on the patient's beliefs and perceptions, some take a more traditional approach and attempt to measure the patient's psychological functioning through the use of psychological tests and questionnaires. The Minnesota Multiphasic Personality Inventory (MMPI), the Rorschach Inkblot Test, the Thematic Apperception Test, or the Beck Depression Inventory are some of the tests that may be used. An example of how one would study psychological variables using this method is given in an investigation in which physiological and psychological variables among patients entering a structured cardiac rehabilitation program were assessed to determine whether a relationship between these variables and noncompliance existed (Blumenthal, Sanders, Wallace, Williams, & Needles, 1982). Patients recovering from myocardial infarction can increase functional work capacity and reduce risk factors associated with recurrent infarction by participating in a graduated program of exercise conditioning. These exercise programs are readily available; however, compliance rates are low, ranging between 13% and 60%.

The Blumenthal et al. study included 35 patients, 32 men and 3 women, aged 36 to 70 years (mean, 53.7) who had experienced a myocardial infarction one to six months before entering the exercise program. For each patient, physical assessment, individual measures of blood pressure, body weight, serum lipids, treadmill testing, and pars radionuclide angiography in an upright position at rest and during maximum exercise in a standing bicycle ergometer were used to assess cardiac dysfunction. Left ventricular ejection fraction (LVEF), the fraction of the end-diastolic volume ejected with each heart beat, was used in the analyses. Psychological assessment included the MMPI, using the ten standard clinical scales and three experimental scales (anxiety, repression, ego strength). In terms of physiological factors, noncompliance was associated with significantly lower left ventricular ejection fractions, suggesting that the noncompliant patient had sustained larger infarcts.

However, there was no difference between drop-out and compliant cases in the change in ejection fraction from rest to exercise. Other physiological variables distinguished compliant cases from drop-outs, including self-report of activity at entry of the program, age, weight, blood pressure, and serum lipids. Functional work capacity was only slightly lower, and MMPI data indicated that noncompliance can be distinguished from compliance in terms of psychological functioning. Noncompliers were more depressed, anxious, and concerned about health, and had lower ego strength. The multivariate analyses revealed that LVEF, ego strength, and social introversion scores on the MMPI were statistically significant in predicting noncompliance. Low ego strength, which was characteristic of the noncompliers, suggests deficits in self-restraint, environmental mastery, and cognitive capacities that limit a person's ability to deal with life events that are stressful. Social introversion, which drop-outs tended to score high on, indicate uncomfortableness in social interactions and withdrawal from social situations. Blumenthal *et al.* (1982) suggest that subjects who dropped out of the program did so because the program included working with others in groups and required motivation to master and cope with stress, characteristics these noncompliant subjects were deficient in.

In summary, the research investigating the predictive value of attitudes, perception, and psychological functioning has contributed to an understanding of compliance. The perceptions and attitudes of individuals, as proposed by the health belief model, appear to be useful in the prediction of compliance. The exact nature of the relationship between these attitudes and compliance remains to be specified. Problems to be encountered include differences in definition and measurement of "compliance." The definition of compliance can vary greatly, from keeping an appointment to injecting oneself 3,000 times with insulin for several years. Most studies have relied on self-report of patient compliance, although biomedical, psychological, and behavioral measures are now being used to a greater extent.

*Clinical Intervention.* The second major area of interest in compliance is the development of approaches and techniques to facilitate compliance. Approaches to the management of noncompliance include patient education, accommodation, modification of environmental and social factors, changes in therapeutic regimen, and enhancement of provider–patient interaction. At present, certain conclusions regarding the effective management of compliance can be made and include the following approaches:

1. *Education.* Patient education can have an impact if it is an active type of education rather than a passive one, in which the patient is the

recipient of information. Examples of active educational strategies include the use of self-help books and tapes.

2. *Accommodation.* This approach attempts to deal with the personality characteristics that appear to hinder compliance. For example, an autonomous patient is made to feel he or she is an active participant in treatment. For an anxious or fearful patient, reassurance and other techniques are used to reduce fear and anxiety to levels that can be constructive in motivating him or her to follow advice. If the anxiety level is too high or too low, the patient will be less likely to comply.

3. *Modification of environmental and social factors.* Social support can be created by enlisting family and friends. Significant others can provide cues for, as well as learn to reinforce, compliant behaviors. The establishment of problem-oriented groups or peer groups can be helpful in providing encouragement and motivation and in establishing new attitudes. Groups can be designed for compliance of various medical regimens, such as a weight reduction group, a diabetic group, and a stop smoking group.

4. *Changes in therapeutic regimen.* The regimen can be made as simple as possible, and the patient should be involved in designing it. If patient input is used, a realistic program can be designed. Compliance from the patient's view represents a series of trade-offs in which the patient gives up or takes on certain behaviors in return for promised benefits. The patient's compliance can be shaped by first having him or her follow simple components of the therapy regimen and reinforcing success, then gradually adding the other components of the regimen.

5. *Enhancement of physician– or health professional–patient interaction.* Tactics health professionals can utilize to increase compliance are to avoid flat rejection of the patient's wishes and provide the patient with feedback after eliciting historical and diagnostic information. Patients have a great need for explanations about the nature of their condition, its cause, and the therapeutic measures undertaken. For example, a patient with chronic headache (migraine type) may wonder if he or she has a tumor or whether something is wrong with his or her brain. An explanation of why migraines occur and how the medication prescribed will help may increase a belief in treatment efficacy and, consequently, medication compliance. And finally, clear explicit communication in words the patient or caretaker can understand facilitates compliance, particularly if it is written down so that the patient can refer to it.

Let us look at a clinical study of specific ways to facilitate compliance or health behavior in a particularly resistant group of patients (Baile & Engel, 1978). In a small clinical series, Baile and Engel evaluated the effect of a behavioral strategy for promoting treatment compliance following myocardial infarction in seven men. These men were referred by nursing staff and house staff of the cardiac care unit because of their recent and past compliance problems. These patients not only had a recent and past history of noncompliance, but they also tended to deny the occurrence of infarct and, therefore, treated their problem lightly. They also possessed a high degree of job involvement, expressing urgency to return to work.

The treatment strategy involved three phases. The first phase consisted of having the patient self-plan a rehabilitation program that included an activity hierarchy. The second phase involved self-monitoring of biobehavioral data. The patient was instructed to record symptoms before and after activity. Self-monitoring of symptoms included recording shortness of breath, chest pain, fatigue, and heart rate. The third phase consisted of weekly feedback visits to review the data and to decide on what new activities to begin. The program lasted 12 to 23 weeks, depending on patient progress.

Compliance rates with the rehabilitation program ranged from 86% to 100%. Compliance was assessed with heart rate monitoring and patient diaries of activities in which they recorded required tasks performed. Only one patient missed one appointment; all the other patients kept their appointments for the rehabilitation program and the general medical clinic. The authors suggest that the rehabilitation program was effective for several reasons. First, the health care system returned control to the patient. Second, the program was task-oriented and kept patients "doing things" in a period when certain aspects of their behavioral repertoire needed to be restricted. Third, there was frequent positive reinforcement for engaging in the program, including the surprise and delight reported by many patients over the fact that their pulse rates did not jump during activities and returned to baseline during rest (a sign that they were progressing). Fourth, the weekly visits provided support and encouragement when patients became discouraged about their progress. And fifth, the therapeutic regimen was individualized, and there was a great deal of interaction with the health care professionals. This strategy may be useful with overcomplainers as well as individuals who become so distressed by their myocardial infarction that they overly restrict their behaviors, retarding progress. The behavioral data can reassure such cases that they can extend their range of activities without "injuring their heart."

As a case in point, the study of compliance demonstrates the complexity of investigating issues related to health behavior. In order to assess a person's likelihood of engaging in health behavior, one must consider attitudes and perceptions of health and illness; interaction with family, peers, and medical professionals; the type of illness; and the complexity and duration of the medical regimen the patient must follow.

Consider our fictitious Mr. Jones. What is the likelihood he will call his physician for a checkup after his next episode of chest pains? If he is seen, and if his physician informs him that currently he is not suffering from any medical problem, but is at risk for developing heart disease and must begin to lose weight, eat proper foods, and abstain from smoking, what is the likelihood that he will begin engaging in health behavior? What are some suggestions you can provide to help Mr. Jones to acquire and comply with behaviors recommended by his physician?

## DIABETES: A CHALLENGE IN COMPLIANCE

Compared to most other diseases, the complexity of the treatment regimen for the diabetic patient constantly challenges the health practitioner, as well as the patient. The substantial amount of responsibility placed on the patient for treatment is often the cause of much distress and often results in noncompliance. This section will provide examples of the type of approaches used to enhance the diabetic's adherence to self-measurement of blood glucose level and to dietary requirements.

Education of the patient as to the nature of diabetes and its treatment has commonly been used to encourage adherence. Evidence as to the effectiveness of an educational approach to adherence in the diabetic patient is limited (Sackett & Haynes, 1976), and research in this area is complicated by the fact that patients with poor metabolic control may receive the greater education. The lack of evidence that educational programs increase adherence has led clinicians to utilize behavioral approaches that focus on increasing self-care behaviors. One area in which such approaches have been applied is in the self-measurement of blood glucose (SMBG) in the treatment of Type I diabetes. The most accurate measurement of SMBG levels below the renal threshold is through the use of test strips with reagent-impregnated pads. Typically, the patient obtains a whole blood sample with a finger prick and places the sample on the strip, where a glucose-oxidase/peroxidase reaction measures glucose concentration in the blood. The immediate feedback from SMBG allows patients to monitor blood glucose control and increases their awareness of the effects of different behaviors on blood glucose (Walford, Gale, Allison, & Tattersall, 1978). The positive relationship between frequent SMBG and improvements of blood glucose control have been reported by Gardner, Mehl, Eastman, and Merimee (1983), yet many patients find it difficult to perform this demanding procedure over a long period of time.

Several behavioral procedures have been utilized to increase patient's adherence to SMBG. Carney, Schechter, and Davis (1983), for example, found that a contingency management program implemented by parents using a point system and praise contingent on SMBG increased the frequency of measurement. Following four months of treatment, two out of three youths who had previously been nonadherent were testing close to 90% of the targeted frequency and showed improved metabolic control. Goal setting and behavioral contracting have also been found to promote SMBG in juveniles (Epstein, Figueroa, Farkas, & Beck, 1981b). Finally, frequent contact with health care professionals (i.e., telephone calls) appears to have a positive influence on patient adherence to SMBG and insulin adjustments (Schafer, Glasgow, & McCaul, 1982).

The role of diet in the treatment of diabetes is well established (American Diabetes Association, 1979). The importance of dietary adherence in patients with Type I and Type II diabetes has further been reported in a review of recent studies in which behavior modification has been used to improve adherence to dietary goals (Wing, Epstein, & Nowalk, 1984). In a study by Epstein, Beck, Figueroa, Farkos, Kazdin, Daneman, and Becker (1981a), a traffic-light diet was used in a sample of adolescents with Type I diabetes. The traffic-light technique utilizes a diet in which foods are divided into red (stop!) foods to be avoided; yellow (caution!) foods to be eaten in moderation; and green (go!) foods to be eaten without any restriction. The emphasis in this study was the reduction of red foods consumed, with no restriction placed on yellow or green foods. Intake of red foods was continously monitored by the subjects throughout the program, and they were awarded points for compliance. In addition to dietary adherence, the program emphasized exercise, insulin adjustment, and compliance with urine monitoring. Epstein *et al.* found that although blood sugar measurement and glycosylated hemoglobin were not affected, the treatment program did increase the number of negative urines obtained.

The role of dietary adherence has also been studied in patients with Type II diabetes, which is commonly associated with obesity. In view of such a relationship, it may be considered pertinent to apply behavioral weight control techniques to diabetic patients. In a study by Rabkin, Boyko, Wilson, and Streja (1983), for example, 40 adult Type II diabetic patients were randomly assigned to either individual counseling or a behavior modification program. Patients in individual counseling were seen by a nutrition counselor for an initial 1-hour session and then six weeks later for a 15-minute session. Patients were required to reduce their caloric intake by 500 to 1000 calories by means of an individualized meal plan. The behavioral condition consisted of weekly small group meetings for six consecutive weeks and was run by the same nutrition counselor. Included in the behavioral program were self-monitoring of caloric intake and stimulus control techniques for changing the home environment. The findings from the study show that weight losses were greater for the individual counseling patients then for the behavior modification patients, both at the 6-week and the 12-week follow-up. Significant reductions in fasting blood sugar from pretreatment to the 12-week follow-up were noted for both groups, although no significant differences between the two groups were found.

In summary, although there is some evidence on the effectiveness of behavioral techniques to increase adherence to treatment in diabetic patients, there is a need for further refinement of such techniques as contingency management and contracting in SMBG and of cueing, self-monitoring, and reinforcement in improving dietary adherence. It is also apparent, considering recent theoretical and empirical work on mechanisms of health behavior, that the current clinical approaches do not address the range of possible factors influencing health behavior. Further, interventions based on such knowledge should prove more effective. General guidelines with potential for maximizing clinical effectiveness are discussed in the following section.

## MODIFYING HEALTH BEHAVIOR

The modification of health-related behaviors is one of the prerequisites for preventing major chronic disease and hastening recovery. Stopping cigarette smoking, for instance, directly reduces the risk of coronary heart disease, many respiratory diseases, and certain types of cancer. An obese hypertensive individual who changes to a diet low in saturated fats, decreases his or her sodium (salt) intake, and regularly uses antihypertensive medication should reduce the risk of developing cardiovascular disease, including stroke.

Jenkins (1979) has provided guidelines to deal with the problems of health-related behavior. Before an effective treatment plan is implemented, information regarding the problem of health-related behavior at hand needs to be gathered. The suggested steps to arrive at a behavioral diagnosis and the design of a treatment plan for a health-related behavior would consist of a full description of the problem, its history (e.g., duration of failure of adherence), assessment of current psychosocial dynamics of the health behavior (e.g., lack of correct health beliefs or misinformation resulting in inhibition of performance), a behavioral diagnosis, design of a treatment plan in cooperation with the recipient, and an evaluation of the effectiveness of the plan for behavior change.

According to Jenkins, it is necessary to change the health regimen and elements of health-care delivery as one of the first steps to effective intervention. Such changes would take into consideration (1) providing continuity of personalized medical care; (2) changing the patient's expectations of treatment or attempting to meet them; (3) maximally simplifying the health regimen; (4) providing health knowledge sufficient to operationalize the recommended behavior and support it; (5) communicating to the patient and his or her significant other(s) the importance of the health behaviors and motives; (6) maximizing the rewards for the prescribed health-related behavior, including devising new rewards; (7) minimizing the "costs" potentially associated with "being a patient" or maintaining the health regimen, that is, expenditure of time and effort, experience of negative feelings, reduction of self-esteem; (8) gradually easing the patient into the medical regimen, and finally; (9) instilling in the patient a sense of personal responsibility for his or her own health maintenance. This type of approach emphasizes the patient's active *informed participation* in his or her medical care.

Identification of the obstacles to health-promoting behavior is made from the behavioral diagnosis. If, for instance, the patient lacks appropriate information or has an incorrect belief system, the task of the health provider is to facilitate successful communication by two-way interchange or a multi-way discussion. Another obstacle to appropriate health behavior may be lack of sufficient motivation on the part of the patient. The health care provider may then need to activate the patient's social support systems to provide the patient with group motivation for behaviors for which individual motivation was previously insufficient. Skill deficits are yet another potential obstacle to engaging in appropriate health behaviors. The patient may need to be taught a variety of skills and tactics to help him or her maintain the desired behavioral changes. Such a learning process should include a program of self-monitoring, goal-setting, and contracting; opportunities for frequent feedback, support, and positive reinforcement; a training program for the spouse or family members to provide positive encouragement; development of a self-reward system; stimulus control of the environment; modeling of correct health behaviors by the health provider; guided participation, self-presented consequences, and cognitive strategies (e.g., patients are encouraged to practice imagining the positive consequences of adhering to the health regimen and the negative consequences of not adhering); and last, training in systematic desensitization and relaxation. A final step in dealing with the obstacles to adherence may be to change the balance of rewards and costs associated with following the recommended health behaviors.

## HEALTH RISK ASSESSMENT AND PROMOTION

The increasing interest in health promotion has prompted the development of assessment instruments aimed at encouraging the modification of life-style parameters. The health hazard/health risk appraisal (HHA/HRA) is one such health promotion technique that compares an individual's health-related behaviors and personal characteristics to mortality statistics and epidemiological data. The goal of the HHA/HRA is to estimate the individual's risk of developing some illness or dying by some specified future time, along with the amount of that risk that could be eliminated by making appropriate behavioral changes. Once these measurements of risk are ascertained, the individual is presented with these findings as well as with the potential benefits of behavioral changes to motivate activities aimed at changing life-style and improving health. The rise in popularity of the HHA/HRA has been attributed to several factors (Wagner, Beery, Shoenbach, & Graham, 1982). First, this instrument may serve as a teaching aid to stimulate discussions of health and behavior. In view of its reliance on self-report questionnaires, simple physiological measurements (e.g., blood pressure, cholesterol level), and computer-assisted calculations, it can also be readily administered to large groups at relatively low cost. Further, it reflects the current thinking and publicity on the role of life-style in disease etiology. Finally, the type of data-gathering devices, computer software, and other aspects of the program can be easily marketed as a package, which has, in turn, attracted the interest of commercial firms.

Little evidence is currently available for how well HHA/HRA motivates individuals for behavioral change. One of the first large-scale studies evaluating the utility of the health hazard appraisal (HHA) was reported by Rodnick (1982). A HHA and a counseling session were conducted for 292 employees at a glass products company in Santa Rosa, California. As part of the program, the company offered its full-time employees a comprehensive health examination, which consisted of health history, weight, height, and blood pressure; SMA-17 (a blood chemistry panel including cholesterol, triglycerides, creatinine, calcium, protein, uric acid, fasting blood sugar, and liver enzyme levels); urine analysis; complete blood count; TB skin test; stool test; and screening physical exam, which included a Pap smear and a pelvic examination for women. The HHA was designed to use much of the above data to give the individual feedback in graphic form of their risk of dying from various causes (e.g., cardiovascular disease, accidents, specific cancers) over the next 10 years. Testing sessions were conducted on groups of 40 subjects over a period of 10 months at monthly intervals. Approximately two weeks after each testing, group meetings were held in which the health instructor interpreted for the group members their respective health risk profiles, based on the results of lab tests and HHA reports. These meetings lasted for one hour, and the participants also received educational pamphlets on hypertension, heart disease, and cancer. Any participant whose results appeared abnormal was advised to consult a physician and was later personally contacted by the plant nurse. A second testing session was conducted approximately one year later and involved essentially the same procedures. Results from this study show that there were significant changes in risk factors over the one-year period. These included (1) a decrease in blood pressure (particularly in individuals with mild hypertension); (2) reduction in cholesterol levels in men; (3) a decrease in cigarette smoking; (4) an increase in exercise (particularly in men and women who initially reported a sedentary pattern); (5) an increase in the number of women performing breast self-examination, as well as receiving physician breast examinations; (6) a decline in alcohol consumption among men; and (7) an increase in seat belt use by men. It would appear, therefore, from these findings that a health promotion program such as that reported by Rodnick (1982) and targeted at a high-risk population (middle-class, middle-aged, sedantary men who have a low rate of physician office visits) can bring about potentially beneficial effects in an occupational setting.

Despite the growing enthusiasm by health psychologists to assist in the promotion of life-style changes assumed to enhance and maintain health, the health benefits reasonably to be expected from behavioral programs designed to implement such changes need to be carefully evaluated. In a recent critical review of the field, Kaplan (1984) has identified several problems facing the clinical practice of health promotion, specifically with regard to four assumptions underlying many of the interventions used. First, the assumption that specific behaviors create risks for serious illnesses is debatable. Both the lack of empirical data and the presence of conflicting findings as to the relationship among dietary and exercise modifications, serum cholesterol levels, and prevention of heart disease provide one example in which such an assumption may be questioned. The earlier finding from the Framingham heart study suggesting that serum cholesterol was the best single predictor of heart disease has recently been disputed. In a major Italian study, for instance, Avogaro (1984) found that in a sample of survivors of myocardial infarctions, 75% of the heart attack victims had normal lipid-cholesterol patterns.

A second assumption made by clinicians involved in health promotion is that behavior and disease are positively correlated and that a subsequent modification of the risk-related behavior will reduce the incidence of the disease. Although plausible on the surface, this assumption is not consistently supported by empirical evidence. Kaplan points out that although it may hold true for certain types of behaviors (e.g., smoking, alcohol abuse) the assumption is not as well supported in the case of other risk factors, such as obesity. For example, much evidence indicates that obesity increases the risk of heart disease (Hubert, Feinleib, McNamara, & Castelli, 1983), yet a report by the Society of Actuaries (1959) claimed that total mortality rates are, in essence, lowest for individuals between −14% and +15% of ideal body weight. Further, in a review of 16 studies by Andres (1980) that examined the causal link between obesity and total mortality, there was no evidence to suggest that moderate obesity is a risk factor. Clearly, such inconclusive evidence for the correlation between risk-related behavior and incidence of disease warrants closer investigation.

A third assumption discussed by Kaplan regards the ease with which behavior is modified. Despite the claims of social psychologists and behaviorally oriented clinicians for the successful modification of certain risk-related behaviors, recent evidence indicates that many health behaviors are very hard to change. One of the main problems is that of adherence by individuals to prescribed treatment regimens (e.g., physical exercise in weight loss programs and relapse prevention in stop smoking programs). In general, the beneficial effects of behavioral interventions tend to be short term, with long-term maintenance of treatment gains currently remaining low. Continued evaluation of the long-term efficacy of specific behavioral intervention in modifying health behaviors is needed.

The fourth assumption presented by Kaplan relates to the cost-effectiveness of behavioral programs in health promotion. Kaplan and Bush (1982) suggest that the most reasonable approach to evaluating the effectiveness of health programs is to express the benefits derived from them in terms of extra years of life they produce. Adjustments may be made in the years of life figure to take into account diminished quality of life. An example of such an approach would be to view a program that improves the quality of life by 10% (or .1 units) on a 0 to 1.0 scale for 10 years as producing the equivalent of 1 life year. The use of such a general health outcome measure would clearly facilitate comparisons between different types of health programs.

A related issue raised by Kaplan was the frequent observation that although significant reductions in mortality from the specific disorder to which the risk reduction was targeted have been reported, differences between treatment and control groups in total mortality are not frequently observed. An example of such a finding is that observed in the coronary primary prevention trial. The study was a randomized experimental clinical trial in which high-risk men were either assigned to a cholestyramine (substance to reduce cholesterol) group or placebo group. Follow-up at ten years indicated that the cholestyramine had lowered cholesterol by an average of 8.5% and that the active drug group experienced 24% fewer heart disease deaths and 19% fewer heart attacks than the placebo group. However, a difference in *total* mortality between the groups was not observed. The total mortality rate for the treatment group was 1.6%, for the placebo group 2.0%. These findings question the value of such interventions, particularly if treatment is relatively aversive (cholestyramine is a grainy substance with an unpleasant taste) and costly ($150/month). The intervention, however, did reduce cardiovascular-related deaths. Clearly, health promotion/risk reduction is an area with much promise, despite its many complexities.

## SUMMARY

A recent focus on preventive health care has generated increased interest in the promotion of health behaviors. As a consequence the need to define what is meant by health and health behavior has become more critical. The first section of this chapter attempted to provide a definition of health behavior as distinguished from illness behavior and sick-role behavior. Examples of health preventive behaviors were discussed as they relate to the health belief model, and research examining acquisition of habits in the context of health behaviors was reviewed.

The next section provided a discussion of factors influencing health behavior. The health belief model and the conflict theory model were described to illustrate the potential role of social, psychological, and cognitive factors in explaining health behavior and/or compliance. The next section of the chapter focused on noncompliance or lack of adherence to medical therapies—a major problem in health care. In this area, the research evaluating behavioral approaches to promote adherence to health care regimens was reviewed. In order to illustrate the complexity of the compliance problem, the chapter focused on the case of diabetes and reviewed some of the research on strategies to facilitate compliance with treatment in the diabetic patient.

Finally, the last section of this chapter reviewed the modification of health-related behaviors and discussed health risk assessment and health promotion practices.

## REFERENCES

American Diabetes Association. (1979). Principles of nutrition and dietary recommendations for individuals with diabetes mellitus. *Diabetes Care, 2,* 520–523.

Antonovsky, A. (1979). *Health, stress, and coping*. San Francisco: Jossey-Bass.

Avogaro, P. (1984). Apolipoproteins, the lipid hypothesis and ischemic heart disease. In R. M. Kaplan & M. H. Criqui (Eds.), *Behavioral epidemiology and disease prevention* (pp. 49–59). New York: Plenum Press.

Baile, W. F., & Engel, B. T. (1978). A behavioral strategy for promoting treatment compliance following myocardial infarction. *Psychosomatic Medicine, 40*(5), 413–419.

Becker, M. H., & Maiman, L. A. (1975). Sociobehavioral determinants of compliance with health and medical care recommendations. *Medical Care, 13*(1), 10–24.

Becker, M. H., Drechman, R. H., & Krischt, J. P. (1972). Predicting mothers compliance with pediatric medical regimens. *Journal of Pediatrics, 81*, 843–854.

Becker, M. H., Haefner, D. P., Kasl, S. V., Kirscht, J. P., Maiman, L. A., & Rosenstock, I. M. (1977). Selected psychosocial models and correlates of individual health-related behaviors. *Medical Care, 15* (Suppl. 5), 27–46.

Belloc, N. B., & Breslow, L. (1972). Relationships of physical health status and health practices. *Preventive Medicine, 1*, 409–421.

Berg, R. L. (1976). The high cost of self-deception. *Preventive Medicine, 5*, 483–495.

Blumenthal, J. A., Sanders, W., Wallace, A. G., Williams, R. B., & Needles, T. L. (1982). Physiological and psychological variables predict compliance to prescribed exercise therapy in patients recovering from myocardial infarction. *Psychosomatic Medicine, 44*, 519–527.

Califano, J. A., Jr. (1979). *Healthy people: The Surgeon General's report on health promotion and disease presentation*. Washington, DC: Superintendent of Documents, U.S. Government Printing Office, Stock Number 017-001-00416-2.

Carney, R. M., Schechter, K., & Davis, T. (1983). Improving adherence to blood glucose testing in insulin-dependent diabetic children. *Behavior Therapy, 14*, 247–254.

Carver, C. S., & Scheier, M. F. (1982). Control theory: A useful conceptual framework for personality—social, clinical, and health psychology. *Pschological Bulletin, 92*, 111–135.

Davidson, P. D. (1982). Issues in patient's compliance. In T. Millon, C. Green, & R. Meagher (Eds.), *Handbook of clinical health physiology*. New York: Plenum Press.

Davis, M. S. (1968). Physiologic, psychosocial, and demographic factors in patient compliance with doctors' order. *Medical Care, 6*, 115–122.

Elling, R., Whittemore, R., & Green, M. (1960). Patient participation in a pediatric program. *Journal of Health and Human Behavior, 1*, 183.

Epstein, L. H., Beck, S., Figueroa, J., Farkas, G., Kazdin, A. E., Daneman, D., & Becker, D. (1981a). The effects of targeting improvements in urine glucose on metabolic control. *Journal of Applied Behavior Analysis, 14*, 365–375.

Epstein, L. H., Figueroa, J., Farkas, G. M., & Beck, S. (1981b). The short-term effects of feedback on accuracy of urine glucose determinants in insulin-dependent diabetic children. *Behavior Therapy, 12*, 560–564.

Folkman, S., & Lazarus, R. (1980). An analysis of coping in a middle-aged community sample. *Journal of Health and Social Behavior, 21*, 219–239.

Gardner, D. F., Mehl, T., Eastman, B., & Merimee, T. J. (1983). Psychosocial factors: Importance for success in a program of SGM. *Diabetes, 32*,(11) (Abstract).

Harris, D. M., & Guten, S. (1979). Health protective behavior: An exploratory study. *Journal of Health and Social Behavior, 20*(1), 17–29.

Hartman, P. E., & Becker, M. H. (1978). Non-compliance with prescribed regimen among chronic hemodialysis patients: A method of prediction and educational diagnosis. *Dialysis and Transplantation, 7*, 978–985.

Haynes, D. L., & Sackett, R. B. (Eds.). (1976). *Compliance with therapeutic regimens*. Baltimore: Johns Hopkins University Press.

Hubert, H. B., Feinleib, B. M., McNamara, P. M., & Castelli, W. P. (1983). Obesity as an independent risk factor for cardiovascular disease: A 26-year follow-up of participants in the Framingham Heart Study. *Circulation, 67*(5), 968–977.

Hunt, W. A., Matarazzo, J. D., Weiss, S. M., & Gentry, W. D. (1979). Associative learning, habit, and health behavior. *Journal of Behavioral Medicine, 2,* 111–123.

Janis, I. L. (1984). The patient as decision maker. In W. D. Gentry (Ed.), *Handbook of behavioral medicine.* New York: Guilford Press.

Janis, I. L., & Mann, L. (1977). *Decision making: A psychological analysis of conflict, choice, and commitment.* New York: Free Press.

Jenkins, C. D. (1979). An approach to the diagnosis and treatment of problems of health related behavior. *International Journal of Health Education, 22* (Suppl. 2), 1–24.

Kaplan, R. M. (1984). The connection between clinical health promotion and health status. A critical overview. *American Psychologist, 39*(7), 755–765.

Kaplan, R. M., & Bush, J. W. (1982). Health related quality of life measurement for evaluation research and policy analysis. *Health Psychology, 1,* 61–80.

Kasl, S. V. (1975). Issues in patient adherence to health care regimens. *Stress, 1,* 5–17.

Kasl, S. V., & Cobb, S. (1966a). Health behavior and illness behavior: I. Health and illness behavior. *Archives of Environmental Health, 12,* 246–266.

Kasl, S. V., & Cobb, S. (1966b). Health behavior; illness behavior, and sick role behavior: II. Sick role behavior. *Archives of Environmental Health, 12,* 531–541.

Kegeles, S. S. (1969). A field experimental attempt to change beliefs and behavior of women in an urban ghetto. *Journal of Health and Social Behavior, 10,* 115–124.

Kimble, G. A., & Perlmutter, L. C. (1970). The problem of volition. *Psychological Review, 77,* 361–384.

Leventhal, H., & Cleary, P. D. (1980). The smoking problem: A review of the research and theory in behavioral risk-reduction. *Psychological Bulletin, 88,* 370–405.

Leventhal, H., & Nerenz, D. (1983). A model for stress research and some implications for the control of stress disorder. In P. Meichenbaum & M. Jaremko (Eds.), *Stress prevention and management: A cognitive behavioral approach.* New York: Plenum Press.

Leventhal, H., Meyer, D., & Nerenz, D. (1980). The common-sense representation of illness-danger. In S. Rachman (Ed.), *Medical Psychology* (Vol. 2). New York: Pergamon Press.

Levine, D. M., Green, L. W., Deeds, S. G., Chwalow, J., Russell, R. P., & Finlay, J. (1979). Health education for hypertensive patients. *Journal of the American Medical Association, 241*(16), 1700–1703.

Levy, R. L. (1980). The role of social support in patient compliance: A review. In R. B. Haynes, M. E. Mattson, & T. O. Engebretson (Eds.), *Patient compliance to prescribed antihypertensive medical regimens: A report to the National Heart, Lung, and Blood Institute.* Bethesda, MD: National Heart, Lung and Blood Institute.

Logue, P. E., Gentry, W. D., Linnoila, M., & Erwin, C. W. (1978). The effect of alcohol consumption on state anxiety changes in male and female nonalcoholics. *American Journal of Psychiatry, 135,* 1079–1081.

Marlatt, G. A., & Gordon, J. R. (1980). Determinants of relapse: Implications for the maintenance of behavior change. In P. O. Davidson, & S. M. Davidson (Eds.), *Behavioral medicine: Changing health lifestyle.* New York: Brunner/Mazel.

Matarazzo, J. D. (1983). Behavioral health: A 1990 challenge for the health sciences professions. In J. D. Matarazzo, N. E. Miller, S. M. Weiss, & J. A. Herd (Eds.), *Behavioral health: A handbook of health enhancement and disease prevention.* New York: Wiley.

Mausner, B., & Platt, E. S. (1971). *Smoking: A behavioral analysis.* New York: Peragamon Press.

McNamee, H. B., Mello, N. K., & Mendelson, J. H. (1968). Experimental analysis of drinking patterns of alcoholics: Concurrent psychiatric observation. *American Journal of Psychiatry, 124,* 81–87.

Mischel, W. (1973). Toward a cognitive social learning reconceptualization of personality. *Psychological Review, 80,* 252–283.

Nerenz, D. R., & Leventhal, H. (1983). Self-regulation theory in chronic illness. In T. Burish & L. Bradley (Eds.), *Coping with chronic disease: Research and applications.* New York: Academic Press.

Pohorecky, L. A. (1981). The interaction of alcohol and stress: A review. *Neuroscience and Biobehavioral Reviews, 5*(2), 209–229.

Rabkin, S. W., Boyko, E., Wilson, A., & Streja, D. A. (1983). A randomized clinical trial comparing behavior modification and individual counseling in the nutritional therapy of non-insulin-dependent diabetes mellitus: Comparison of the effect on blood sugar, body weight, and serum lipids. *Diabetes Care, 6*(1), 50–56.

Rodnick, J. E. (1982). Health behavior changes associated with health hazard appraisal counseling in an occupational setting. *Preventive Medicine, 11,* 583–594.

Rosenstock, I. M. (1966). Why people use health services. *Milbank Memorial Fund Quarterly, 44,* 94.

Schachter, S. (1973). Nesbitt's paradox. In W. C. Dunn, (Ed.), *Smoking behavior: Motives and incentives.* Washington, DC: Winston.

Schafer, L. C., Glasgow, R. E., & McCaul, K. D. (1982). Increasing the adherence of diabetic adolescents. *Journal of Behavioral Medicine, 5,* 353–362.

Society of Actuaries. (1959). *Build and blood pressure study* (Vols. 1 & 2). Chicago: Society of Actuaries.

Stunkard, A. J. (1979). Behavioral medicine and beyond: The example of obesity. In O. F. Pomerleau & J. P. Brady (Eds.), *Behavioral medicine: Theory and practice.* Baltimore, MD: Williams & Wilkins.

Suchman, E. A. (1977). Preventive health behavior: A model for research on community health campaigns. *Journal of Health and Social Behavior, 8,* 197.

Wagner, E. H., Beery, W. L., Schoenbach, V. J., & Graham, R. M. (1982). An assessment of health hazard/health risk appraisal. *American Journal of Public Health, 72*(4), 347–352.

Walford, S., Gale, E. A., Allison, S. P., & Tattersall, R. B. (1978). Self-monitoring of blood glucose. Improvement of diabetic control. *Lancet, 1*(8067), 732–735.

Wing, R. R., Epstein, L. H., & Nowalk, M. P. (1984). Dietary adherence in patients with diabetes. *Behavioral Medicine Update, 6*(1), 17–21.

# ILLNESS BEHAVIOR

## CLINICAL VIGNETTES

The following clinical vignettes (Pilowsky, 1978) illustrate the range of behavioral response to illness that is possible.

> A 40-year-old female is admitted to a surgical ward complaining that she has coughed up blood. Her right leg is somewhat swollen and painful. While in the ward she produces further amounts of blood in her sputum and complains of pains in her chest. A diagnosis of deep vein thrombosis with pulmonary embolism is made and a decision taken to ligate the right iliac vein. At operation, the surgeon, to his surprise, finds that the vessel had

already been ligated at a previous operation. The patient later admits that she simulated the illness and at an interview tells of long-standing feelings of depression related to rejection by her mother. (p. 131)

A 50-year-old man being treated for Hodgkin's disease stops taking all medications. He insists that he is perfectly well and that this realization has been vouchsafed to him by some superior force. After treatment in a psychiatric ward he is gradually able to accept the reality of the situation and resumes his treatment program. His physical condition is in fact under excellent control. (p. 131)

*In 1964, Norman Cousins, former editor of* Saturday Review, *flew home from a trip abroad with a slight fever and achiness. Within a week, it became difficult for him to move his neck, arms, fingers, and legs. He was hospitalized and his sedimentation rate (a measure of collagen disease) was found to be 80 mm per hour; it subsequently climbed to 115. He continued to experience difficulties moving his limbs and even turning over in bed. Nodules appeared on his body, gravel-like substances under the skin, and, at the low point of his illness, his jaws almost locked. He had been stricken with a collagen disease—diagnosed as ankylosing spondylitis. A specialist indicated that Cousins had one chance in 500 for recovery. Cousins reports, "All this gave me a great deal to think about. Up to that time, I had been more or less disposed to let the doctors worry about my condition. But now, I felt a compulsion to get into the act. It seemed clear to me that if I was to be that 'one case in 500,' I had better be something more than a passive observer" (Cousins, 1976). Working with Selye's model of stress and illness, Cousins began considering what effect positive emotions would have on his body chemistry. He also had read that vitamin C helps oxygenate the blood. Believing that he could stand pain as long as he knew progress was being made in meeting the basic need of restoring his body's connective tissue, he asked his physician to consider the following treatment plan:*

1. *Discontinue all pain-killing medications*
2. *Administer large doses of vitamin C*
3. *Deep belly laughter or recreation of the positive emotions (Cousins chose to watch Candid Camera films.)*

*His physician agreed to the plan. Cousins found that 10 minutes of genuine belly laughter had an analgesic effect and would result in two hours of pain-free sleep. It was also noted that this laughter affected his sedimentation rate. Following each laughter episode, there was a drop of at least 5 points. The drop itself was not significant, but it was stable and cumulative. The vitamin C therapy was associated with a drop of 9 points. He continued with laughter and vitamin C therapy for 8 days, at the end of which he was able to move his thumb without pain. The sedimentation rate was in the 80s and dropping fast, and the gravel-like nodules on his neck were shrinking. He was now convinced that he was going to make it back all the way. Two weeks later, he was in Puerto Rico recovering. It was a slow recovery. His neck was limited in its turning radius, his knees were wobbly, and he occasionally had to wear a brace, but he was soon back at his job at the* Saturday Review.

Considering the illness behaviors described above, one wonders what an adaptive, or normal, response to illness is. What is illness behavior? What can be considered abnormal? What factors help explain the variations observed in response to illness? This chapter will present definitions of illness behavior and describe the etiological factors that may contribute to abnormal and/or chronic illness behavior. Finally, the modification and prevention of illness behavior are discussed.

## DEFINITIONS

### Illness Behavior

Sociology has played a particularly important role in the study of the concept of *illness behavior*. One of the more widely accepted definitions of illness behavior is that of Mechanic, (1978a), a sociologist, who concluded that illness may be thought of in two ways: *Illness* can refer to "a limited scientific concept or to any condition that causes or might usefully cause an individual to concern himself with his symptoms and to seek help" (p. 249). Illness behavior, then, refers to any behaviors relevant to the second interpretation of illness. Mechanic was particularly interested in the subset of illness behaviors that involves help-seeking and in behaviors that lead up to contact with a health care provider, as well as why some people seek help and others do not.

Mechanic described several determinants of illness behavior. In general, these determinants involve the perception and salience of the symptoms, the disruptive and persistent nature of the symptoms, individual needs and the available alternate interpretations of the symptoms, and treatment availability and cost. He also noted that the determinants can operate at two different levels: other-defined and self-defined. *Other-defined* refers primarily to situations in which people other than the individual of interest evaluate that person's illness behaviors; this would most likely apply to children and psychotic persons. *Self-defined* refers to situations in which the individual perceives and evaluates his or her own symptoms. When self-defined and other-defined levels differ significantly, the individual of concern may be forced into treatment. The significance of Mechanic's discussion of illness behavior lies in the emphasis he placed on how cultural influences and social learning directly affect what illness behavior an individual will engage in. These determinants of help-seeking behavior, then, reflect the major decisions a person will make when choosing to seek or not seek help, and each decision will be influenced by cultural and social learning factors.

Mechanic's theory of help-seeking has not been adequately tested. One problem with his theory is that it does not include information on the independence of each of the determinants of illness behavior. Although the theory discusses the decision process of seeking or not seeking care, it only explains factors that lead to the inital contact with health care professionals. Another problem with Mechanic's definition of illness behavior is the use of the term *symptom*. *Symptom* suggests dysfunction. However, many people react with illness behavior when no pain, or other sign of organic malfunction, is reported. A good example of this is illustrated in the first vignette, in which the patient complained of pain and swelling in her right leg, although no organic malfunction was present.

## Sick Role

Parsons (1964) formulated the concept *sick role* in order to describe illness behavior without focusing on symptoms *per se*. Parsons believed that social roles are important for the maintenance of any society, but noted that there are times when a person cannot fulfill social roles adequately. When this occurs, society deals with this by allowing the individual to adopt a sick role. Parsons' sick role theory specifies the different types of behavior adopted by the sick person. There are four basic components to the sick role. The first component is the absence of responsibility for the condition. The patient's inability to perform social roles and associated tasks is not considered to be under that person's volitional control. It is understood that the person cannot simply decide to get well, but rather that some type of treatment or curative process is necessary before he or she can engage in expected social roles. Second, because the person is considered sick, he or she is exempt from performing social roles. The type of exemption depends on the severity and nature of the illness and continues only as long as the third and fourth components are present. Third, being sick is thought of as undesirable to the person. Because the sick role is undesirable, the person is obligated to seek help and cooperate with others to recover. Thus, although the person is exempt from social roles, there is the new responsibility of getting well *as soon as possible*. The fourth component is seeking adequate help. The person adopting the sick role must seek out and comply with the prescribed treatment. The individual usually sought out is a physician. In summary, the sick role entails a possible new benefit, the exemption from role obligations and tasks, and two new obligations, to return to a state of health by seeking out and complying with treatment.

A major criticism of Parsons' sick role concept is that it applies most readily to middle-class sick role behaviors; sick role behaviors in other cultures or subcultures may take different forms. There is also evidence that some social groups respond differently to illness (Zola, 1966). Zborowski (1952) reported different responses to pain among three different social groups (Jews, Italians, and second-generation, white Protestant Americans), finding that Jews and Italians were more sensitive to what were assumed to be the same level of pain associated with similar neurological ailments. Also, when patients returned home from the hospital, the Italian patients resumed their masculine and authoritarian behavior, whereas the Jewish patients continued to react very emotionally to the pain. This study illustrates that different social groups may evaluate the same symptoms differently, which determines the type of sick role behavior in the respective subculture.

A second major criticism is that although the sick role concept is applicable to easily identified or acute medical problems, it does not predict such role behavior for illnesses that are incurable, chronic, not easily identified, or not organically based. Parsons (1975) reported that for incurable illnesses, such as cancer or diabetes, the person must attempt to "manage" the illness so that he or she can engage in expected social roles. Although these criticisms elucidate potential problems, the sick role concept remains useful in emphasizing the sociological factors involved in illness.

Using the concept of Parsons' sick role, Pilowsky (1978) modified it by defining illness as "a state of the organism which fulfills the requirements of an appropriate reference group for admission to the sick role." An appropriate reference group is any social group most able or willing to underwrite the social cost of the sick role. This group may vary with the stage of the illness. In the early stages, the individual may underwrite the social cost, in the expectation that the illness is self-limiting (i.e., short lived). That is, at the onset of illness, the individual may adopt the sick role, deciding to rest until health is returned. However, if the illness is prolonged, it typically affects others, such as family, friends, and work associates and, subsequently, society. Therefore, these others play a role in sanctioning the sick role. Pilowsky further defines illness behavior as "the ways in which individuals *react* to aspects of their own functioning which they evaluate in terms of health and illness." Going one step further, he indicates that when an individual's illness behaviors do not follow the socially accepted sick role process, as in the case where illness behaviors are associated with an illness with no apparent organic cause or in cases in which the sick role is no longer adaptive, the term *abnormal illness behavior* must be applied.

### Abnormal Illness Behavior

A diagnosis of abnormal illness behavior (AIB) is made definitively by a physician. The physician may use such terms as *hypochondriac* or *conversion reaction* or may indicate to the patient that the problem is "all in your head" or related to "nerves." In whatever way the physician chooses to indicate AIB, the main message to the patient is that the sick role sought or adopted by the patient is not appropriate to the objective physiological pathology evaluated. More precisely, Pilowsky (1978) defines AIB as

> the persistance of an inappropriate or maladaptive mode of perceiving, evaluating and acting in relation to one's own state of health, despite the fact that a doctor (or other appropriate social agent) has offered a reasonably lucid explanation of the nature of the illness, and the appropriate course of management to be followed, based on a thorough examination and assessment of all parameters of functioning (including the use of special investigations where necessary), and taking into account the individual's age, educational and sociocultural background. (p. 133)

With this definition to guide him, Pilowsky developed a classification system of AIB. Table 9-1 lists the categories for syndromes that are characterized by a discrepancy between organic pathology and patient behavior. Note that Pilowsky considers both "illness-affirming" and "illness-denying" syndromes as equally important categories of AIB. Illness-affirming syndromes are disorders in which the patient becomes convinced of the disease underlying the disorder. In contrast, patients displaying an illness-denying type of syndrome either minimize or negate the existence of a significant illness. For example, the patient with chronic nonspecific gastrointestinal discomfort who, despite multiple medical assurances as to the benign nature of the symptom, continues to maintain he is suffering from cancer exemplifies the illness-affirming variant of abnormal illness behavior. On the other hand, the patient diagnosed as having lung cancer who refuses to visit his physican or to begin a stop smoking program because he attributes his cough to the dampness in the air, is engaged in illness-denying behavior.

An example of abnormal illness behavior can be found in a study by Lavey and Winkle (1979) and, more recently, Wielgosz, Fletcher, McCants, McKinnis, Haney, and Williams (1984). Lavey and Winkle conducted a retrospective analysis of 45 consecutive patients with chest pain (angina) who had normal arteriograms based on reviews by a car-

## TABLE 9-1
Variations of Abnormal Illness Behavior

I. Illness affirming
   A. Motivation predominantly conscious
      1. Malingering, e.g., in military context; compensation seeking
      2. Munchausen's syndrome
   B. Motivation predominantly unconscious
      1. Neurotic conversion reaction; hypochondriacal reaction
      2. Psychotic hypochondriacal delusions associated with
         (a) psychotic depression
         (b) schizophrenia
         (c) monosymptomatic hypochondriacal psychosis
II. Illness denying
   A. Motivation predominantly conscious
      1. Illness denial in order to obtain insurance coverage; employment
      2. Denial to avoid feared therapies
   B. Motivation predominantly unconscious
      1. Neurotic
         (a) "flight into health"; e.g., relief of symptoms (pain, nausea) soon
            after administration of antidepressant
         (b) counterphobic behavior, e.g., risk-taking associated with hemophilia
      2. Psychotic denial of somatic pathology, e.g., as part of hypomanic reaction
   C. Neuropsychiatric
      Anosognosia: denial of hemiparesis

*Note.* From "A General Classification of Abnormal Illness Behaviors" by I. Pilowsky, 1978, *British Journal of Medical Psychology, 51*, 134–135. Copyright 1978 by the British Psychological Society. Adapted by permission.

diologist and a cardiovascular radiologist. The normal arteriograms indicated that the chest pain was most likely *not* the result of large-vessel coronary artery disease. The purpose of the study was to evaluate continuing disability in this patient group despite the absence of pathology.

Patients with evidence of arrhythmias or other cardiovascular disease were excluded from the study. The subject sample consisted of 14 males and 31 females (age range 25–70, mean age 48). Their charts were reviewed, and the patients were described as follows: (1) No patient was felt to have chest pain from anxiety; however, this was not formally determined and is a flaw in the study; (2) treadmill tests for the majority of the cases (36 out of 45) were negative, three were positive, and six were inadequate for evaluation; (3) the electrocardiogram was normal in 39 patients and borderline for an old infarction for 3 patients, and there were atrial premature beats in one, incomplete right bundle branch block in one, and left anterior fascicular and right bundle branch block in one; and (4) no previous myocardial infarction was documented.

Subjects were requested to answer the following questions on their disability *before* the arteriogram: (1) Are activities limited by the heart problem? (2) If so, in what way? (3) How long had activity been limited? (4) Had an emergency room been visited for chest pain without hospitalization? (5) Was the patient ever hospitalized for chest pain? (6) Was a physican seen regularly for the heart problem? (7) Is cardiac medication being taken?

In addition, the following questions covering the period between the normal arteriogram and the present follow-up were asked: (1) What is the degree of current chest pain? (2) Has there been a return to certain activities? (3) If activities are still limited, in what way? (4) Has there been emergency room hospitalization or hospital admission for chest pain? (5) Is a physician seen regularly for the heart problem? (6) Is cardiac medication being taken? (7) Have there been subsequent invasive cardiac studies?

Results of the evaluation, which took place on an average of 3½ years following the initial arteriography, included several interesting findings. First, chest pain was reduced in 66% of the patients. However, 79% (27 of 34) of those who were initially limited by cardiac symptoms continued to be limited behaviorally to the same or *greater* degree at the time of follow-up; 82% continued to visit physicians regularly because of cardiac complaints; 56% continued to use cardiac medications; 26% were admitted to hospitals to rule out myocardial infarctions, an event that did *not* develop in any instance; and 9% underwent a second arteriogram, which was normal. The results of this study indicate that despite a tendency toward improvement in chest pain, a good prognosis for longevity, and the absence of subsequent infarction, these patients continued to be disabled to a remarkable degree.

Wieglosz *et al.* (1984) also studied a group of patients with chest pain and insignificant or no coronary artery disease. Of the 821 patients, 28% reported similar or worse pain in the first year after angiography (suggesting a significant narrowing of the luminal diameter of the coronary artery). Predictors of this continued pain included sex (female), chest pain descriptions, and hypochondriasis as reflected by the MMPI. Hypochondriasis was the strongest determinant of continued pain, indicating that an exaggerated preoccupation with personal health is *prospectively* associated with continued chest pain, despite insignificant or no coronary disease.

These studies illustrated that a group of patients with no "rational" reason (although recent evidence indicates angina can be triggered by coronary artery spasm, which would not show on an arteriogram) continue to seek medical assistance. Why? How can these cases be identified and what management efforts can be developed to assist with such cases? These questions will be addressed in the following sections.

## Somatoform Disorders

Somatoform disorder is a term currently used to describe a variety of abnormal illness behaviors. The term describes a group of disorders, the symptomatic manifestation of which is primarily physical, yet the etiology is primarily presumed to be psychological in origin. It is important to emphasize that although patients typically present with a multitude of symptoms for which there is no obvious medical basis, this does not exclude the possibility of a pathophysiological basis for such symptoms. Indeed, biomedical theory and technology may not be adequate to identify certain processes at present. The somatoform disorders do, however, differ from those physical disorders and symptoms that can be affected by psychological factors (e.g., nausea, asthma, angina). Patients with this latter group of disorders are not considered as having variants of abnormal illness behavior.

The group currently referred to as somatoform disorder includes somatization disorder (formerly hysteria), conversion disorder, psychogenic pain disorder, and hypochondriasis. Another group of disorders somewhat related to abnormal illness behavior are the factitious disorders. The main difference between this set of disorders and the somatoform disorders is that, in the somatoform disorder, symptom production is considered to be involuntary, whereas in the factitious disorders, symptoms are viewed to be voluntarily produced and fabricated. Table 9-2 presents a summary of the various somatoform disorders, according to the Diagnostic and Statistical Manual of Mental Disorders (American Psychiatric Association, 1980).

Figure 9-1 illustrates the approach to conceptualizing various health disorders developed by the authors. The purpose of this 2 × 2 contingency table is to categorize the various illness behaviors within a general framework. The figure indicates four major types of disorders, each with a different pattern of psychological/environmental and pathophysiological input. The four patterns involve the identification or nonidentification of psychological factors contributing to the disorder, as well as pathological or organic factors. Whereas the inability to identify pathological sources of input may be a limitation of current diagnostic technologies, in the 2 × 2 schema we have assumed that all reasonable medical diagnostic procedures were conducted in an effort to identify pathophysiological input.

Type I disorders represent relatively clear psychological and patho-

## TABLE 9-2
### Somatoform Disorders

Somatization Disorder
  History of physical symptoms of several years duration
  Onset before age 30
  Multiple symptom complaints requiring
  (a) medication or
  (b) alteration of life pattern or
  (c) physician consultation
  Symptoms not adequately explained by physical disorder, injury, or side effects of
    medication, drugs, alcohol
  Report of symptom is sufficient, not direct observation

Conversion Disorder
  Predominant disturbance is loss of or alteration in physical functioning suggesting
    physical disorder
  Etiological role of psychological factors as suggested by one of the following:
  (a) temporal relationship between environmental stimulus (related to conflict or
    need) and initiation or exacerbation of symptom
  (b) symptom enables individual to avoid some activity that is noxious
  (c) symptom enables individual to obtain support from environment that otherwise
    would not be readily available
  Symptom *not* under voluntary control
  Symptom cannot be accounted for by a known physical disorder or
    pathophysiological mechanism
  Symptom not limited to pain or disturbance in sexual functioning
  Symptom not due to somatization disorder or schizophrenia

Psychogenic Pain Disorder
  Severe and prolonged pain as prominent disturbance
  Pain as symptom inconsistent with nerve distribution
  After *extensive* evaluation, no organic pathology or pathophysiological mechanism can
    be found to explain pain
  When related organic pathology exists, complaint of pain is grossly in excess of what
    would be expected from physical findings
  Psychological factors etiologically involved according to same criteria, as specified
    with conversion disorder (see conversion disorder)
  Not due to another mental disorder

Hypochondriasis
  Predominant disturbance is unrealistic interpretation of physical signs or sensations
    as abnormal, resulting in preoccupation with fear or belief of serious disease
  Complete physical evaluation does not support existence of physical disorder that can
    account for symptoms
  Persistent unrealistic fear or belief of having a disease despite medical reassurance
    causing impairment in social or occupational functioning
  Absence of schizophrenia, affective disorder, or somatization disorder

*Note.* From *Diagnostic and Statistical Manual of Mental Disorders* (3rd ed.) by the American Psychiatric
Association. Copyright 1980 by the American Psychiatric Association. Adapted by permission.

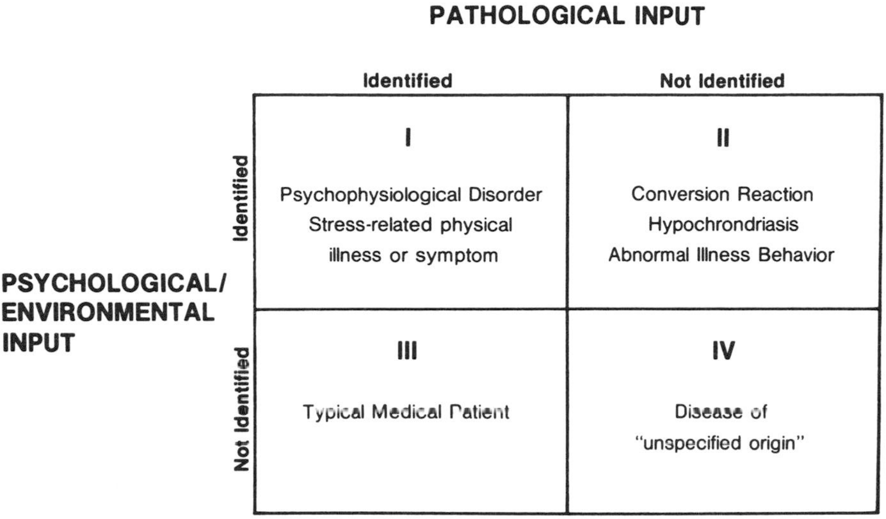

**PATHOLOGICAL INPUT**

|  | Identified | Not Identified |
|---|---|---|
| **Identified** | **I**<br><br>Psychophysiological Disorder<br>Stress-related physical<br>illness or symptom | **II**<br><br>Conversion Reaction<br>Hypochrondriasis<br>Abnormal Illness Behavior |
| **Not Identified** | **III**<br><br>Typical Medical Patient | **IV**<br><br>Disease of<br>"unspecified origin" |

**PSYCHOLOGICAL/ ENVIRONMENTAL INPUT**

FIGURE 9-1. Schema for categorizing illness.

logical sources of input, Type II disorders comprise the various problems discussed in the present chapter, and Type III the common illnesses frequently seen by the family physician (i.e., colds, and other viral infections, bacterial infections). Type IV disorders, however, present with an extremely complicated clinical picture, in which the persistent symptoms are not associated with a specific psychological or pathological input. Patients with these disorders of unspecified origin can, however, present with psychological symptoms secondary to the primary symptoms. An example might be the patient with recurrent episodes of nausea with no apparent cause who then develops secondary anxiety in anticipation of becoming nauseated. Another example is the individual who periodically experiences vertigo (dizziness) in a variety of situations, with no apparent pathological or physiological cause, who begins to feel uncertain about his or her ability to engage in certain physical activities.

If most patients in the general category of somatoform disorders (Type II disorders) do not have a clear-cut medical basis for their physical symptoms, what then are the factors responsible for the development, exacerbation, and maintenance of these complex variants of illness behavior? Etiological factors can be divided into cognitive-perceptual processes, social learning factors, emotional factors, and psychosocial factors.

## MEASUREMENT OF ABNORMAL OR MALADAPTIVE ILLNESS BEHAVIOR: ONE APPROACH

Several studies have been directed at describing and measuring the various characteristics or dimensions of abnormal illness behavior over the past decade. Pilowsky (1978), using chronic pain patients, developed a 52-item questionnaire, the Illness Behavior Questionnaire (IBQ) to investigate this issue. Over a two-year period, Pilowsky collected data on a sample of 100 unselected chronic pain patients. Subjects were an average age of 49.1 years, the pain was experienced for an average of 7.4 years, and the patients were resistant to traditional medical treatment. Based on their response to the IBQ, the following clusters or factors were observed.

1. *General hypochondriasis.* Patients are characterized by a diffuse anxious concern with health, "disease phobia," or fear of contracting disease.
2. *Disease conviction.* There is the conviction that disease is present, and this is often associated with bodily preoccupation and rejection of medical opinion. Patients with high scores tend to be certain as to the presence of the disease rather than phobic about the possibility of contracting it.
3. *Psychological versus somatic perception of illness.* High scorers are more willing to attribute the disorder to psychological determinants or their own behavior; low scorers reject this possibility.
4. *Affective inhibition.* High scorers indicate a reluctance to express feelings to others, especially when the feelings are negative ones, such as anger. This characteristic can be described as low assertion.
5. *Affective disturbance.* This scale indicates a dysphoria dimension: High scorers are anxious and depressed, low scorers tend to deny such affects.
6. *Denial of problems.* Patients scoring high on this dimension tend to deny financial or family problems and perceive their illness as the only difficulty in their lives.
7. *Irritability.* High scorers are aware of strains in interpersonal relationships, as well as a tendency to anger easily.

The seven factors that emerged from the study provided a basis for assigning scores to patients on each of the seven factor scales. Pilowsky (1978) then studied the scale profiles of the 100 patients by cluster analysis, and was able to classify six principal types of patients, as follows:

1. *Capacity for using denial adaptively.* This characterizes persons who minimize stress at times, and even resist medication for pain. This is not rare in those suffering from malignant disease.
2. *Use of denial, but less effective in employing strategy.* Subjects report some anxiety and/or depression, but ascribe it to their pain.
3. *Irritability and interpersonal friction with denial of problems other than physical health.* Patients here are characterized by somatizing (displacing) interpersonal problems and prefer to communicate distress in physical terms.
4. *Somatic preoccupation and rejection of reassurance.* This type of patient denies life problems other than bad health. They report little dysphoria or irritability and cling to the sick role.
5. *High disease conviction and many life problems.* This type of patient takes a depressive and masochistic stance to life situations. They often develop hostile-dependent relationships.
6. *Anxious hypochondriacal concern with health.* These patients report difficulty in communicating their feelings to others, and express a sense of affective disturbance.

Patient types 1 through 3 represent relatively adaptive forms of illness behavior. These types of illness behavior are not surprising because of the complex nature of the pain problem. Patient types 4 through 6 represent maladaptive forms of illness behavior. Although the IBQ does not allow one to predict abnormal illness behavior, it does appear to distinguish between various patterns or styles in patients and may be useful in planning appropriate treatments for different patients.

The magnitude of maladaptive illness behavior may be partly a function of the *duration* and *severity* of the illness. Chapman, Sola, and Bonica (1979) indicated that Pilowsky's descriptions of illness behavior in chronic pain patients referred to Pain Centers may not be applicable to patients from private practice. They found that private practice patients who were experiencing pain for a shorter duration and who were not referred for refractory, multiple pain problems were less depressed; showed less conviction of disease, less general hypochondriasis, and less affective disturbance; and were less somatically focused, with a greater tendency to accept the possibility of a psychological component. The Chapman *et al.* (1979) study also illustrates the difficulties in generalizing across various patient types (private versus clinic). The characteristics described by Pilowsky provide a potentially useful classification of abnormal illness behavior. In Chapter 12, the phenomenon of chronic pain will be addressed more fully. It is worth noting here that the behavior of many chronic pain patients can be categorized as abnormal illness behavior. Chronic pain patients maintain illness behavior over a long period of time and typically do not return to their earlier roles. Additional approaches to measuring illness behavior are discussed in the chapter on pain.

### ETIOLOGICAL CONSIDERATIONS: HYPOCHONDRIASIS

Much of illness behavior can be characterized by a preoccupation with one's body, disease, and health, although as discussed, this hypochondriasis is not the only clinical feature. This section will review recent hypotheses regarding illness behavior, with an emphasis on hypochondriasis as a working model and point of departure. Hypochondriasis was chosen for further discussion because of its central role in illness behavior.

*Hypochondriasis* is typically defined as "an unrealistic interpretation of one's bodily sensations as abnormal, leading to the fear and belief that one has a serious disease" (Barsky & Klerman, 1983, p. 274). According to the DSM III, the disorder is generally considered to include the following characteristics: (1) physical symptoms disproportionate to demonstrable organic disease, (2) fear of disease and the conviction that one is ill, (3) preoccupation with one's body, and (4) persistent and unsatisfactory pursuit of medical care ("doctor shopping"). Physical complaints are typically of a vague, variable, and generalized nature, although in certain cases the symptoms can be very specific. Other typical clinical features are listed in Table 9-3.

In a review of hypochondriasis, bodily complaints, and somatic styles, Barsky and Klerman (1983) discussed three major etiological hypotheses: intrapsychic, cognitive-perceptual, and social learning. Since these hypotheses can often be generalized to other aspects of illness behavior, they will be discussed in detail.

### Psychodynamics of Hypochondriasis

Psychodynamic conceptualizations of hypochondriasis relate to an unconscious gratification and meaning for bodily symptoms and physical suffering. The symptoms and suffering can represent (1) an alternative channel to deflect sexual, aggressive, or oral drives or (2) an ego defense against guilt or low self-esteem (Nemiah, 1980). The first "mechanism" (i.e., aggressive wishes directed at others transformed into physical complaints) can involve anger resulting from past rejec-

**TABLE 9-3**
Clinical Features of Hypochondriasis

1.  Pain as most common symptom
2.  Bowel and cardiorespiratory complaints frequent
3.  Head, neck, abdomen, and chest most common body regions affected
4.  Gastrointestinal, musculoskeletal, and central nervous system organ systems most frequently implicated
5.  Multiple symptoms from several different organ systems that wax and wane over long periods of time
6.  Tendency toward greater concern regarding authenticity, meaning, and etiological significance of symptoms rather than unpleasant sensations
7.  Fear of disease and profound disease conviction with psychological factors frequently rejected
8.  Bodily preoccupation and fascination
9.  Symptoms as response to life events and situational stressors
10. View of self as afflicted, suffering, accomplishment has been to endure misery
11. Relentless search for medical care—extensive history of prior medical care

tion, losses, or loneliness expressed in the present by reproaching others for one's pain and suffering. A family member might volunteer to help in response to a request by the patient, yet that assistence is rejected as ineffective. The concept of suppressed anger in hypochondriasis has been tentatively supported (cf. Barsky & Klerman, 1983). The hypothesis of hypochondriasis as a defense against low self-esteem argues that it is more tolerable for the patient to take the position that a problem exists within his or her body than with the self. Somewhat related to this hypothesis is the position that physical suffering can serve as a defense against guilt, providing well-deserved punishment for past wrongdoing. Support for these mechanisms are searched for in the early developmental stages of life, and such factors as parental care during illness or identification with a chronically disabled sibling or parent are important candidates for research.

The psychodynamic hypotheses require more operationally based terminology and validation with rigorous research designs. Whereas the majority of the concepts are supported by anecdotal reports, these concepts could be empirically studied (Barsky & Klerman, 1983). As pointed out by the reviewers, longitudinal designs, with adequate measurement devices, would be needed to determine whether periods of somatic exacerbation are *preceded* by diminished self-esteem, increased anger, or guilt. The temporal relationship between anger and symptoms would assist in understanding whether anger (inner or outer) preceded symptom exacerbation or was a consequence of such symptoms.

## Cognitive-Perceptual Abnormalities

A second, perhaps more scientifically acceptable or verifiable set of hypotheses relate to a *perceptual or cognitive abnormality* as the basis for hypochondriasis. This explanation is represented by three possible mechanisms: (1) patients amplify and augment normal bodily sensations; (2) patients misinterpret bodily symptoms of emotional arousal and normal bodily function; and (3) a constitutional predisposition to thinking and perceiving in physical and concrete terms in contrast to emotional terms, sets the stage for symptom preoccupation. According to Barsky and Klerman, these mechanisms suggest that a *perceptual defect* is the primary underlying disorder, not the illness behavior itself. The components of hypochondriasis as depicted in Table 9-3 are only manifestations of this primary perceptual defect, which results in abnormal bodily perceptions.

The hypothesis that hypochondriacal patients amplify and augment normal bodily sensations is supported by a number of observations. These patients do tend to report normal bodily sensations as more noxious and intense than controls. Hanback and Revelle (1978) found that a subgroup of students who scored high on a hypochondriasis scale tended to report heightened arousal and heightened perceptual sensitivity to bodily sensations. Although the arousal measure did not include physiological indices, additional research on the relation of heightened sensation would contribute considerably to our understanding of the amplication hypothesis.

The hypothesis that patients *misinterpret* normal bodily sensations is based on sociopsychological concepts of misattribution. The main point in the explanation is that normal bodily sensations or the minimal symptoms of daily living (e.g., indigestion) and somatic correlates of emotional arousal (increased heart rate, stomach flutter, etc.) are seen as representing serious disease. The attribution of these sensations, emotional correlates, and bodily symptoms is inaccurate in the patient with hypochondriacal characteristics. It is argued that this misattribution can occur more readily when the symptoms are diffuse, ambiguous, common, and in a body part that is not directly observable. Such symptoms as weakness, fatigue, nausea, or diffuse pain represent such nonspecific bodily experiences and also characterize patients with illness behavior. The patient with such illness behavior tends to attribute such symptoms to disease, whereas the normal healthy adult might relate such symptoms to job stress, aging, etc. The misattribution process can become a self-perpetuating, self-validating process in which the attribution of disease or illness is recurrently evoked in the presence of the symptoms, thus creating a closed loop. The misattribution itself can increase emo-

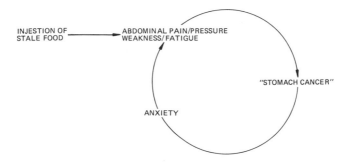

FIGURE 9-2. Example of the closed loop misattribution process.

tional arousal, which, in turn, exacerbates the symptoms and continues the cycle. Figure 9-2 illustrates the misattribution of abdominal pain resulting from the ingestion of spoiled food. Rodin (1978) argues that the attribution of an internal perception to a disease depends on (1) external cues, (2) interpersonal communication, and (3) context or information regarding the situation.

The final hypothesis used to explain hypochondriasis from a cognitive-perceptual perspective is that these patients have an innate abnormality in internal perception and expression, particularly relative to emotion. Consequently, the individual focuses on bodily symptoms or sensations rather than on emotions. This latter hypothesis is related to the misattribution hypothesis, with the addition of the assumption of an innate abnormality. This abnormality in awareness of emotion, observed in patients with classic psychosomatic disorders, is *alexithymia*. Unfortunately, as discussed earlier, illness behavior is *not* equivalent to the classic psychosomatic disorders, and such a generalization to illness behavior is highly speculative. The innate nature of alexithymia is also unsubstantiated.

## Social Learning

The social learning hypothesis postulates that hypochondriasis represents a complex set of behaviors that evolve and are maintained through such learning processes as modeling and operant and respondent (classical) conditioning. The social learning model generally conceptualizes chronic illness as a function of two major factors: the consequences of illness behavior and the premorbid state of the individual. In terms of the consequences of behavior, the concept of reinforcement or secondary gain is crucial. The patient who adopts or develops the illness behavior pattern may receive environmental support for

this continuing disability or sick role. For instance, compensation payments may be such that the extrinsic rewards for working are simply not
sufficient to motivate or maintain "working behavior." Other aspects
involve attention from and care by others for sick role behavior, thus
maintaining or enhancing behavior. There is also the case of patients
with minimal social support for whom illness provides a meaning in life
and permits contact with "caring" people, that is, health care professionals. One example is the pain patient with no husband and few
friends, whose activity is limited to bridge and "existing," and who
spends most of her time discussing her symptoms with health care
professionals. Another aspect of AIB is that these behaviors may be a
means of avoiding negative or aversive consequences. Here, the individual can effectively avoid unpleasant situations or experiences by engaging in certain illness behaviors. An example might be the middle-
aged cardiac patient who experiences chest pains or unusual sensations
in and around the chest in the early morning when he and his wife
usually engage in sexual activities. The chest pain may be real, but its
intensity may be magnified or the effect of the pain on his behavior may
be intensified in order to avoid the sexual involvement he finds increasingly unsatisfactory as his wife continues to gain weight. Here, the
disability is partially maintained to avoid unpleasant sexual activity, not
necessarily by the existing cardiac pathology.

Another major hypothesis that the social learning model proposes
is that abnormalities in the individual *before* the report of the symptoms
or disorder may play a role in maintaining the illness behavior. That is,
the premorbid state of the individual or his or her behavioral style may
affect the types of illness behavior the individual subsequently engages
in. A common clinical observation with patients experiencing chronic
disability uncorrelated with organic disease is that these patients very
often lack the social skills that would assist in facilitating recovery.
Somewhat related is the presence of social anxiety, which could lead to
an avoidance of social activities (Wooley, Blackwell, & Winget, 1978).
For example, the young man who finds it difficult to relate to his female
peers would feel more comfortable sitting at home with persistent back
pain than attending social events with friends for fear of meeting a
woman he would have to interact with. This last explanation also involves the persistence of maladaptive cognitions or "self-statements."
Specifically, the presence of such self-defeating attitudes regarding
oneself and one's ability to deal effectively with certain situations can
increase anxiety and lead to an avoidance of the situation. A common
finding among individuals who display chronic illness behavior is low
self-esteem, or what was reported in the early literature as low ego-

strength. The sick role is a socially acceptable way for an individual to avoid situations in which self-esteem could be challenged.

Research related to the social learning model tends to support the above assumptions. An example of this type of research was reported in a study by Wooley and Blackwell (1975), in which they determined how caretaking responses were elicited and maintained in a group of hospitalized patients with a variety of chronic illnesses before behavioral treatment was introduced. Each patient was given ten blank token forms. Patients were told to reward other patients for behaviors he or she thought should be encouraged or to request another person to change his or her behavior. After the tokens were collected, their contents were analyzed. It was discovered that patients gave over 70% of the tokens for care-taking responses, 22% for socializing, and hardly any for achievement and communication. In contrast, the staff control group, who were to deliver tokens to other staff, showed an inverse distribution of behaviors that were rewarded. Social learning mechanisms as related to pain itself are discussed in Chapter 12.

## Illness Behavior and Depression

The role of depression in illness behavior is complex. Frequently, it is difficult to determine whether an underlying depressive disorder co-exists in patients with illness behavior, particularly in those patients who do not report a mood disturbance. It is also difficult to determine definitively whether a depressive disorder preceded the development of the chronic illness behavior, co-occurred with the illness behavior, or is a reaction to prolonged illness and disability. Somatic complaints are quite high in depressed cases, and depression is highly correlated with pain in patients with a variety of chronic pain disorders (Roy, 1982).

Blumer and Heilbronn (1982) have suggested that chronic pain and its associated illness behaviors represent a major expression of a muted depressive state or a variant of depressive illness with a set of associated psychobiological factors. The chronic pain is viewed as a *synchronous* expression of depression. In a review of a large number of cases ($n = 900$), Blumer and Heilbronn observed many clinical features, referred to as pain-prone disorder, characteristic of this group. These clinical features are presented in Table 9-4. As the table indicates, many of these characteristics are related to general features of hypochondriasis and other forms of illness behavior. In particular, the almost exclusive focus on pain and the desire for a surgical or other medical solution were highly characteristic of this group. Evidence for the depressive component of the disorder, as reported by Blumer *et al.*, includes positive

## TABLE 9-4
Clinical Characteristics of the Pain Prone Disorder

Somatic complaint
  Continuous pain of obscure origin
  Hypochondriacal preoccupation
  Desire for surgery
Solid citizen
  Denial of conflicts
  Idealization of self and of family relations
  Ergomania (prepain): "workaholism," relentless activity
Depression
  Anergia (postpain): lack of initiative, inactivity, fatigue
  Anhedonia: inability to enjoy social life, leisure, and sex
  Insomnia
  Depressive mood and despair
History
  Family (and personal) history of depression and alcoholism
  Past abuse by spouse
  Crippled relative
  Relative with chronic pain

Note. From "Chronic Pain as a Variant of Depressive Disease: The Pain Prone Disorder" by D. Blumer and M. Heilbronn, 1982, *Journal of Nervous and Mental Disease, 170*, 386. Copyright 1982 by Williams & Wilkins, Co. Reprinted by permission.

dexamethasone suppression test findings (assumed to represent a biological marker of depression) and a positive clinical response to antidepressants. The work of Blumer is intriguing and represents an important psychobiological approach to understanding the possible emotional contributions to chronic benign pain and associated illness behavior.

## Psychosocial Adaptation to Illness

The concept of viewing physical illness as a stressor and understanding the patient's ability to adjust to the crisis of illness represents a somewhat different perspective. Moos and Tsu (1977) presented a model that views physical illness as a major life crisis. A life crisis is one that causes physical and/or psychological disorganization and must be resolved within a short time span. A crisis may be resolved to the disadvantage or the advantage of the individual. The person is also vulnerable and open to input from others during the crisis period. A serious physical illness is seen as a threat to the individual. A person who is ill may be separated from family, lose key life roles, and undergo changes in appearance and bodily functions, as well as such unpleasant feelings as anger, guilt, and helplessness. (See Chapter 6, Table 6.)

Moos and Tsu outlined seven major adaptive tasks for the sick individual. They also noted that a person's cognitive appraisal of the tasks, and the choice of coping skills, will determine how a person recovers from illness. In turn, a person's cognitive appraisal and coping skills are determined by three main factors that include (1) background and personal characteristics, (2) factors related to the illness, and (3) physical and social environment.

The patient and the family encounter special problems or tasks, as categorized by Moos and Tsu (see Table 9-5). The first three tasks are considered illness-related. The first task involves dealing with a wide range of physical symptoms, including pain, disfigurement, and weakness. The second task deals with treatment procedures and hospitalization. Examples are coping with aversive treatments, such as chemotherapy and dialysis, and separation from family, and particularly children. The third deals with relationships with health care professionals. Neither patient nor family may know what questions to ask—there may be problems in asking for medication or expressing such feelings as sadness, anger, and hopelessness relative to the illness, treatment, or staff. The second group of tasks involves issues related to the crisis in general. These tasks include achieving a reasonable emotional balance, perceptions of an adequate self-image, and feelings of competency and mastery. Readjustment in terms of goals, expectations, and dependency must also take place. An example is a patient who, following surgery, continues to experience symptoms, but is encouraged to be independent, look for work, and take less medication. Another task is maintaining relationships with friends and family. This can be particularly difficult for patients who are seriously ill or dying, yet these patients require social support. The final task, according to the model, includes prepara-

### TABLE 9-5
#### Adaptive Tasks Related to Illness

Illness-related
1. Dealing with pain and incapacitation
2. Dealing with the hospital environment and special treatment procedures
3. Developing adequate relationships with the professional staff

General
4. Preserving a reasonable emotional balance
5. Preserving a satisfactory self-image
6. Preserving relationships with family and friends
7. Preparing for an uncertain future

Note. From "The Crisis of Physical Illness: An Overview" by R. H. Moss and V. D. Tsu in *Coping with Physical Illness* (p. 9) edited by R. H. Moss. Copyright 1977 by Plenum Publishing Corporation. Reprinted by permission.

tion for an uncertain future, with the possibility of significant losses. An example is the diabetic who may lose his eyesight if the disease worsens.

In order to deal with the various tasks described above, different individuals will use different coping skills. Coping skills may be adaptive or non-adaptive, depending on a particular task. Moos and Tsu (1977) described several major types of coping skills. The first type of coping skills includes denying or minimizing the seriousness of a crisis. An example is a myocardial infarct patient who thinks of his heart attack as just being "severe indigestion." A second set of coping skills is seeking relevant information. For instance, learning about the cause and course of a kidney disease can help a patient feel more in control and know better what to expect. A third set of coping skills includes requesting reassurance and emotional support from family, friends, and health care professionals. Joining special groups may be one way of achieving support; for instance, most communities offer coping-with-cancer groups. Learning specific illness-relevant procedures is a fourth set of coping skills. Being able to take care of certain of one's own health care needs may foster pride and feelings of independence. Setting concrete goals, rehearsing alternative outcomes, and finding a general purpose or pattern of meaning are also skills that can help patients cope with tasks.

Different patients will cope with the varying tasks adaptively or nonadaptively, using some of the coping skills described or idiosyncratic coping skills. The patient's journey to recovery will be influenced by many factors; as mentioned earlier, three general determinants can be distinguished. Age, intelligence, beliefs, and past coping experience all fall under the general, but particularly important background and personal characteristics of the individual patient. For example, strong religious beliefs may help a patient accept the idea of death. A highly intelligent patient may be able to understand medical procedures and cooperate more readily than a patient with intellectual deficits. Developmental factors need to be considered in the case of a young child who may not have developed the coping skills an adult would possess. A second group of factors are illness-related ones. Is the disease painful or will it cause disfigurement? Is the patient extremely weak? Can the disease be cured, or is there no cure, as with diabetes? Finally, the general physical and social environment is critical. Adjustment to the hospital may be facilitated by a supportive staff. Is the family providing emotional and physical support? The model provided by Moos and Tsu is a general schema for understanding the phases and factors of dealing with illness. It provides a framework that can be tested, as in examining the relationship between the staff's interactions with the patient and the patient's coping with illness. It also is a cogent reminder that an individual's response to illness is *idiosyncratic*. It is a response that depends on a variety of biopsychosocial factors, and although a general framework can be useful in studying general relationships, in order to understand a particular patient, individual assessment is mandatory.

## PSYCHOLOGY OF SYMPTOMS: TOWARD AN INTEGRATED MODEL

Pennebaker (1982) has conducted a series of studies directed at understanding the role of psychological factors in the experience of physical symptoms. Although some of the issues were briefly reviewed in the cognitive-perceptual section of etiological considerations, Pennebaker's work represents one of the few systematic research programs in the area of physical symptom experience, and therefore it will be discussed in greater detail in this section. The work of Pennebaker extends beyond the problem of hypochondriasis to symptom experience in a number of health problems (e.g., diabetes).

Pennebaker argues that the study of physical symptoms or sensations must differentiate between encoding awareness and a reporting of internal state because each can be affected by different processes. Although we are constantly processing information (sensation encoding), not all such information is consciously processed. The awareness and reporting of such sensations are influenced by a variety of psychological processes. Factors that influence our awareness of internal sensation include (1) the relative magnitude of internal receptor stimulation, (2) the degree of available external information, (3) cognitions that influence selective attention to internal state, and (4) a general tendency to attend internally (Pennebaker, 1982). Shift from symptom awareness to symptom reporting is hypothesized to be a function of the potential consequences of such a report (reinforcement, punishment). The individual may report a symptom accurately or overreport a specific symptom. The distorted symptom report can be influenced by concerns regarding self-image.

A number of demographic and cultural factors can influence the report of symptoms. These include age (older), sex (female), marital status (unmarried), occupational status (unemployed), socioeconomic status (lower SES), and race (black). The descriptions in parentheses indicate increased symptom reporting. Subcultural and cross-cultural differences in reporting have also been observed. These factors must be considered in any attempt to understand the mechanisms of symptom reporting. Also, individuals differ greatly in their labels for bodily experiences, and detailed descriptions of such symptoms clarify the definition of the symptom. Of particular interest is Pennebaker's observation that psychological factors appear to alter the perception of a variety of symptoms, despite the fact that the symptoms are based on different anatomical substrates. This suggests a common final pathway for such perception.

Pennebaker (1982) hypothesized that the perceptual processes necessary for encoding physical symptoms or internal sensory information are similar to those proposed in the processing of external or sensory events (e.g., audition). He applied concepts from perception and cognitive psychology to understand the psychobiological basis of physical symptom reporting. Perception involves three facts: *orienting, schemas,* and *selective search,* and *inference.* All these facts are subject to distortion and bias. This general perceptual process is based upon the following assumptions: (1) The organism is limited in the amount of information that can be processed at a given time; (2) the search for information can oscillate between external and internal stimuli; and (3) the organism can actively seek out information *and* passively encode information. The active approach is related to learning, expectation, and sets; the passive approach is related to the understanding of stimulus characteristics.

Empirical research supports the hypothesis that when the external environment does not yield information, the tendency to encode internal sensations, symptoms, and emotions increases, and that such processes can occur at a very low level of awareness. In addition, Pennebaker's work (1982) supports the assumption that the schemas or hypotheses we adopt influence our perceptions of symptoms and behavior. These schemas guide our search for additional information and help organize sensory input. The schemas are subject to biases and distortions in perception. The more ambiguous the information, the more important the role of schemas in filtering out irrelevant information. Such selective filtering is particularly relevant to bodily sensations, given a diverse set of possible sensations and competing hypotheses to explain them. Body schemas represent an important component in Pennebaker's model. He argues that although body schemas can be adopted and revoked quite quickly, they can also evolve over several years and be used frequently. Such schemas can be very persistent, particularly in light of frequent confirming sensory information. The patient with a "cancer schema," who is receiving confirmatory sensory information in the form of rectal pain, despite repeated normal work-ups, provides an example of a potentially highly resistent schema. Although a schema cannot be precisely defined, it is a useful construct, and when carefully applied, it has an important explanatory function.

A naturally occurring phenomenon that can perhaps be influenced by schemas and selective search is *mass psychogenic illness.* This has been reported in industrial settings, schools, and churches, to name but a few settings and occurs when large numbers of people are gathered at times of stress (Colligan, Pennebaker, & Murphy, 1982). The sequence is one in which several individuals become ill, with such diffuse symptoms as nausea, headache, and fatigue for which no pathophysiological basis is found. Subsequently, one person will then become overtly ill (faint, vomit), and other people, who are friends, will begin to notice that they have similar symptoms; the symptoms then "spread." The schema may relate to the experience of job stress or occupational exposure to a toxic substance (e.g., vinyl chloride), and the diffuse symptoms occur within such a schema.

In sum, symptom reporting, according to this model, is a function of a competition of cues from external and internal environments and the development of schemas, with selective search and influence processes operating to confirm or negate such schemas.

## MODIFICATION OF ILLNESS BEHAVIOR

Several strategies can be used to modify illness behavior as well as to help the patient cope more effectively with the crisis of illness to prevent *maladaptive* illness behavior. The treatment strategies discussed in the following section are aimed at modifying the cognitive-perceptual processes (e.g., misattribution, heightened sensitivity to somatic input), social learning factors (e.g., reinforcement of illness behavior, avoidance behavior), emotional factors (e.g., depression, anxiety), and psychosocial factors (e.g., facilitating social support) presumed to be involved in the development and maintenance of illness behavior. Although all these components of illness behavior may be interrelated in any given patient, a careful evaluation of the individual patient's illness behavior help the clinician target specific components for modification.

### Cognitive-Perceptual Processes

The use of such cognitive therapies as rational emotive therapy (RET) in the modification of illness behavior is based on the rationale that faulty or irrational patterns of thinking modulate maladaptive emotions and behaviors. Rational emotive therapy is aimed at helping the patient identify irrational thoughts or beliefs that have self-defeating or self-destructive consequences and testing or challenging these beliefs in therapy sessions and in actual extratherapeutic situations (Ellis, 1977). According to Ellis, irrational thoughts or beliefs are either empirically false or cannot be empirically verified. A patient with chronic abdominal pain, for example, may amplify and augment such normal bodily sensations as abdominal pressure or tightness and attribute a negative valence to these sensations, which results in the experience of distress and pain. This heightened perceptual sensitivity to bodily sensations, and their subsequent misinterpretation by the patient, may lead the patient to believe that he or she is the victim of some disease process (e.g., stomach cancer). Such a conviction may often precede the development of illness behavior. Rational emotive therapy, therefore, would focus on the therapist first eliciting the precipitating external stimulus events, then determining the specific thought patterns (and underlying beliefs) that constitute the internal response to these events that generate negative emotions (e.g., anxiety, depression), and finally helping the patient modify these beliefs and thought patterns.

Another example of the cognitive procedures used to alter the patient's heightened sensitivity to somatic input is described by Melzack and Wall (1982). A patient with chronic pelvic pain, for instance, may be trained to ignore his pain by evoking imagery that is incompatible with pain. Such imagery may involve the patient imagining himself in the peaceful surroundings of a secluded lake, laughing at the jokes of his favorite comedian, or out at a party. Alternatively, the patient may be instructed in interpreting the subjective experience in terms other than "pain" (e.g., tingling or buzzing) or to reduce the significance of the experience. The patient may also be taught to acknowledge the pain, while at the same time imagining it to occur within a different setting or context (e.g., cramps from a 24-hour viral infection). Other strategies may involve redirecting the patient's attention to various situations in the environment (e.g., focusing on noises), diverting the patient's attention to self-generated thoughts (e.g., composing a tune), or training the patient to view the painful area in a detached way. The relative effectiveness of cognitive strategies for coping with the sensory component of the pain experience has been demonstrated in recent reviews (McCaul & Malott, 1984; Tan, 1982).

Finally, cognitive-behavioral approaches have been utilized in the form of *stress/pain inoculation training* (Meichenbaum & Turk, 1976) to help patients manage their pain experience. Typically, a patient would initially be given information to enhance his or her understanding of the pain and the stressors that accompany it. The patient would then be trained in a variety of coping strategies (e.g., relaxation, distraction, imagery techniques) and finally would be asked to rehearse these strategies while conceptualizing the pain and stress at each phase of the total pain experience. In a study comparing group progressive-relaxation training and cognitive behavioral group therapy (stress inoculation) for chronic low back pain, Turner (1982) found that at a one-month follow-up, posttreatment patients treated with cognitive behavioral therapy showed significantly more improvement on measures of pain, depression, and disability than patients trained in progressive relaxation, although both treatment groups had a marked reduction in health-care use at a two-year follow-up. Additionally, the cognitive behavioral therapy patients improved markedly in time spent working. Although the relative effectiveness of cognitive and cognitive-behavioral strategies has been demonstrated in the modification of the sensory experience of pain, the need to establish their efficacy in altering heightened sensitivity to other types of somatic input (e.g., the premenstrual syndrome, respiratory constriction, gastrointestinal sensations) requires further investigation.

## Social Learning Factors

The preceding discussion on etiological considerations in illness behavior indicated that one approach to conceptualizing illness behavior, and the increased disability often seen in patients exhibiting it, is in the context of a learned social role. Based on such a hypothesis, illness behavior is seen to develop as a result of (1) vicarious learning through models, particularly in childhood; (2) direct social reinforcement of illness behavior by family, friends, and physicians; and (3) avoidance learning (secondary to a social skill deficit or social anxiety).

Wooley, Blackwell, and Winget (1978) reported a treatment program that focused on enhancing the patient's ability to take independent action in coping with his or her illness. Wooley et al. (1979) targeted specific goals to alter a patient's illness behavior. These goals included (1) having the patient assume responsibility for his or her care, (2) decreasing the care-taking responses by others, especially physicians and family members, (3) altering the social contingencies that supported illness behavior, (4) decreasing the frequency of complaints throughout hospitalization and increasing achievement orientation, and, finally, (5) collecting one-year follow-up data on the generalization of success from target to nontarget behaviors. The treatment program emphasized the elimination of social reinforcement for illness behavior (through group therapy) by teaching the patient techniques directed at reducing physical symptoms (e.g., relaxation, distraction, biofeedback, and self-control programs), initiating therapy directed at helping family members reconstruct the learning process that led to the development of illness behavior in the patient, and establishing contingencies to support the patient's emerging sense of autonomy and independence.

Several important implications for the treatment of illness behavior may be derived from the findings of Wooley et al. (1978). Patients who underwent family therapy and who returned to intact families, for ex-

ample, showed more improvement throughout the course of hospitalization and maintained this improvement in the year after discharge.
In contrast, those patients who did not have adolescent or adult family
members who had been instructed in methods of how to support independence tended to relapse and to re-enter the health care system. The
return to intact families, therefore, is one possible predictor of positive
treatment outcome. Another predictor of positive outcome that emerged
from the findings of these studies was the degree to which patients were
able to attribute their improvement to the self-help components of the
program. The ability to derive satisfaction from accomplishment was
observed more frequently in successful patients. Finally, use of psychoactive medications did not differentiate successful and unsuccessful patients at the one-year follow-up. Neither group of patients differed on
this dependent variable, suggesting that the use of psychoactive drugs is
not necessarily associated with maintenance of illness behavior. The
unsuccessful patients, who reverted to the illness role, were those who
had received a new diagnosis and a new regimen of care.

A clinical example of the operant conditioning approach (Table 9-6)
may be drawn from a case report by Levenkron, Goldstein, Adamides,
and Greenland (in press). The patient was a 38-year-old assembly line
worker with no major health or work problems during his 14 years of
employment until he suddenly experienced a burning axillary pain after
pushing heavy objects at work. One month following the initial onset of
pain, the patient was in an auto accident and experienced substernal
burning and pulling discomfort that persisted for several hours. Substernal pain upon exertion, which was experienced for several weeks, became more frequent. The pain was associated with rapid heart beat and
trembling and resulted in an inability to work. Various medical diagnostic procedures, including coronary arteriogram and an extensive
blood work-up, were completed following admission to a coronary care
unit. All tests were negative, yet the patient continued to experience
chest pain and persisted in the belief that he had an undetected heart
disease (i.e., a disease conviction). Upon his second hospitalization for
additional diagnostic work, the patient was referred to the Behavior
Therapy Unit, an inpatient unit that emphasized the behavioral treatment of medical disorders.

Levenkron *et al.* identified several problematic illness behaviors including (1) chest pain that prevented the patient from leaving home and
allowed him to remain in bed or to recline on a couch all day; (2) the
cessation of all household and child care activities; (3) the cessation of
recreational and social activities with his spouse; and (4) a decrease in
energy and increased fatigue, sleep disturbance, weight loss, and diurnal mood variation indicative of a depressive disorder. Levenkron *et al.*

## TABLE 9-6
Treatment Program for a Patient with Chronic Chest Pain and Illness Behavior

| Target behaviors | Skill development |
|---|---|
| **Functional/physical** | |
| Increase daily productivity | Follow daily schedule of therapy appointments, activities, and independent self-care responsibilities |
| Increase physical activity and body strength | Self-monitor daily activity level; follow exercise protocol |
| **Emotional/Psychological Experience** | |
| Increase awareness of emotions and their physical connection | Self-monitor mood, emotional experience, and change |
| Increase direct expression of feelings and communication | Assertiveness training; family sessions |
| Increase feelings of well-being and relaxation | Progressive muscle relaxation training; group therapy sequence |
| **Social performance generalization** | |
| Prepare for discharge | Weekend therapeutic pass to carry out activity plan; return to work from hospital; reestablish social ties |

*Note.* From "Chronic Chest Pain with Normal Coronary Arteries: A Behavioral Approach to Rehabilitation" by J. C. Levenkron, M. G. Goldstein, O. Adamides and P. Greenland, in press, *Journal of Cardiac Rehabilitation.* Reprinted by permission.

also noted that rest and diazepam were used contingent upon pain, which provided a potential reinforcing relationship between pain and these illness behaviors. Apparently, pain and illness behavior were also associated with an avoidance of conflict with the patient's adolescent son, which again served to reinforce the illness behavior. The treatment is described in Table 9-6. Following a 6 ½-week hospitalization, the patient increased his activity level and reported the resolution of the depressive symptoms. A five-month follow-up indicated that the time spent walking/standing exceeded time sitting. The patient reported only two episodes of chest pain, resulting in six days of lost work, over a one-year period.

## Emotional Factors

Depression is often seen as a manifestation of illness behavior, and chronically ill patients may show many of the features of a major depressive episode. Feelings of sadness (dysphoria) in some patients with a major depression are accompanied by the experience of anxiety, irritability, tension, and upset. In addition to dysphoria, the DSM-III requires that four of the eight following symptoms be present to meet the criteria for a major depression:

1. Poor appetite or a significant weight loss, or increased appetite or significant weight gain
2. Insomnia or hypersomnia
3. Psychomotor agitation or retardation
4. Loss of interest (withdrawal) or of pleasure (anhedonia) in usual activities or decrease in sexual drive
5. Loss of energy or easy fatigability
6. Feelings of worthlessness or self-reproach, or excessive or inappropriate guilt
7. Poor concentration, slow thinking, or indecisiveness not associated with incoherence or loosening of associations
8. Recurrent thoughts of death, suicidal ideation, wishes to be dead, or suicidel attempts

Although there are many approaches to the treatment of depression (pharmacotherapy, interpersonal psychotherapy, brief psychodynamic therapy), only illustrative examples of Beck's cognitive therapy and Lewinsohn's social learning model in the treatment of depression will be presented here.

The cognitive approach described by Young and Beck (1982) comprises four major processes: (1) eliciting automatic thoughts, (2) testing automatic thoughts, (3) identifying maladaptive underlying assumptions of such thoughts, and (4) analyzing the validity of such maladaptive assumptions. Initially, the therapist and patient work together to identify the specific antecedent cognitions triggering such emotions as anger, sadness, and anxiety. The therapist typically asks the patient a series of questions designed to explore some of the possible reasons for the patient's emotional reactions. The patient may also be urged to elicit the automatic thoughts by imagining in detail the distressing situations that trigger the emotional response and then role-playing them with the therapist, for instance, if they are interpersonal. Testing automatic thoughts by operationally defining a negative construct, reattributing it, and generating alternatives is the next stage of therapy. The therapist and patient define, in operational terms, what the patient means by a particular word or expression (e.g., failure). Once the patient and therapist agree upon the criterion for "failure," they examine past evidence to assess whether the label "failure" is indeed a valid one. The goal of this procedure is to teach the patient to *recognize the arbitrary nature of his or her self-appraisal* and to make the patient more aware of more common-sense definitions of these negative terms. Another technique used at this stage of therapy is that of reattribution, whereby patient and therapist may review the situations in which patients unrealistically blame themselves for unpleasant events and explore other factors that may explain what happened other than, or in addition to, the patient's behavior. Finally, a problem-solving approach may be adopted, whereby the patient and therapist work to generate solutions to the problems that had not been considered previously.

The therapist also attempts to identify, with the patient's help, underlying assumptions responsible for automatic thoughts. Underlying assumptions may be viewed as the rules or the "rights" and "wrongs" of the patient in judging himself or herself and other people. One of the major goals of therapy is to *identify* and *challenge* these rules, which are typically couched in absolute terms, are unrealistic, or are used inappropriately or excessively. One strategy, for example, used in testing the validity of maladaptive assumptions may be for the therapist and patient to generate lists of the advantages and disadvantages of changing an assumption and then discuss and weigh these lists. In order for the therapy to become a more active, involving process, the patient is also assigned homework to facilitate the transfer of learning of new skills from therapy sessions to the home environment.

Another approach to the treatment of depression is based on social learning theory, as described by Lewinsohn, Sullivan, and Grosscup (1982). In this type of approach, it is assumed that a low rate of response-contingent reinforcement constitutes a critical antecedent for the occurrence of depression. There are a number of reasons that can explain the low rates of positive reinforcement and/or high rates of punishment experienced by an individual: (1) the limited availability of positive reinforcers or the number of punishing aspects in the person's immediate environment; (2) the lack of a skill that prevents the individual from obtaining available positive reinforcing and/or coping effectively with aversive events; and (3) a diminishment of the potency of positively reinforcing events and/or a heightening of the negative impact of punishing events.

Lewinsohn *et al.* (1982) have provided guidelines for implementing a treatment program that attempts to assist the patient in (1) decreasing the frequency and the subjective aversiveness of unpleasant events in his or her life and (2) increasing the frequency of pleasant events in his or her life. The five steps suggested in accomplishing this goal include (1) daily monitoring of unpleasant and pleasant events, (2) relaxation training, (3) managing aversive events, (4) time management, and (5) increasing pleasant activities. The treatment program is presented to the patient as problem solving, task oriented, and educational. Compliance with the program is facilitated through the use of contingency contracts, and an effort is made throughout treatment to keep the intermediate goal meaningful and specific for the therapist and the patient. The final stage of the treatment program involves the therapist and patient planning tactics that would help the patient resist the pressure of the old environment and facilitate the practice of new skills. In order to gradually fade out therapist support, and to assist the patient in an easier transition to the home environment, sessions toward the end of the treatment program are spread out over several weeks. This latter approach is a common procedure in clinical behavior therapy.

## Psychosocial Factors

Illness behavior is often accompanied by attempts on the part of the patient to adapt to a persistent somatic input. Equally, the patient is faced with the task of adapting to the numerous changes in his or her social and physical functioning. In order to alleviate the impact of such changes on the patient, a multidisciplinary (physician, social worker, psychologist, nurse) approach aimed at assisting the patient adapt to these psychosocial changes is often helpful. As discussed in the preceding section on the etiological considerations in illness behavior, Moos and Tsu (1977) have delineated a model of coping with chronic illness in which psychosocial intervention may be beneficial. These psychosocial interventions may be targeted at helping the patient both with illness-related and general adaptive tasks, as listed in Table 9-5. Often in the context of medical settings, psychosocial teams are consulted (consultation–liaison teams) to facilitate the patient's coping within this framework. Such an approach is believed to serve as a preventive measure for further medical complications as well as the occurrence of illness behavior. Studies to evaluate the effects of the psychosocial approach are still lacking, and future research will need to validate the effectiveness of such interventions.

## ADDITIONAL PROCEDURES

Additional approaches to the management of maladaptive illness behavior include techniques directed at reduction of anxiety or stress, enhancement of social or interpersonal skills, job skills training, and group therapy approaches.

### Management of Anxiety or Stress

The careful assessment of a patient's behavior may indicate that anxiety is relevant to the maintenance of the observed chronic illness behaviors. For example, avoiding such anxiety-provoking situations as interviewing for a job may contribute to the line worker's continued preoccupation with multiple diffuse symptoms. If this is the case, a decrease in anxiety should be targeted. Anxiety may also be a consequence of the illness or the symptom itself. An example of this condition may be the development of an intense fear of death each time a specific symptom (e.g., unusual stomach pain) occurs. Regardless of the cause of anxiety, several procedures may be used to help decrease such anxiety, including progressive muscle relaxation training, systematic desensitization, and hypnosis.

Progressive muscle relaxation is used by clinicians for a variety of psychological as well as health-related disorders (see Chapter 7 for a detailed discussion). Progressive muscle relaxation training is used to decrease muscle tension that is thought to be associated with the experience of anxiety. The general procedure is to teach patients to distinguish between tense and relaxed muscles. The patient is instructed to practice daily until he or she can relax on self-command. Thus, when feeling anxious, the patient counteracts tension by eliciting a relaxation response.

Systematic desensitization employs the relaxation procedure in such a way as to help the patient cope with a particular problem. The therapist has the patient construct a hierarchy of a variety of situations that would produce varying levels of anxiety. The patient is instructed to relax when asked to imagine a scene that elicits the least amount of anxiety. If the patient expresses no anxiety, the next scene is imaged. When anxiety is experienced, the patient is instructed to relax, and, once relaxed, the scene is again imaged. If the patient experiences no anxiety, he or she progresses up the hierarchy of scenes until he or she can imagine the most anxiety-provoking scene with no anxiety. Systematic desensitization can also be accomplished *in vivo*, whereby the patient actually confronts situations in the hierarchy in a systematic sequence, as with the imagery-based approach.

Hypnosis is also widely used to help reduce anxiety. Hypnotic procedures facilitate a state of suggestibility in the patient, often utilizing suggestions of relaxation and the increased ability to cope with stressful situations. The patient can also be trained in self-hypnosis, which generalizes the effectiveness of this procedure. A more detailed review of stress reduction procedures was provided in Chapter 7.

## Social Skills Training

Often a patient will have poor social skills, which hinders his or her ability to have social and emotional needs met by health care professionals and family and friends. Social skills training is aimed at increasing the person's effectiveness in interacting with others by teaching appropriate conversation skills and assertiveness.

## Job Skills Training

Oftentimes a patient will have to reevaluate the suitability of his or her career. For instance, a construction worker may suffer a serious injury that will prevent return to a job that requires manual labor. If he or she has no other skills, career counseling and retraining is useful in helping the patient set new goals and gain a sense of independence. Without such training, a patient may spend the rest of his or her life receiving disability payments, a situation that serves to reinforce illness behavior.

## Group Therapy

Group therapies can have several functions, including enhancing interpersonal skills and providing an emotionally supportive situation. A patient may benefit from attending "special groups" that accept only patients with the same type of problem (e.g., arthritis group). Patients can share their fears, problems, and successes. Sometimes, the patient's family also attend to enhance their understanding of the patient's problem and to learn how to better support the patient.

## SUMMARY

Responses to symptoms and illness can vary considerably across individuals and for the same individual at various points in life. When such a response is disproportionate to the extent of symptoms or illness, the presence of maladaptive illness behavior or somatoform disorders is presumed. Such illness behavior can take many forms, although a common component of most maladaptive illness behavior is a persistent preoccupation with bodily concern. Explanations for such illness behavior include psychodynamic factors, cognitive-perceptual deficits, and social learning mechanisms. Emotional factors, particularly depression and anxiety, also play a significant role. Although modification of maladaptive illness behavior is extremely difficult, various approaches based on hypothesized mechanisms are available to assist with the task.

Maladaptive illness behavior represents a major problem to society, the health care system, and the family of the patient. The financial cost of such overuse of health care is considerable, and the emotional impact on the family can be significant as well. Solicitous behavior of family members is often transformed into resentment and anger and, if no change in condition is achieved, helplessness and depression. Theoretically, the prevalence of such illness behavior could rise substantially, given the increased prevalence, of chronic illness and the increasing number of older individuals. Both these conditions are conducive to the development of maladaptive illness behavior, in that persistent symptom reporting characterizes both groups, and such symptoms, given the necessary and sufficient conditions, could lead to maladaptive illness behavior with its multiple components. Clearly, given the developmental, cognitive-perceptual, social psychological, psychophysiological, and clinical components of illness behavior, health psychology has a considerable potential for furthering our understanding, management, and subsequent prevention of this major health problem. The problem requires careful analysis at the basic mechanism and clinical outcome levels, but much remains to be determined regarding the development of such behaviors and the factors contributing to their maintenance. The psychobiology of symptom experience remains a virtually untapped area. More research on factors that contribute to the preoccupation with somatic input or heightened sensitivity to bodily sensations is required, and the different mechanism(s) that are operable in patients with no organic pathology, in contrast to those with clear organic pathology, must be determined. The principles and techniques used in health psychology can be of great use here.

## REFERENCES

American Psychiatric Association. (1980). Committee on nomenclature and statistics. *Diagnostic and statistical manual of mental disorders* (3rd ed.). Washington, DC: American Psychiatric Association.

Barsky, A. J., & Klerman, G. L. (1983). Overview: Hypochondriasis, bodily complaints, and somatic styles. *American Journal of Psychiatry, 140*(3), 273–283.

Blumer, D., & Heilbronn, M. (1982). Chronic pain as a variant of depressive disease: The pain prone disorder. *Journal of Nervous and Mental Disease, 170*(7), 381–406.

Chapman, C. R., Sola, A. E., & Bonica, J. J. (1979). Illness behavior and depression compared in pain center and private practice patients. *Pain, 6*(1), 1–7.

Colligan, M. J., Pennebaker, J. W., & Murphy, L. (Eds.). (1982). *Mass psychogenic illness: A social psychological analysis.* Hillsdale, NJ: Erlbaum.

Cousins, N. (1976). Anatomy of an illness (as perceived by the patient). *New England Journal of Medicine, 295*, 1458–1463.

Ellis, A. (1977). The basic clinical theory of rational-emotive therapy. In A. Ellis & R. Grieger (Eds.), *Handbook of rational-emotive therapy.* New York: Springer.

Hanback, J. W., & Revelle, W. (1978). Arousal and perceptual sensitivity in hypochondriacs. *Journal of Abnormal Psychology, 87*, 523–530.

Lavey, E. B., & Winkle, R. A. (1979). Continuing disability of patients with chest pain and normal coronary arteriograms. *Journal of Chronic Disease, 32*(3), 191–196.

Levenkron, J. C., Goldstein, M. G., Adamides, D., & Greenland, P. (in press). Chronic chest pain with normal coronary arteries: A behavioral approach to rehabilitation. *Journal of Cardiac Rehabilitation.*

Lewinsohn, P. M., Sullivan, J. M., & Grosscup, S. J. (1982). Behavioral therapy: Clinical applications. In A. J. Rush (Ed.), *Short-term psychotherapies for depression.* New York: Guilford Press.

McCaul, K. D., & Malott, J. M. (1984). Distraction and coping with pain. *Psychological Bulletin, 95*(3), 516–533.

Mechanic, D. (1978a). *Medical Sociology* (2nd ed.). New York: Macmillan.

Mechanic, D. (1978b). Effects of psychological distress on perceptions of physical health and use of medical and psychiatric facilities. *Journal of Human Stress, 5,* 26–32.

Meichenbaum, D., & Turk, D. C. (1976). The cognitive-behavioral management of anxiety, anger, and pain. In P. O. Davidson (Ed.), *The behavioral management of anxiety, depression and pain.* New York: Brunner/Mazel.

Melzack, R., & Wall, P. D. (1982). *The challenge of pain.* New York: Basic Books.

Moos, R. H., & Tsu, V. D. (1977). The crisis of physical illness: An overview. In R. H. Moos (Ed.), *Coping with physical illness.* New York: Plenum Medical.

Nemiah, J. C. (1980). Somatization disorder. In H. I. Kaplan, A. M. Freedman, & B. J. Sadock (Eds.), *Comprehensive textbook of psychiatry* (Vol. 2, 3rd ed.). Baltimore, MD: Williams & Wilkins.

Parsons, T. (1964). *Social structure and personality.* London: Collier-Macmillan.

Parsons, T. (1975). The sick role and the role of the physician reconsidered. *Milbank Memorial Fund Quarterly, 53,* 257–258.

Pennebaker, J. W. (1982). *The psychology of physical symptoms.* New York: Springer.

Pilowsky, I. (1978). A general classification of abnormal illness behaviours. *British Journal of Medical Psychology, 51*(2), 131–137.

Rodin, J. (1978). Somatopsychics and attribution. *Personality and Social Psychology Bulletin, 4,* 531–540.

Roy, R. (1982). Many faces of depression in patients with chronic pain. *International Journal of Psychiatry in Medicine, 12,* 109–119.

Tan, S. Y. (1982). Cognitive and cognitive-behavioral methods for pain control: A selective review. *Pain, 12*(3), 201–228.

Turner, J. A. (1982). Comparison of group progressive-relaxation training and cognitive-behavioral group therapy for chronic low-back pain. *Journal of Consulting and Clinical Psychology, 50*(5), 757–765.

Wielgosz, A. T., Fletcher, R. H., McCants, C. B., McKinnis, R. A., Haney, T. L., & Williams, R. B. (1984). Unimproved chest pain in patients with minimal or no coronary disease: A behavioral phenomenon. *American Heart Journal, 108*(1), 67–72.

Wooley, S. C., & Blackwell, B. (1975). A behavioral probe into social contingencies on a psychosomatic ward. *Journal of Applied Behavior Analysis, 8,* 337–339.

Wooley, S. C., Blackwell, B., & Winget, C. (1978). A learning theory model of chronic illness: Theory, treatment and research. *Psychosomatic Medicine, 40,* 379–401.

Young, J. E., & Beck, A. T. (1982). Cognitive therapy: Clinical applications. In A. J. Rush (Ed.), *Short-term psychotherapies for depression.* New York: Guilford Press.

Zborowski, M. (1952). Cultural components in response to pain. *Journal of Social Issues, 8,* 16–30.

Zola, I. K. (1966). Culture and symptoms: An analysis of patients presenting complaints. *American Sociological Review, 31,* 615–630.

# PART THREE

# PROBLEM AREAS
Etiology and Intervention

*Part III uses specific health problems to illustrate the application of the techniques and concepts discussed in Parts I and II. Three major problem areas were chosen (coronary heart disease, smoking, pain) to provide detailed "case studies" of how health psychologists attempt to tackle these health problems.*

# CORONARY HEART DISEASE

Despite considerable advances in research and practice over the past three decades, cardiovascular disease and, in particular, coronary heart disease (CHD) remains the primary cause of premature death in the United States. This chapter will illustrate the various methods and concepts within health psychology that have been applied to further our understanding of the factors that contribute to CHD and the various prevention and intervention strategies used to reduce the risk of CHD morbidity and mortality. This chapter will first provide an overview of etiological considerations, including a definition of CHD and specification of risk factors. The remainder of the chapter will focus on "coronary-prone behavior pattern," or the Type A behavior pattern, as it relates to the development and maintenance of CHD. As was discussed in Chapter 1, this behavior pattern represents the first well-defined *psychological* or *behavioral* risk factor in the history of risk factor research in health and illness. Therefore, the Type A behavior pattern will be emphasized, with a focus on (1) defining the pattern and presenting it in historical perspective, (2) describing the pattern and the methods used to measure and identify it, (3) reviewing the research validating the Type A construct and providing an overview of the psychological aspects of the behavior pattern, and (4) reviewing the psychophysiological research related to the pattern and discussing the possible physiological mechanisms accounting for the Type A–CHD relationship. The developmental aspects of Type A behavior will also be reviewed. Finally, the Type A behavior pattern will be considered within the work environment, a common trigger of the Type A behavior pattern. After considering the various factors contributing to Type A behavior, the final section will focus on means of modifying this behavior pattern with a review of the prevention research on efforts to modify Type A behavior and its subsequent potential negative health consequences and a review of intervention studies with patients displaying the Type A behavior pattern with CHD (postmyocardial infarction—MI patients).

## DEFINITION AND ETIOLOGY

In the majority of cases, disease of the coronary arteries is the result of atherosclerosis, although other etiological factors can contribute to the clinical presentation of coronary artery disease (e.g., coronary artery spasm, the occlusion of coronary artery by a dissecting aneurysm, and congenital abnormalities) (Julian, 1978). The terms *coronary heart disease* (CHD), *atherosclerotic heart disease*, and *ischemic heart disease* are frequently used interchangeably to refer to cardiac disease producing myocardial ischemia. In general, CHD refers to a condition in which atherosclerosis is the primary characteristic. The clinical complications associated with CHD include angina pectoris, sudden arrhythmic death, and myocardial infarction (MI).

Prospective research has identified a set of variables associated with CHD. These risk factors include elevated serum cholesterol, hypertension, smoking, physical inactivity, obesity, age, sex, diabetes mellitus, and familial history. Certain of these factors are associated with specific manifestions of CHD to a greater degree than others, and many of these factors are related to CHD in an exposure-dependent manner. However, research indicates that the classical risk factors account for only about one-half of the CHD incidence in middle-aged American men and that other variables contribute significantly to this incidence (Keys, Aravanig, Blackburn, Van Buchem, Buzina, Djordjevic, Fidanza, Karvonen, Menotti, Puddu, & Taylor, 1972). Although the likelihood of CHD is greater when more of the risk factors are present, the best combination of these factors still fail to identify most new cases of the disease (Jenkins, 1971). Also, considerable debate exists regarding the specific contribution of some of these factors. Statistically and clinically, these factors do not tell the entire story; they do not perfectly predict the incidence of CHD. Let us now consider an additional risk factor, which was proposed as early as 1892 by Osler who described a relationship between a certain type of behavior pattern or style and CHD.

## FULL SPEED AHEAD: THE TYPE A BEHAVIOR PATTERN

Osler (1892) described the individual susceptible to CHD as "not the delicate, neurotic person . . . but the robust, the vigorous in mind and body, the keen and ambitious man, the indicator of whose engine is always at full speed ahead." Some 50 to 60 years later, a more general interest in this subject began to develop and such attributes as compulsive, restless, hard-working, striving, needful of authority, and passively hostile were added to Osler's description of the coronary-prone individual. In the mid-1950s, cardiologists Friedman and Rosenman, who were at first quite convinced that cholesterol level was the major factor contributing to coronary heart disease, noted, after an investigation of dietary habits of a representative group of volunteers from the San Francisco Junior League and their husbands, that the women in the study had an *identical* dietary intake of cholesterol to their husbands, yet their husbands' rate of CHD was higher. Why, then, these cardiologists asked, were their husbands demonstrating CHD to a greater extent? What was protecting these women? While Friedman and Rosenman were pondering these results, the then-president of the San Francisco Junior League suggested that they look in a different direction. The women argued that it was the stress at work that was contributing to their husbands' CHD and, after some consideration, Rosenman and Friedman decided to investigate this factor. They mailed out questionnaires to 150 businessmen actively involved in the San Francisco business community, requesting that they indicate what habits they believed had preceded a heart attack in a friend of theirs. Approximately 70% of these men indicated that overindulgence, excessive competitive drives, and meeting deadlines were the outstanding characteristics exhibited. Interestingly, less that 5% reported that a friend's heart attack was preceded by excessive ingestion of fatty foods, smoking cigarettes, or failure to exercise. The investigators also surveyed 100 internists who treated coronary patients. The majority of these internists reported excessive competitive drives in meeting deadlines as also frequently preceding the heart attack. These observations, among others, motivated these investigators to conduct a matched cohort study in which they compared two groups of males matched on age, diet, and exercise. One group displayed the coronary-prone behavior pattern, the other group did not. These investigators reported an increased prevalence of clinical CHD in the group that exhibited the overt behavior pattern in contrast to the group that did not (Friedman & Rosenman, 1959). This behavior pattern, called Pattern A, involved a constellation of overt behaviors, including (1) expressive facial and body gestures, (2) rapidity and explosiveness of speech, and (3) hyperalertness and general restlessness. These behaviors were also related to such characteristics as being time-urgent, impatient, hard-driving, ambitious, competitive, and hostile. Friedman and Rosenman (1974) described the Type A behavior pattern as follows:

> An action–emotion complex that can be observed in any person who is aggressively involved in a chronic, incessant struggle to achieve more and more in less and less time, and if required to do so against the opposing efforts of other things or other persons. It is not psychosis or complex of worries or fears or phobias or obsessions, but a socially acceptable—indeed often praised—form of conflict. Persons possessing this pattern also are quite prone to exhibit a free-flowing but extraordinarily well-rationalized hostility. As might be expected, there are degrees in the intensity of this behavior pattern. Moreover, because the pattern represents the reaction that takes place when particular personality traits of an afflicted individual are challenged or aroused by a specific environmental agent, the results of this reaction (that is, the behavior pattern itself) may not be felt or exhibited by him if he happens to be in or confronted by an environment that presents no challenge. For example, a usually hard-driving, competitive, aggressive editor of an urban newspaper, if hospitalized with a trivial illness, may not exhibit a single sign of Type A behavior pattern. In short, for Type A behavior pattern to explode into being, the environmental challenge must always serve as the fuse for this explosion. (p. 84)

Although, as discussed in the chapter on research methods, cohort studies are important first steps for determining the role of a specific risk factor in a hypothesized disorder, prospective longitudinal studies provide more convincing evidence. In 1960, Friedman and Rosenman, along with a number of collaborators (including psychologists and epidemiologists), initiated such a prospective epidemiological investigation — the Western Collaborative Group Study (WCGS). This study investigated CHD incidence in 3,524 men, aged 39 to 59 years at intake, who were currently employed by ten California companies. A comprehensive set of data was obtained at intake and annually until this study was terminated eight to nine years later. The data included education; annual income; medical history for CHD and diabetes; physical activity at work; exercise habits; smoking habits; current cigarette smoking; systolic and diastolic blood pressure; serum total cholesterol; fasting serum triglycerides; serum beta/alpha lipoprotein ratio; and behavior pattern (Type A or Type B), as measured by a structured Type A interview. Since only 45 subjects were lost to the study because of early relocation, non-CHD death, or self-exclusion, 3,154 subjects were evaluated. Coronary heart disease occurred in 257 subjects during the follow-up period, and death occurred in 140 subjects, 31 of their initial CHD event, 19 of a recurring CHD event, and 90 of non-CHD causes. The 3,154 subjects at risk included 1,589 assessed as exhibiting Type A behavior pattern and 1,565 assessed as exhibiting Type B behavior pattern. This study indicated that the relative risk ratio (see Chapter 3 for definition) prior to adjustment for other risk factors in males, aged 39 to 49, was 2.21, whereas after correction for the contribution of other classical risk factors it was 1.87. For males 50 to 59, the ratio was 2.31 before adjustment and 1.98 after statistical removal of other risk factors. This $8\frac{1}{2}$-year prospective study indicated that the majority of the risk that the pattern carries is independent of such standard risk factors as smoking, blood pressure, and serum cholesterol. The results from this study indicated that those judged Type A at the *onset* of this study had twice the rate of heart disease at $8\frac{1}{2}$ years then those originally judged Type B (opposite of the Type A subject). It should be emphasized, however, that these data came from employed men only.

In the well-known Framingham Heart Study, 1,674 men and women in the cohort, aged 45 to 77 years and free of CHD, were requested to complete a 300 question psychosocial interview. The interview measured behavior Types (A or B), reactions to anger, situational stress, somatic strains, and psychosocial immobility. The behavior types considered in this study included the Framingham Type A behavior, emotional lability, ambitiousness, and non-easygoing scales. The reaction-to-anger scales measured ways of expressing or coping with anger, such as keeping it in, or to oneself, (anger-in), taking it out on others (anger-out), or talking with a friend or relative (anger-discuss). The situational-stress scales measured situations in one's job, marriage, or life that posed potential threats to the individual. Examples of such potential threats include non-support from one's boss, job overload, marital disagreements, and dissatisfaction, as well as aging and personal worries. The somatic-strain scales provided an index of physiological or behavioral responses indicative of response to stress, including tension, anxiety, and anger symptoms. Mobility in one's occupational career was measured by requesting participants to indicate changes in one's job or line of work and times promoted over the previous 10 years. Differences between the respondents' education or occupation and that of their fathers were also noted, using the educational and occupational mobility scales. Participants were free of CHD at the onset of the study. No manifestation of CHD, including MI, angina pectoris, or coronary insufficiency syndrome was diagnosed before or at the initial examination.

The findings from the Levine, Scotch, Feinleib, and Kannel (1978) study indicate that women, aged 45 to 64, who developed CHD scored significantly higher on the Framingham Type A behavior scale, suppressed hostility (not showing or discussing anger), and scored higher on the tension and anxiety symptoms scales than women remaining free of CHD. Type A women had twice as much CHD and three times as much angina as Type B women over the eight-year study period. Multivariate analyses indicated that Framingham Type A behavior and suppressed hostility were *independent* predictors of CHD incidence when controlling for standard coronary risk factors and other psychosocial scales. The findings for males indicated that the Framingham Type A behavior score, work overload, suppressed hostility, and frequent job promotions were associated with an increased risk of developing CHD, particularly for those between 55 and 64 years of age. For males aged 45 to 64, Type A behavior was associated with a two times greater risk of angina, MI, and CHD, in general, in contrast to Type B individuals. This association was found only for white collar workers and was also independent of the standard coronary risk factors in other psychosocial scales. This study, which is prospective in nature, further supports the relationship between Type A behavior and suppressed hostility in the pathogenesis of CHD for both men and women.

Although epidemiological studies are important, the question remains as to the link between Type A behavior, the clinical manifestations of CHD, and its underlying pathophysiology. More specifically, few measures of Type A behavior relate to the incidence of MI and its antecedents. Scores on Type A behavior ratings relate to uncomplicated coronary atherosclerosis, atherosclerotic complications in other vascular beds (for example, thrombotic strokes or gangrene), and uncomplicated atherosclerosis. Although research on these issues is limited, certain investigations have indicated that the Type A behavior pattern is more prevalent in those individuals who have experienced an MI or angina (Jenkins, 1978). Studies have also indicated that the severity of coronary atherosclerosis, as measured by coronary arteriography, is correlated with Type A behavior, although it should be emphasized that all the individuals in the population studied had some symptoms of CHD. This finding suggests that the Type A behavior pattern may not be sufficient to explain the findings. The Type A behavior pattern was also correlated with peripheral vascular disease. As suggested by a review committee from the National Heart, Lung, and Blood Institute of the National Institute of Health, much work remains to be done to relate the Type A behavior pattern to specific aspects of CHD (Cooper, Detre, & Weiss, 1981). That is, the relationship between Type A and MI, uncomplicated coronary atherosclerosis, and atherosclerosis in cerebral and peripheral vascular beds, as well as the coronary bed, needs to be investigated.

Despite these limitations, there appears to be an association between Type A behavior and clinical CHD as well as between Type A behavior and certain pathophysiological indices of CHD. Given the potential importance of the Type A behavior pattern, how can it be recognized?

## HOW IS THE TYPE A BEHAVIOR PATTERN DIAGNOSED OR MEASURED?

Before we consider the actual measurement of Type A behavior, it is important to point out the need to clarify the difference between the coronary-prone behavior pattern and the Type A behavior pattern. It is often argued that the use of the coronary-prone behavior pattern suggests a linkage between certain behavioral characteristics and the risk of CHD; however, the existence and nature of such an association, despite what was previously reviewed, remains a matter of empirical investigation rather than a fact. If we also consider the possibility that the Type A behavior pattern may be related to a number of health problems, our use of the term *coronary-prone behavior pattern* interchangeably with Type A is misleading. The National Heart, Lung and Blood Institute's review panel on coronary-prone behavior and CHD suggests that behavior characterized by the qualities previously discussed be referred to as the *Type A behavior pattern*, and that the term *coronary-prone behavior pattern* should not be discarded, but rather reserved for those behaviors that are shown to be specifically related to CHD. This makes it possible, then, to focus on the behavioral data independent of its relation to CHD. For the purposes of this chapter, however, Type A behavior is discussed in relation to CHD because the majority of research conducted thus far relate Type A to CHD.

Any discussion of how such a complex construct as the Type A behavior pattern is measured requires a clear conceptualization of the construct. As we briefly indicated in a earlier section, the Type A behavior pattern involves a constellation of overt behaviors. Table 10-1 illustrates the various characteristics of Type A and the counterpart Type B as reviewed by Chesney, Eagleston, and Rosenman (1981). The actual validation of the Type A construct will be discussed in a later section.

The measurement of Type A behavior falls into two general categories: structured clinical interview and self-report inventories. The major Type A assessment technique is the *structured interview* (SI). The SI was developed during Friedman and Rosenman's early studies of the prevalence of the Type A behavior pattern. Subject selection for these research studies involved first describing the Type A and Type B behavior patterns in detail to individuals who then identified colleagues who most closely

**TABLE 10-1**
Characteristics of Type A and Type B Behavior

| Characteristics | Type A | Type B |
|---|---|---|
| Speech | | |
|   Rate | Rapid | Slow |
|   Word production | Single-word answers; acceleration at the end of sentences | Measured; frequent pauses or breaks |
|   Volume | Loud | Soft |
|   Quality | Vigorous; terse; harsh | "Walter Mitty" |
|   Intonation/inflection | Abrupt; explosive speech; key word emphasis | Monotone |
|   Response latency | Immediate answers | Pauses before answering |
|   Length of responses | Short and to the point | Long; rambling |
|   Other | Word clipping; word omission; word repetition | |
| Behaviors | | |
|   Sighing | Frequent | Rare |
|   Posture | Tense; on the edge of the chair | Relaxed; comfortable |
|   General demeanor | Alert; intense | Calm; quiet attentiveness |
|   Facial expression | Tense; hostile, grimace | Relaxed; friendly |
|   Smile | Lateral | Broad |
|   Laughter | Harsh | Gentle chuckle |
|   Wrist clenching | Frequent | Rare |
| Responses to the interview | | |
|   Interrupts interviewer | Often, particularly on question 13 | Rarely, even on question 13 |
|   Returns to previous subject when interrupted | Often | Rarely |
|   Attempts to finish interviewer's questions | Often | Rarely |
|   Uses humor | Rarely | Often |
|   Hurries the interviewer ("yes, yes," "m-m," head nodding) | Often | Rarely |
|   Competes for control of the interview | Wide variety of techniques— interruptions; verbal | Rarely |

fit the Type A description. Rosenman or Friedman then interviewed each of these peer-selected subjects to evaluate the degree of Type A behavior. Assessment of behavior pattern was based on both the content of the individual's responses and the presence or absence of Type A behavior displayed during the course of the interview. The focus was on both

**TABLE 10-1** (*continued*)

| Characteristics | Type A | Type B |
|---|---|---|
| Hostility | duets; extraneous comments; lengthy or evasive answers; questioning or correcting the interviewer Often demonstrated during the interview through mechanisms such as boredom, condescension, authoritarianism, challenge | None |
| Typical content | | |
| Satisfied with job | No, wants to move up | Yes |
| Hard-driving, ambitious | Yes, by own and others' judgements | Not particularly |
| Feels a sense of time urgency | Yes | No |
| Impatience | Hates waiting in lines; will not wait at a restaurant; annoyed when caught behind a slow-moving vehicle | Takes delays of all kinds in stride and does not become frustrated or annoyed |
| Competition | Enjoys competition on the job; plays all games (even with children) to win | Does not thrive on competition and rarely engages in competitive activities |
| Admits to polyphasic thinking and activities | Often does or thinks two (or more) things at the same time | Rarely does or thinks two things at once |
| Hostility | In content and stylistics— argumentative responses; excessive qualifications; harsh generalizations; challenges; emotion-laden words; obscenity | Rarely present in any content |

*Note.* From "Type A Behavior: Assessment and Intervention" by M. A. Chesney, J. R. Eagleston, and R. H. Rosenman in *Medical Psychology: Contributions to Behavioral Medicine* (pp. 21 )edited by C. K. Prokop and L. A. Bradley. Copyright 1981 by Academic Press, Inc. Reprinted by permission.

content and observable behavior. A standardized interview that could be administered by a trained interviewer was developed, based on the questions Rosenman and Friedman had asked in previous research. Three basic themes conceptualized as characteristic of the behavior pattern were emphasized. These three themes included (1) degree of drive

## TABLE 10-2
### The Type A Structured Interview

I would appreciate it if you would answer the following questions to the best of your ability. Your answers will be kept in the strictest confidence. Most of the questions are concerned with your superficial habits and none of them will embarrass you. (Begin taping now.)

Your code number is _____ .

1.  May I ask your age?
2.  What is your job here at _____?
    (a) How long have you been in this type of work?
+3. Are you SATISFIED with your job level?
    (a) Why? Why not?
+4. Does your job carry HEAVY responsibility?
    (a) Is there any time when you feel particulary RUSHED or under PRESSURE?
    (b) When you are under PRESSURE does it bother you?
+5. Would you describe yourself as a HARD-DRIVING, AMBITIOUS type of person in accomplishing the things you want, OR would you describe yourself as a relatively RELAXED and EASY-GOING person?
    (a) Are you married?
    (b) (If married) How would your WIFE describe you in those terms—as HARD-DRIVING and AMBITIOUS or as relaxed and easy-going?
    (c) Has she ever asked you to slow down in your work? Speed up?
    (d) (If no) NEVER?
    (e) How would SHE put it in HER OWN words?
    (f) Do you like to get things done as QUICKLY as possible?
+6. When you get ANGRY or UPSET, do people around you know about it?
    (a) How do you show it?
    (b) Do you ever pound on your desk? Slam a door? Throw things?
+7. Do you think you drive HARDER to ACCOMPLISH things than most of your associates?
8.  Do you take work home with you?
    (a) How often?
    (b) Do you really do it?
9.  Do you have children? (If no children—Have you every played with small children?) With your children, when they were around the ages of 6 and 8, did you EVER play competitive games with them, like cards, checkers, Monopoly?
    (a) Did you ALWAYS allow them to WIN on PURPOSE?
    (b) Why or why not?
10. When you play games with people YOUR OWN age, do you play for the FUN of it, or are you REALLY in there to WIN!
11. Is there any COMPETITION in your job?
    (a) Do you enjoy this?
*12. When you are in your automobile, and there is a car in your lane going FAR TOO SLOWLY for you, what do you do about it?
    (a) Would you MUTTER and COMPLAIN to yourself? Honk your horn? Flash your lights?
    (b) Would anyone riding with you know that you were ANNOYED?
13. Most people who work have to get up fairly early in the morning, in your particular case, uh-what-time-uh-do-you-uh, ordinarily uh-uh-uh-get-up?
*14. If you make a DATE with someone for, oh, two o'clock in the afternoon, would you BE THERE on TIME?
    (a) Always? Never?
    (b) If you are kept waiting, do you RESENT it?

TABLE 10-2 (*Continued*)

(c) Would you SAY anything about it?

(d) Why or why not?

15. If you see someone doing a job rather SLOWLY and you KNOW that you could do it faster and better yourself, does it make you RESTLESS to watch him?

(a) Would you be tempted to STEP IN AND DO IT yourself?

(b) Have you ever done that?

(c) What would you do if someone did that to you?

16. Do you OFTEN do two things at THE SAME TIME—like reading while watching TV, shaving while taking a shower, writing or reading while talking on the telephone?

(a) Never? Always?

17. Do you OFTEN find that while you are listening to ONE thing you are also THINKING about something ELSE?

(a) Never? Always?

18. What IRRITATES you most about your work, or the people with whom you work?

(a) Why is that so bad?

19. Do you EAT rapidly? Do you WALK RAPIDLY? After you've FINISHED eating, do you like to sit around the table and chat, or do you like to GET UP AND GET GOING?

*20. When you go out in the evening to a restaurant and you find 8 or 10 people WAITING AHEAD OF YOU for a table, will you wait?

(a) Most of the time, how long will you wait?

(b) What will you do while you are waiting?

(c) Are you impatient while you are waiting?

21. What would you do if you had made a reservation at a restaurant and upon arriving the hostess tells you that there will be a 20-minute wait?

(a) What if after waiting 20 minutes the hostess says that it will be another 20 minutes?

22. Would you EVER ask another person in a restaurant to stop smoking?

(a) What would you say? How would you do it?

(b) (If no) What if your companion asked you to ask the man smoking a cigar to stop: How would you do it?

(c) If no, Why not?

23. How do you feel about WAITING in lines—bank lines, supermarket lines, post office lines?

(a) How long would you wait?

(b) What will you do while you are waiting?

(c) Are you frustrated while waiting?

*24. Do you ALWAYS feel anxious to GET GOING and FINISH whatever you have to do?

(a) Always? Never?

25. Do you have the feeling that TIME is passing too RAPIDLY for you to ACCOMPLISH all the things that you THINK you should GET DONE in one day?

(a) Do you OFTEN feel a sense of TIME URGENCY or TIME PRESSURE?

26. Do you HURRY in doing most things?

That completes the interview. Thank you very much.

Closure: This completes the interview of Subject (give code numbers).

*Note.* From "Type A Behavior: Assessment and Intervention" by M. A. Chesney, J. R. Eagleston, and R. H. Rosenman in *Medical Psychology: Contributions to Behavioral Medicine* (pp. 24–25) edited by C. K. Prokop and L. A. Bradley. Copyright 1981 by Academic Press, Inc. Reprinted by permission.

and ambition; (2) degree of past and present competitive, aggressive, and hostile feelings; and (3) degree of time-urgency. In the WCGS study, interviews were audiotaped for later blind ratings. Interviewers also noted such nonverbal behaviors as mental and emotional alertness, speed of motion, gesturing, body restlessness, and facial grimaces. Table 10-2 shows the structured interview protocol used to assess the Type A behavior pattern. Although most descriptions of the Type A construct refer to either Type A or Type B behavior patterns, the score obtained from the structured interview is actually more complicated and is represented by a five-point scale. Interviewees receive one of five scores: A–1 — fully developed pattern; A–2 — several Type A characteristics present, but not the complete pattern; X — an even mix of Type A and Type B characteristics; B–3 — several Type B characteristics, but some Type A characteristics also; and B–4 — relative absence of Type A characteristics.

During the structured interview, the interviewer creates a challenge situation, presenting a standardized environmental stimulus that will evoke Type A behavior from the subject if the pattern is part of the individual's behavioral repertoire. As Chesney, *et al.* (1981) indicate, the interview is a structured experimental situation, and the theory and technique must be mastered before a researcher can successfully conduct an interview. The interviewer must be able to conduct the interview while concurrently evaluating the various behavioral patterns seen. A number of interviewer behaviors need to be consistent, including voice style, overall length of the interview, the content of the questions, and actual behavior. Although the structured interview represents the most widely used form of assessing Type A behavior, and has been validated by the Western Collaborative Group Study, a number of problems characterize this assessment procedure. It is difficult to train interviewers to an acceptable level of reliability, thus limiting the technique to a few highly trained interviewers. The interview is also transparent, as can be seen in the Table 10-2. It is quite clear what the interviewer is trying to assess. This transparency, then, could result in response bias on the part of the interviewee whereby the expected responses are provided. Such transparency also results in a problem with repeated use, particularly in intervention studies in which pre–post measures of Type A behavior would be required. In this situation, participants who have completed a program and invested time and energy in such a program could very well respond in the expected direction, given the explicit nature of the questions. Last, the categorization of Type A behavior is fairly global, providing only five categories. This global characterization only specifies the dimensions of Type A or B and does not specify a pattern of problem areas within Type A behavior. For example, it is unclear which characteristics of Type A are highly prevalent in a given individual (e.g., time-urgency, hostility, or competitiveness). Such a specification, in addition to the various cognitive aspects of Type A and the physiological correlates for a given individual, could be of assistance in the modification of the Type A constellation.

A number of self-report inventories, some developed directly from the SI (e.g., Jenkins Activity Survey, JAS), have also been developed to measure the Type A behavior pattern. The JAS contains approximately 50 items similar to those used in the SI. Scoring of the items is based upon the findings of various psychometric studies used to differentiate large groups of men based on the SI. In other words, the JAS was developed to provide as close a discrimination between Type A and Type B individuals as determined by the SI, as possible. Of the 21 items that are weighted substantially to differentiate between Type A and Type B, one item deals with hostility at an earlier age, five items are directed at assessing hard-driving, competitiveness, eight items relate to immediate quick action (for example, eating quickly and being told that one is too active), and seven items relate to pressured style of working (e.g., not taking vacations). The Framingham Type A scales, as discussed in the earlier Haynes *et al.* study (1978) are a third measure of Type A. This is a self-report measure of 10 items that evaluate the individual's competitive drive, time-urgency,and perception of job pressure (Haynes *et al.* 1978). These items were selected from a 300-item inventory by a panel of experts to closely approximate those of Type A. Matthews (1977) developed a Type A behavior pattern scale for children. The instrument, the Matthews Youth Test for Health (MYTH), uses teachers' observations of children's behaviors. This scale is an interesting development in the evaluation of Type A behavior.

In general, the various Type A measures used have only a modest degree of overlap; however, all three measures (structured interview, Jenkins Activity Survey, Framingham Type A Scale) appear to be reliable. Of the men in the WCGS study, 80% displayed similar interview-based classifications over periods ranging from 12 to 20 months. Evaluations of recorded interviews of men by two independent raters revealed agreement rates on the order of 75% to 90%; this rate, however, may be lower for middle-aged women. Test–retest scores for the various forms of the JAS ranged from .6 to .7 across a one- to four-year interval; the Framingham Type A scale had an internal reliability of .70. These findings suggest that, within a given measure of Type A, there is some consistency in the scores across time; however, measures that supposedly assess the same construct do not appear to be related to each other. The JAS and the Framingham Type A scale agree with the SI classification in only 60% to 70% of middle-aged white collar men and undergraduate men. This represents only a 10% to 20% increase over chance in the classification of Type A. Unfortunately, at present, there are no data available for blue collar or lower socioeconomic status men. In regard to women, the structured interview and Framingham Type A scale were related in an undergraduate sample, but not in a sample of the adult populations. In sum, a number of methods for assessing the Type A pattern have been developed over the past two decades. Although individual measures appear reliable, correlation with other measures of Type A behavior is somewhat low. This situation may be the result of an inadequate conceptualization or definition of the Type A construct obtained before the development of an assessment device. A well specified operational definition of the Type A construct is also necessary to further our understanding of the psychobiological mechanisms of Type A behavior and the relationship between Type A behavior and CHD. Operational definitions are, in fact, a function of the types of methods used to measure a given construct and, therefore, consideration of the characteristics or dimensions of Type A, as measured by the various instruments discussed, represents an important first step to the ⌣ understanding of Type A behavior.

## BEHAVIORAL AND PSYCHOPHYSIOLOGICAL DIMENSIONS OF TYPE A BEHAVIOR

Matthews (1982) reviewed the literature on the Type A behavior pattern and noted that the research on the characteristics of Type A fall into several categories: (1) experimental studies on the behavior of Type A and Type B individuals; (2) self-reports of how Type A and Type B individuals behave; and (3) Type A and Type B responses during psychophysiologic studies. The psychophysiological research was reviewed by Matthews to identify environmental events that elicit physiological differences between Types A and B, rather than to focus on the suspected psychobiological mechanisms and their implications. This latter issue will be discussed later in this chapter. The Matthews (1982) review was divided into findings based on the SI, the JAS, and the Framingham Type A scale. Given the lack of convergence among these measures, it was decided that it was more informative to consider the findings for each of the measures separately.

There have been only a few studies on the actual behavior of individuals classified by the structured interview as Type A or Type B. When instructed to read a paragraph describing a battle aloud, A's and B's differ in their speech patterns. Type A's spoke quickly, loudly, and explosively, particularly when asked to take the role of commander of the battle unit. More recent research has indicated that Type A's also speak quickly, loudly, and explosively during the SI itself. This speech behavior is highly correlated with scores on the interview, but only modestly related to a self-report measure of Type A behavior. A number of other studies measured a variety of behaviors including reaction time and parent–child interactions, and therefore, to summarize results across findings is not possible. What appears to be a consistent finding, however, is that Type A's speak in a distinctly different manner than Type B's. When considering *self-report* and survey data from Type A's measured by the SI, it appears that Type A's report that they are more aggressive, angry, achievement-oriented, shrewd, active, quick, dominant, sociable, lacking in self-control, and hard-working than Type B's. These findings are based on middle-aged, middle-class Caucasian men. Whereas Type A women report greater self-confidence and a high status occupation, they also report symptoms indicative of stress, as well as a dissatisfaction with life achievement and marriage. The correlations between the SI measure and the various indices discussed are statistically significant, yet not large, which indicates a reliable relationship, yet one that only accounts for a small percentage of variance.

In the physiological studies, the findings based on Type A interviews indicate that Type A's exhibited increased serum triglyceride activity before and following digestion of a fat meal and elevated norepinephrine levels during a contest, in contrast to Type B's. Matthews (1982) reviewed 16 physiological studies in which the SI assessment of Type A were used, and reported that 10 out of the 14 studies indicated that the male Type A exhibited elevations relative to a resting baseline in systolic blood pressure, in plasma epinephrine or norepinephrine, and at times, in heart rate in response to specific environmental events. These events were characterized as frustrating, difficult, and moderately competitive. Interestingly, in highly competitive situations, Type B's blood pressure and catecholamine levels rose to the extent of Type A's. When differences emerged, they were differences in *reactivity*, and not *resting* levels. High resting blood pressures were reported for A's in job environments without autonomy and peer support and for B's in job environments with autonomy, peer support, and low physical comfort. Three studies did not observe A, B differences in blood pressure and heart rate; a fourth study indicated no A, B differences in urinary catecholamines and heart rate throughout the working day for white-collar men in Belgium. Procedural differences between these and the previous studies may account for the differences in the results. Psychophysiological studies with women indicated that in one of three experiments, A, B blood pressure differences were observed.

Although the various psychophysiological studies based upon the SI indicated cardiovascular and neuroendocrine differences between

Type A and B subjects, performance differences were reported in only two experiments. The absence of Type A differences in performance is unusual and may reflect the differential objectives of the studies. These investigations focused on psychophysiological difference measures and only secondarily on differences in performance. The experimental protocol, therefore, was not designed to identify performance differences. It is interesting, however, that in two studies in which patients were under general anesthesia, Type A's responded with greater blood pressure elevations than Type B's. This suggests that the Type A behavior itself is not necessary for cardiovascular and neuroendocrine hyperreactivity, but rather that this hyperreactivity is *independent* of the overt behavior pattern.

The various findings based upon the SI assessment of Type A reviewed identify a number of important issues. What is the psychological significance of the Type A speech behavior, a behavior that is highly related to the SI assessment and covaries with physiological arousal? Is loudness of voice somehow related to anger or contempt? Matthews also points to a second possible meaning of speech behavior, that is, it may represent the more general index of reactivity to a challenging event, the provocative interview. A second issue highlighted by these findings is the low association between Type A assessment and self-reported Type A behaviors; perhaps it is unreasonable to assume that a global measure of Type A, such as the interview, would correlate with a very specific measure of the Type A construct as measured by single psychometric tests. Further work on relating Type A interview scores with observable and self-reported Type A behaviors is required to obtain a more precise picture of the actual, empirically measured constellation of dimensions comprising Type A.

The results from the JAS primarily come from studies on college undergraduates exposed to a number of tasks thought to evoke relevant components of the Type A behavior pattern. Most notable is the work of Glass and colleagues (Glass, 1977), in which he attempted to validate the Type A construct in a series of experiments over several years. Glass focused on three components: excessive and relatively constant achievement striving, time-urgency, and competitive aggressiveness. He attempted to determine whether these characteristics are observed to a greater degree in Type A's than in Type B's using controlled laboratory studies. Glass developed a measure of Type A in college students (student version of the JAS) and conducted a series of studies comparing A's and B's on a number of dimensions in an attempt to clarify the Type A construct. Type A's outperformed Type B's in difficult situations that required persistance or endurance. Situations that induced fatigue, provided external distractions, or required continued performance after a brief salient failure are the types of environmental conditions in which Type A's outperformed Type B's. However, Type B's outperformed Type A's on tasks that require slow, careful responses, a broad focus of attention, or continued performance following a prolonged salient failure. Interestingly, when the failure experience was not highly salient, the reverse occurs: Type A's outperform Type B's. No Type A – B differences were found on tasks that had an explicit time deadline or on tasks performed following successes. These findings, taken as a whole, indicate that the superior performance of A's on tasks requiring speed and persistence are consistent with the achievement-striving aspect of Type A behavior. In spite of fatigue or the possibility of failure, the Type A individual continues to achieve a series of goals as quickly as possible and to work rapidly and persistently. Type A's are also able to ignore potentially interfering distractions. On the other hand, the poor performance of A's in situations that require slow work may be interpreted as consistent with the time urgency and impatience characteristics of the Type A individual. In situations that require slow methodical work, impatience may interfere with adequate performance. It is also possible, however, that these findings indicate a preference in the Type A individual for working at a more rapid pace.

Other studies have attempted to measure aggressive and hostile behavior in both Type A and B individuals. Although no significant differences emerged between Type A and B undergraduates who were interrupted during task performance, the results suggested that A's exhibited more irritation. Glass and his colleagues also observed that working on a frustrating task was sufficient for Type A's to increase the levels of shock subsequently delivered to a cohort. The work on hostility will be discussed in greater detail later in this chapter. In terms of achievement striving, Type A adults, both men and women, reported rapid career advancement, more education, a higher occupational status, and more rewards from their work. Undergraduate men and women reported that they study and work more hours for paid employment and sleep less than do Type B's. Type A undergraduate men also reported receiving more academic and athletic honors and having been more active in high school sports. When looking at the JAS results with regard to personality characteristics, a number of studies indicated that Type A's have *higher* scores than B's on measures of impulsivity, dominance, and activity.

A number of psychophysiological studies using the JAS scale to identify Type A's have been conducted. Approximately one-half the studies that measured blood pressure and heart rate during task performance found that Type A's exhibit elevations in systolic blood pressure, but not in diastolic blood pressure or heart rate. Type A's also exhibit greater decreases in pulse transit time (an indicator of beta-adrenergic activity) when confronted with a difficult stressful condition relative to a minimal stress condition. Type A's were also observed to have higher peak blood pressures during the workday, smaller decreases in blood platelet aggregation in response to exercise, and greater peripheral vasoconstriction during a competitive game. Greater adrenal and cortisol excretion relative to an active stimulation or overstimulation condition was observed during inactivity or understimulation in Type A's in comparison to Type B's. A choice reaction time task in which subjects were actively engaged did not yield A – B differences in either urinary catecholamines or cortisol excretion, although Type A's perform more efficiently. As summarized by Matthews (1982), situations that did elicit physiological and neuroendocrine changes in the expected direction can be characterized as being difficult and moderately competitive or requiring slow careful responses or patience. The psychophysiological studies indicating no Type A – B differences were somewhat different from the studies described, in that they were more likely to include women or cardiac patients. In sum, those individuals categorized as Type A, as measured by the JAS have a sense of time passing rapidly, work quickly, persist in the face of fatigue or the possibility of failure, ignore distractions that can interfere with good performance, and are willing to harm others in the context of helping them learn. Type A's also report that they work hard and achieve success, and, psychophysiologically, male Type A's sometime show elevations in systolic blood pressure during difficult, moderately competitive tasks.

The findings using the Framingham Type A measure are somewhat limited in the total number of studies using the scale. Haynes *et al.* (1978) observed that Framingham Type A scores were related to self-reports of emotional lability, marital disagreement, concerns about aging, personal worries, daily stress, tension, anxiety, and anger (experiencing many bodily sensations when angry). Scales concerning expression of anger, outward or inward, were not correlated with the Type A scale. Chesney, Black, Chadwick, and Rosenman (1981) observed that the Framingham Type A scale measure was related to anxiety, neuroticism, and depression in a sample of employed middle-class men. The single psychophysiological study of the Framingham Type A scale indicated no significant differences between Type A's and B's. The findings on the Framingham Type A scale, in general, suggested that an individual scoring in the Type A range experiences negative affect and adverse symptoms associated with a pressured competitive life-style; however, it is not known how the Framingham Type A scores and observable behavior are related.

In summary, certain behavioral and psychobiological characteristics of individuals who score high or low on measures of Type A have been empirically observed. Unfortunately, because the various measures of Type A are only marginally related, it was necessary to discuss the Type A behavioral and psychophysiological characteristics for each measure separately. In regard to men evaluated by the SI as Type A, it appears that the predominant behavioral characteristic may be a general reactivity to psychological events that are frustrating, difficult, and moderately competitive. This reactivity takes the form of rapid, loud, and explosive speech, in addition to cardiovascular and neuroendocrine changes indicative of sympathetic arousal. When evaluated using the JAS, Type A's are characterized as vigorous achievement strivers who can be aggressive and competitive and who also show some indication of cardiovascular reactivity during difficult, moderately competitive events. When classified using the Framingham Scale, Type A's are reported as dissatisfied and uncomfortable with the competitive orientation and job pressures that characterize their lives. As pointed out by Matthews (1982), the various measures of Type A actually have different behavioral and psychophysiological characteristics, represent different methods, and are frequently used in different studies that are designed to address different aspects of the Type A behavior pattern. The findings discussed in this section, however, do suggest some moderate degree of construct validation. That is, it is now apparent that the overt behavior pattern, at least, consisting of achievement orientation, time-urgency, and aggressiveness, appears to be fairly consistently observed. These characteristics are also associated with heightened sympathetic reactivity.

## APPROACHES TO CONCEPTUALIZING THE TYPE A CONSTRUCT

Matthews (1982) indicates that at least four approaches have been designed to help conceptualize the Type A pattern. These approaches are directed at specifying the psychological dimensions underlying the various behavioral characteristics of the Type A individual. Matthews identifies the four approaches as (1) *component analysis*, (2) *self-involvement*, (3) *uncontrollability*, and (4) *ambiguous standards of evaluation*.

In the component analysis approach, the emphasis is on specifying the core psychological elements of Type A that are specifically related to CHD. This is based upon the assumption that only certain Type A attributes are specifically related to atherosclerosis and CHD, not the general Type A pattern itself. Therefore, this approach argues that it is important to identify these specific components and study them in greater detail. Examples of empirical support for such an approach can be found in the Western Collaborative Group Study, in which factor analysis of the SI responses of a large number of males indicated five major factors of which only *two*, competitive drive and impatience, were statistically related to subsequent onset of clinical heart disease. Also, further study indicated that only 7 items of the total of 40 interview ratings discriminated CHD cases from age-matched healthy controls. Three of these seven items were related to self-reports of impatience and hostility, one was related to self-reported competitiveness, and the additional three were associated with voice stylistics, vigor of response, explosive voice, and potential for hostility. Although this approach to studying Type A is empirical, it does not provide any insight into the psychological basis or factors contributing to the Type A behavior pattern. It may, however, provide a way to focus on specific components of the Type A behavior pattern that are reliably related to clinical manifestations of CHD. In other words, this approach can filter the various characteristics and permit a more precise specification of important components of the behavior pattern.

The second approach is directed at the study of self-involvement and is illustrated by the work of Scherwitz, Berton, and Leventhal (1978). Scherwitz *et al.* have observed that self-references, that is referring to one's self (me, my, mine) in responding to interview questions, were associated with the highest level of systolic blood pressure during baseline and task performance in Type A's in contrast to Type B's who display fewer significant correlations between self-reference and physiological activity. Scherwitz *et al.* (1978) refer to this characteristic as *self-involvement*, or the extent to which "the individual is personally involved in responding to interview themes and intense feelings" (p. 595). These investigators suggested that this characteristic may help explain the various speech characteristics and the autonomic reactivity observed in Type A individuals. They further related these findings to research on self-awareness theory, in which it has been observed that individuals who are highly aware of themselves tend to use personal pronouns frequently and have some behavior patterns in common with Type A's. For example, they tend to be aggressive when provoked and tend to compare their performance to internal standards of excellence while working on a task. It is then further argued that if these internal standards are high, discrepancies between actual performance and goals could lead to considerable striving, frustration, and a sense of helplessness. Advocates of the self-involvement construct argue that it may not only be useful because it could explain the basis for certain Type A behaviors, but, given that self-involvement is also correlated with various cardiovascular and behavior variables, that it is also potentially important in explaining the link between Type A behavior and CHD.

Although the idea of self-involvement as an explanatory construct for certain Type A behaviors seems plausible, the concept, as presented by Scherwitz *et al.* is that of a *moderator* variable, not a psychological dimension of Type A. That is, it is argued that self-involvement can potentiate certain Type A behaviors (e.g., excessive striving). A problem with the concept of self-involvement rests in a number of inconsistent findings regarding the hypothesis that self-referencing potentiates a relationship between Type A behavior and physiological reactivity. It has recently been observed that self-referencing Type A's have high resting levels of blood pressure, but do *not* display a significantly greater elevation in blood pressure in response to a specific task (Lovallo & Pishkin, 1980). Other research indicates that the number of self-references is positively correlated with blood pressure reactivity in Type A's, but not in Type B's, and perhaps, more importantly, self-references are negatively associated with the severity of coronary atherosclerosis in a cardiac catherization sample. Other problems with the self-involvement concept include the lack of studies that test whether Type A's are self-involved, with the majority of research simply assuming self-involvement, based on certain observations. Matthews (1982) suggests that a number of issues need to be addressed in order to clarify the self-involvement construct. These issues include (1) identifying the standards that Type A's place on their behavior and the extent to which they are aware of such standards, (2) using a measure of self-involvement that is independent of scoring from the SI, in order to evaluate the independent contribution of this measure to physiological and behavioral responses assumed to be associated with the Type A pattern, and (3) identifying the relationships between Type A self-involvement, as measured by such an independent scale, and individual differences of self-awareness, to determine the relationship between Type A self-involvement and self-awareness.

Glass (1977) has proposed that the Type A individual engages in various behaviors (i.e., working hard to succeed; suppressing subjective states, such as fatigue; and conducting activities at a rapid rate) as an attempt to maintain a sense of control over stressors in the environment, that is, events that are uncontrollable and perceived as potentially harmful. Therefore, when the Type A individual is confronted with a stressful event, he or she will struggle to control that event. This struggle is characterized by hard-driving, aggressiveness, quick annoyance, and competitiveness. According to Glass, therefore, Type A behaviors represent a style of coping with stressful events within the environment, and Type A's are thus chronically struggling to exert control. It has also been proposed that this active form of coping with stress is associated with greater sympathetic activity, which is, in turn, related to a number of specific cardiovascular and biochemical changes that are assumed to play a role in the pathophysiology of CHD (lipid metabolism, platelet aggregation, cardiac arrythmia). It has also been hypothesized that this control, when perceived as absent (i.e., helplessness), results in a depletion of norepinephrine, with a potential shift to parasympathetic dominance. Some clinicians and investigators have argued that this abrupt shift between sympathetic and parasympathetic activity may contribute to sudden cardiac death.

The work on control represents one of the more comprehensive approaches to understanding the psychology of Type A behavior. The hypothesis relates to perceived loss of control. Perception of loss of control would accelerate Type A's efforts to regain such control. However, if such efforts result in continued failure, Type A's would then reduce their efforts to respond and act helpless. In an attempt to validate this hypothesis, Glass and colleagues conducted a series of studies in which subjects were exposed first to controllable or uncontrollable tasks, followed by another task in which the efforts to control the second task were measured. Uncontrollable tasks were essentially tasks in which there was no relationship between an individual response and subsequent outcome. Glass reasoned that enhanced performance following an uncontrollable event relative to that following a controllable event represented this tendency to enhance control, whereas poor performance represented the tendency to act helpless or give up. His results were quite complicated; however, in general, there was a tendency toward support of the hypothesis. When investigating the cognitions or thoughts of A's and B's in a failure situation, Brunson and Matthews (1981) observed that Type A's used problem-solving strategies that could not lead to a solution, even if one were possible, and attributed their failure in this specific situation to lack of ability, whereas Type B's tended to use problem-solving strategies that were unsophisticated, but could lead to a solution. Type B's indicated that they were bored and attributed their failure not to a lack of ability, but rather to external situations, such as bad luck or task difficulty. As Brunson and Matthews indicated, "type A's appear to lose faith in their ability to exert environmental control. B's, on the other hand, become passive and withdraw from a situation that they deem uncontrollable" (p. 309).

A theory within psychology, *psychological reactance*, has been applied to understand further the uncontrollability dimension. This reactance theory proposes that threatening an individual's freedom initiates or triggers an emotional state called reactance in that individual (Brehm, 1966). This motivational state then facilitates the restoration of and reassurance about this freedom. This freedom can be threatened quite easily, simply by persuasive communications. A strategy to resist the communication would be to simply change one's opinion in an opposite direction from that proposed. Carver (1980) used this reactance notion to test the hypothesis that Type A's would be more easily threatened by a loss of control than Type B's as evidenced by greater resistance to such coercive communications. Indeed, the Type A's perceived a greater threat in a coercive communication and changed their opinion in a direction *opposite* to that proposed. In summary, then, it appears that Type A's respond to threats to control by trying actively to counter the threats and attempt to recreate some sense of control. Interestingly, when failure seems to be inevitable, the Type A individual switches to a strategy that cannot possibly succeed. As pointed out by Matthews (1982), these findings must be considered in light of the fact that the results were observed in highly salient, uncontrollable situations and that the results were based on differentiation of Type A and B as measured by the JAS. The fact that this work was based primarily on the JAS is of some importance given that the psychophysiological and neuroendocrine changes assumed to play a role in the pathogenesis of CHD are not commonly observed when using the JAS. As discussed previously, the SI is the method of identifying Type A that is most closely related to the physiological changes believed to play a role in CHD. Therefore, although the research on controllability appears to be promising, further work on the underlying psychophysiology and psychobiology of controllability of Type A's, as measured by the SI, appears warranted. The final point raised by Matthews in her review relates to the observation that the uncontrollability approach, although conceptualizing Type A behavior as a coping response to uncontrollable stress, has not actually incorporated theory and data from the coping literature as discussed in Chapters 5 and 6. Integrating the coping literature with the concept of uncontrollability for Type A would seem a promising area of investigation.

The final approach to conceptualizing Type A behavior originates in the work of Matthews and Siegel (1982) in their efforts to identify the basis of Type A behavior. Matthews and Siegel have suggested that the etiology of Type A behavior is a function of strongly valuing productivity and the associated ambiguous standards for evaluating this productivity. This combination Matthews believes, is associated with a sense of time passing rapidly and the need for achievement striving. Matthews argues that the complexity of information should increase as the degree of ambiguity for evaluating the task performance increases. An example that Matthews provides is the situation in which someone is hired to complete a job that does not have clear standards for performance evaluation. If the individual values productivity strongly, the combination of this with ambiguous standards would evoke various Type A behaviors (sense of time-urgency) until a clear performance evaluation standard was specified or some external reward was provided to signify that the behavior was adequate. In the absence of such factors, the behavior would continually be evoked.

Dembroski and MacDougall (1978) indicated that Type A's prefer to sit with others rather than to sit alone while waiting for a stressful situation to occur. They argue that Type A's elicit information from others in order to compare their own behavior during the stressful situation. This finding suggests that Type A's may have a greater interest in social comparison information than Type B's. Other findings indicate that Type A's have a greater interest in performing well relative to others, to their own standards, and to the best possible performance. These findings, as a whole, suggest that Type A's value productivity and tend to have vague, albeit high standards. Research with children also tends to support such findings. The developmental approach to Type A will be discussed in more detail later.

As indicated in this section, the psychological explanations for Type A behavior are diverse and complex. Research on the psychology of Type A has been conducted only since the 1970s, which may account for some of the confusion regarding psychological factors in Type A. New research is being published in this area rapidly, and some general consensus and models should emerge within the next decade. At present, however, the constructs of self-involvement, uncontrollability, and ambiguous standards of evaluation remain as the key explanatory factors in the Type A behavior pattern. We will now focus on hostility, a specific component of Type A behavior that appears to play a major role in linking Type A's to CHD. A review of the research on hostility will help illustrate an integrative approach to the study of Type A behavior, with discussions from social psychology, psychophysiology, developmental psychology, psychiatry, and physiology.

## ANGER–HOSTILITY AND CORONARY HEART DISEASE: A PARADIGM

A role for anger and hostility in the development, exacerbation, and maintenance of a number of medical disorders was proposed by earlier investigators in psychosomatic medicine, but most of the empirical research supports the role of anger and hostility in cardiovascular disorders. The current discussion will be directed specifically at anger, hostility, and CHD. The first question to be addressed is whether there is, in fact, a relationship between anger and CHD. Support for such a relationship has been provided by a number of investigators. The relationship between anger and CHD appears to operate both through the Type A behavior pattern, with anger arousability as one of the major characteristics of the Type A individual, and through an independent mechanism whereby anger possesses predictive abilities even after Type A behavior has been removed from equations used to predict CHD.

Jenkins (1966) reported that silent MI cases scored higher on potential for hostility, in contrast to controls, as measured by interviewers' ratings based on voice cues and facial and postural gestures during the structured Type A interview. Additional analyses of the Western Collaborative Group Study data by Matthews, Glass, Rosenman, and Bortner (1977) indicated that four of the seven Type A interview items that were able to discriminate CHD cases from controls were related to anger/hostility. Two of the four items were actual self reports of anger by the respondents, in which they indicated that they became angry more than once a week and that their anger was often directed at others (i.e., anger-out). The remaining two items were based on ratings of explosive voice and potential for hostility as determined by the interviewer. As discussed in the preceding section, the Framingham study observed that anger-*in* was related to CHD incidence in both men and women and that this association was independent of the relationship between Type A behavior and CHD incidence (Haynes, Feinleib, & Kannel, 1980). Additionally, recent prospective studies have indicated a relationship between an MMPI (Minnesota Multiphasic Personality Inventory) measure of hostility and CHD incidence (Barefoot, Dahlstrom, & Williams, 1983; Shekelle, Gale, Ostfeld, & Paul, 1983). Barefoot *et al.* reported on a 20-year follow-up of medical students where hostility scores were predictive of CHD incidence, MI, angina, and CHD death, in addition to mortality from *all* causes after adjusting for other CHD risk factors. Shekelle *et al.*, using the same inventory of hostility over a 20-year period, reported that mortality from CHD and total mortality among initially disease-free employees were related to these hostility scores. This relationship, however, was reduced to nonsignificance when other CHD risk factors were included. The MMPI score of hostility indicated considerable stability across a one- and four-year interval in these studies. Research with Swedish workers, conducted by Theorell, Lind, and Floderus (1975), indicated that self-reported hostility associated with delay predicted all deaths, MIs, and ulcers. These latter studies suggest the nonspecific role of anger in that such anger/hostility tended to be associated with a variety of causes of death. Nevertheless, such research also indicates a relationship between anger and CHD.

Let us consider this anger–CHD relationship more closely. In a review by Diamond (1983), the anger–CHD research was divided into the following categories: (1) psychodynamic studies of coronary patients, (2) personality studies in CHD, and (3) anger and hostility in the Type A behavior pattern. Psychodynamic conceptualizations of coronary patients focus on an aggressive characteristic of these patients and the identification of motives or *drives* for these aggressive characteristics. Concepts of "repressed aggression channelled into the body," proposed by Menninger and Menninger (1936), are examples of such an approach. The clinicians discussed a hostile relation with the mother and a strong emotional attachment to the father, with such a relationship serving to deny *powerful* hostility. Identification with the father was speculated by the Menningers to help explain certain cases of heart attacks in sons of fathers who were similarly stricken. Arlow (1945) further discussed this identification process, indicating that such a process existed with a "feared father," yet the process was faulty in that it led to continuous competing and striving for achievement, with no resolution of anxiety or tension. This psychodynamic literature was based on a limited number of observations or cases and presented a number of problems in terms of empirical verification of the various constructs proposed.

Personality research in patients with CHD utilizes both projective and objective psychometric techniques. The majority of these studies were retrospective, comparing subjects with known cardiac conditions to patient or healthy controls. The findings of personality studies, in general, have indicated that coronary patients tend to be less introspective and less competent in handling their aggressive tendencies. Rorschach protocols of CHD patients were interpreted as indicative of aggressive drives to dominate others, in addition to ambition, extroversion, and limited creativity. Other studies indicated that post-MI cases were described as having rigid control over emotions, obsessive-compulsive defenses, impoverished fantasy lives, and pragmatic thinking (Dongier, 1974). As discussed by Diamond (1983), there were considerable methodological problems with the various personality studies. These problems included the retrospective field nature of the studies and that the studies were not all controlled for age, sex, IQ, and social status. Additional problems included the lack of specificity of a diagnostic entity, for example, angina pectoris, and the frequent use of nonstandardized scales or interviews. However, findings from the various personality studies on coronary patients do tend to present a general picture of the coronary patient as having such attributes as aggressiveness, hard-driving behavior, and achievement striving. It is aggressiveness, rather than hostility or anger, that is often discussed in this literature. Diamond suggests that perhaps this aggressiveness indicates that emotional arousal is translated into goal-directed activities. Diamond also suggests that the process involved in anger and hostility may be more difficult to evaluate using self-report techniques. Diamond assumed that this is the result of rigid control of affective expression and the excessive use of denial characteristics noted by some investigators. The final area that Diamond discusses is the research on anger and hostility in the Type A behavior pattern.

A reanalysis of the Western Collaborative Group data from interview ratings on CHD cases and matched controls indicated that competitive drive and impatience were associated with CHD incidence. Four items — explosive voice modulation, vigorous answers, potential for hostility, and irritation at waiting in line — were those that differentiated the two groups. The items, "competitive in games with peers," "feel that the time passes too slowly," "anger directed outward," and "gets angry more than once a week" were also endorsed more frequently for the CHD cases. Chesney et al. (1981), found that the aggression scale of the Adjective Checklist was the best discriminator of Type A behavior as measured by the interview. This suggested that aggression represents a major component of the Type A behavior pattern and implies that this aggression/physiological reactivity and CHD itself should be further clarified.

In psychophysiological research on Type A's, potential for hostility was most strongly related to systolic blood pressure and heart rate increases in response to challenge tasks. Competitive drive and rapid accelerated speech were significantly associated with systolic blood pressure elevation only (Dembroski, MacDougall, Shields, Petitto, & Lushene, 1978). In a later investigation of cardiovascular response, Type A, and level of challenge, the greatest physiological differences observed between A's and B's were under conditions of high challenge. Interestingly, a subset of Type A's, who were categorized as high hostile/competitive on the basis of component analysis of the structured interview protocols, reacted to *both* high and low challenge with the physiological elevations seen in the full Type A sample for high challenge only. Dembroski, MacDougall, Herd, and Shields (1979) hypothesized that the high hostile Type A's may perceive a variety of situations as challenging (even mild challenging circumstances) and, therefore, respond frequently and excessively with heightened cardiovascular reactivity. The relationship between the potential for hostility and physiological reactivity was replicated in a sample of women (MacDougall, Dembroski, & Krantz, 1981). The hostility component of Type A correlated significantly with systolic blood pressure increases during a reaction time task, interpersonal interview, and quiz.

Using a different approach, Glass, Krakoff, et al. (1980) evaluated the relationship between harrassment and physiological reactivity in Type A and B adult male transit workers. Blood pressure, plasma catecholamines, and heart rate were measured while the subject was working at a video game in competition with a trained confederate. Marked increases in blood pressure, heart rate, and epinephrine was observed during the harassment/competition condition only. During this condition, the confederate delivered a series of derogatory remarks related to performance. The comparison condition was one in which the confederate, who controlled the game outcomes, remained silent during play (competition only condition). In a second study reported by Glass *et al.* (1980), subjects competed singly against the computer; however, this time, a monetary incentive was also provided. The investigators observed that direct competition elicited comparable results in Type A's and B's, but that harassment evoked more extreme physiological arousal only among the Type A subjects. If simple harassment can elicit greater physiological reactivity in Type A's, what might occur when a goal that the Type A individual is trying to achieve is blocked? It has been suggested by Glass (1977) that Type A's might be more susceptible to goal blocking, considering their habitual goal orientation and assumed need for control. Other questions relating to harassment, anger, Type A, and physiological reactivity include, To what extent do such harassment situations actually evoke hostility? and What is the relationship between measures of hostility and physiological reactivity observed within the context of the anger-provoking situation? These questions relate to the identification of certain situations or stimulus conditions that elicit enhanced physiological reactivity among Type A's, and their concomitant emotional consequences. A study by Diamond, Schneiderman, Schwartz, Smith, Vorp, and DeCarlo-Pasin (1984) recently addressed some of these issues.

Diamond *et al.* (1984), using male undergraduates, investigated anger-related variables of harassment and goal blocking and the expression of anger and psychophysiological reactivity in Type A's. Using the SI to identify Type A's and B's, Diamond *et al.* tested Type A's and B's under three conditions: (1) *competitive control,* in which the subject and the confederate merely competed for 15 minutes; (2) *goal blocking,* in which a programmed series of distractions was delivered to impede a subject's efforts to compete successfully (i.e., interrupting with irrelevant questions, frequently reminding players to remain still, delaying onset of games, accidentally resetting the score); and (3) *harassment,* in which the confederate delivered eight derogatory comments to the subject (i.e., Can't you keep your eye on the ball; You're not even trying; I sign up for an experiment and they pair me up with a retard). In an effort to improve the credibility of his role, the confederate had established himself during the pregame period as a rude, contentious individual. Systolic and diastolic blood pressure was monitored, in addition to heart rate, during baseline, stimulus condition, and recovery period. A number of personality variables were also measured, including a scale of hostility and the anger sections of the Framingham psychosocial survey, consisting of seven questions regarding response to anger arousal. The results of the Diamond *et al.* study included the following: (1) harassment in the context of competition evoked marked elevations in systolic blood pressure and heart rate, compared with goal blocking during competition or just simple competition alone, and Type A subjects displayed the greatest systolic blood pressure increases during the harassment condition (particularly early in the game); (2) Type B's tended toward higher blood pressure reactivity than Type A's in the competition only or control condition; and (3) potential for hostility or stylistic hostility, as measured by the structured interview, outwardly directed anger, as measured by the Framingham psychosocial survey, and Type A were associated with physiological reactivity among highly hostile subjects. The highly hostile subjects were those showing greater scores on a personality scale of hostility. The Diamond *et al.* study illustrates the complexity of relating such factors as anger/hostility (trait hostility), Type A behavior, and physiological reactivity. It appears that there is a complex relationship between outward expression of anger, tendency toward hostility, and physiological reactivity. As Diamond *et al.* argued, if cardiovascular reactivity is associated with increased coronary risk in Type A individuals, it may be associated only in a subgroup of Type A's (i.e., those displaying high anger-out expressiveness and high trait hostility). Clearly, this issue should be studied further before any definitive conclusions can be drawn; however, the research of Diamond *et al.* highlights the complexities involved.

Another approach to studying the anger/hostility–CHD relationship include studies relating anger to atherosclerosis (Williams, Haney, Lee, Hong Kong, Blumenthal, & Whalen, 1980). The Williams *et al.* research investigated measures of Type A behavior, as assessed by the SI, and hostility level, using a subscale of the MMPI. Over 400 patients who underwent diagnostic coronary arteriography for suspected CHD completed the Type A interview and the measure of hostility. A significantly greater number of Type A patients had at least one artery with a clinically significant occlusion of 75% or greater. When looking at the hostility measure, it was found that only 48% of those patients with low scores on hostility displayed a significant occlusion. This contrasted considerably with patients in all groups scoring higher than 10 on the hostility scale — these individuals showed a 70% rate of significant disease. Figure 10-1 illustrates the relationship of Type A behavior pattern, hostility, and sex to the occurrence of significant coronary occlusion. As can

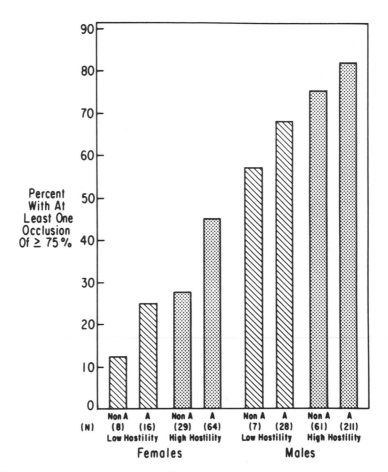

**FIGURE 10-1.** Type A behavior, hostility, sex, and degree of coronary occlusion. From "Type A Behavior, Hostility, and Coronary Atherosclerosis" by R. B. Williams, T. L. Haney, K. L. Lee, Y. Hong Kong, J. A. Blumenthal, & R. Whalen, 1980, *Psychosomatic Medicine, 42,* 545. Copyright 1980 by Elsevier Science Co., Inc. Reprinted by permission.

be seen in the figure, there is a linear relationship between hostility, sex, and Type A scores. There is a considerable increase in the amount of observed atherosclerosis in Type A males with high hostility scores.

The measurement of anger/hostility itself is complex. As with such broad constructs as stress and pain, anger involves a complicated set of psychological, behavioral, and psychophysiological components. A recent investigation of anger and cardiovascular risk factors (including Type A) in adolescents illustrates one well conceived approach to the measurement of anger (Siegel, 1984). Siegel was not directly investigating CHD or hypertension, given that this would have been quite difficult in the population she studied (i.e., adolescents). The relationships between anger and multiple indicators of cardiovascular risk were studied. Of particular importance in this study was the focus on adolescents, as well as Siegel's careful investigation of the construct of anger. It is becoming more obvious that studies during late childhood and adolescence are critical for understanding the atherosclerotic process because of evidence that this process may begin before or during the second decade of life. Also, longitudinal studies of aggression, a behavioral manifestation of anger, have indicated a considerable stability for this behavior during the entire life span. Therefore, early investigations of the relationship of anger and cardiovascular risk factors are an important approach for understanding the role of psychological factors in the development of CHD, as well as the specific relationship between anger and cardiovascular disease risk factors. Siegel's research also focused on determining whether anger, as measured by her index, suggested a *unidimensional construct* or a more complicated *multidimensional construct* (i.e., heterogeneous).

Siegel studied 213 adolescents between the ages of 13 and 18 obtained from a pool of 516 students who participated in a school blood pressure screening. Siegel *et al.* obtained measures of anger (a 19-item anger index), physical variables (blood lipids, blood pressure, smoking, obesity, physical activity level), psychological variables (test anxiety, life satisfaction, life events, self-concept), and Type A behavior pattern (behavior pattern assessed by the adolescent structured interview). The anger index, physical variables, and Type A measures are of particular interest here. The 19 item anger index was developed from three sources: (1) the 15-item "becomes angry" scale of the Edwards Personality Inventory — examples of items include "seldom gets angry about anything" and "becomes angry when having to wait for others"; (2) two items written specifically for the study, including "response to frustration with irritation and anger" and has "frequent feelings of anger"; and (3) two observational ratings, both of which were made by the interviewer during the Type A behavior pattern assessment. These behaviors included showing anger when describing what was most irritating about school and level of hostility manifested during the interview. The 19-item anger index is shown in Table 10-3.

A factor analysis of the anger index indicated two general factors. Siegel defined these factors as *frequent anger-out* and *anger situation*. The various items comprising these factors are listed in Table 10-4. The use of factor analysis for identifying components of anger represent an important methodological approach in health psychology. The procedure allows the investigator to identify empirically specific components of a general construct. The results of the factor analysis suggest that frequent anger directed outward and the range of situations that arouse or trigger anger are dimensions of the anger response. The frequent anger-out factor consisted of such items as difficulty controlling anger when hurt, raises voice when angry, frequent feelings of anger, and two behavioral observations reflecting the extent of manifest hostility. The anger situations factor included a variety of situations such as "gets angry if I can't find something" and "gets angry if feels someone is blocking his plans."

The investigation of the two anger factor scores and their relation to Type A behavior and other CHD risk factors turned up some interesting findings. The frequent anger-out factor was associated with higher systolic and diastolic blood pressure, smoking, and less leisure time for physical activities. Thus, with the exception of serum cholesterol and obesity, all the measures of physical health status were, in part, related to the anger-out factor scores. Analysis of the anger situation factor

## TABLE 10-3
### Anger Index Items and Their Sources

I. Self-Reports
    A. Edwards Personality Inventory "Becomes Angry" Scale
        1. Has difficulty controlling anger when someone hurts him/her.
        2. Becomes angry when sees someone being mistreated.[a]
        3. Is the sort of person who is not difficult to make angry.
        4. Becomes so angry that feels like throwing or breaking things.
        5. Gets angry if feels someone is blocking his/her plans.
        6. Raises voice when gets angry.
        7. Seldom gets angry about anything. (keyed false)
        8. Gets angry easily but gets over it quickly.
        9. Gets angry with anyone who tried to restrict his/her freedom.
        10. Seldom gets angry with others. (keyed false)
        11. Gets over an angry spell very quickly. (keyed false)
        12. Gets angry when can't find something he/she is looking for.
        13. Becomes angry when has to wait for others.
        14. Gets angry if belongings are disturbed by someone.
        15. Gets angry if someone tries to take advantage of his/her friendship.
    B. Additional Items
        1. Responds to frustration with irritation and anger.
        2. Has frequent feelings of anger.

II. Observer Ratings (from Adolescent Structured Interview)
        1. Showed anger when describing irritations at school.
        2. Hostile during interview.
Alpha = 0.75

*Note.* From "Anger and Cardiovascular Risk in Adolescents" by J. M. Siegel, 1984, *Health Psychology,* 3(4)300. Copyright 1984 by Laurence Erlbaum Associates. Reprinted by permission.
[a]Item deleted because of low interitem correlations.

**TABLE 10-4**

Anger and Cardiovascular Risk in Adolescents

| Factor I[a]—Frequent anger out (FAO)—79% of variance | Loading |
|---|---|
| 1. Seldom gets angry about anything. (keyed false) | .66 |
| 2. Seldom gets angry with others. (keyed false) | .56 |
| 3. Raises voice when gets angry. | .47 |
| 4. Has difficulty controlling anger when someone hurts him/her. | .45 |
| 5. Has frequent feelings of anger. | .39 |
| 6. Showed anger when describing irritation at school. | .39 |
| 7. Hostile during interview. | .35 |
| 8. Is sort of person who is not difficult to make angry. | .33 |
| Alpha = .69 | |
| Factor II[a]—Anger situations (AS)—21% of variance | |
| 1. Gets angry with anyone who tried to restrict his/her freedom. | .55 |
| 2. Gets angry if belongings are disturbed by someone. | .50 |
| 3. Responds to frustration with irritation and anger. | .44 |
| 4. Gets angry when can't find something he/she is looking for. | .43 |
| 5. Gets angry if feels someone is blocking his/her plans. | .38 |
| Alpha = .59 | |

Note. From "Anger and Cardiovascular Risk in Adolescents" by J. M. Siegel, 1984, *Health Psychology* 3(4)303. Copyright 1984 by Laurence Erlbaum Associates. Reprinted by permission.
[a]Correlation: Factor I with Factor II, $r(203) = .36$, $p < .001$.

indicated that, controlling for sex and age, higher scores on the anger situation factor were associated with obesity. A significant sex-by-anger situation interaction for smoking indicated that higher scores on this factor were associated with a greater likelihood of smoking, but the relationship was stronger for girls than for boys. Other sex-by-anger situation interactions were observed where higher scores on this factor were associated with an increase in activity for girls and a decrease in activity for boys. With the exception of blood pressure and cholesterol, all the measures of physical health status were, in part, related to the anger situation factor scores.

Given the cross-sectional nature of this study, it is difficult to argue specifically for the predictive role of anger in the various risk factors studied (this was not a prospective study). That is, it is difficult to determine whether anger precedes or is a consequence of the risk factor indicators in the study. However, the important finding here was that frequent anger directed outward was related to a different set of cardiovascular risk factors than were anger situations. This study also indicated that adolescents characterized by frequent anger-out tend to have elevated blood pressure and a relatively sedentary life-style during leisure time, whereas adolescents who get angry in response to a variety of situations tend to be Type A, overweight, and relatively sedentary at school/on the job. Smoking, on the other hand, was reported to be associated with both anger factor scores. This research represents an interesting approach to the study of anger and cardiovascular disease; however, further work is needed to determine whether intensity, magnitude, frequency, or mode of expression of anger (anger-in/anger-out) is most highly related to certain cardiovascular risk factors. This research, in addition to the psychophysiological approach, should help answer key questions relating hostility/anger to CHD in both adolescents and adults.

### Born to Strive?

Is there a subset of individuals who are born to strive? One consideration when the developmental course of the Type A behavior pattern is examined is whether there is an underlying genetic predisposition for such behavior. The genetic contribution to the development of health disorders can be studied, to some extent, in twins. Monozygotic (MZ) (identical) twins are defined as having 100% of their genes in common, as compared to dizygotic (DZ) (fraternal or nonidentical) twins who share an average of only 50% of their genes. The assumption underlying the twin study method is that both types of twins are equally affected by environmental influences, so that any greater similarity within the MZ than within the DZ pairs can be attributed to genetic factors. If both MZ twins exhibit the same trait under investigation, they are said to be *concordant*. The number of concordant pairs divided by the total number of pairs represents the concordance coefficient. *Discordance* in only a single pair of MZ twins who have lived through the period of risk calls into question the role of genetic factors in the etiology of a particular disorder. One method of assessing important environmental etiological factors is to define the nongenetic influences that differentiate the affected proband from the unaffected co-twin. Another method used to separate genetic effects from environmental effects is the study of MZ twins who have been reared apart. This latter method, however, has several shortcomings, since it is rare to find these pairs of twins reared apart and, if they have been, the separation is often incomplete.

There is little evidence to suggest a genetic influence on the global Type A behavior pattern (Matthews & Krantz, 1976; Rosenman, Rahe, Borhani, & Feinleib, 1976). In an attempt to estimate the heritability of coronary-prone behavior, Rahe, Hervig, and Rosenman (1978) studied 93 pairs of MZ and 97 pairs of DZ middle-aged, American male twins. In addition to a SI assessment of Type A behavior, participants were required to complete four psychological test batteries: the Thurstone Temperament Schedule, the Jenkins Activity Survey, the California Psychological Inventory, and the Gough Adjective Check List. Rahe *et al.* (1978) found that Type A behavior, as determined by interview, did not show evidence of heritability. However, psychological test scores that significantly correlated with Type A behavior (e.g., active, impulsive, dominant, sociable, impatient) were found to have generally significant heritability estimates.

Modest genetic input has been found for certain components of the Type A behavior pattern, such as drive, competitiveness, dominance, sociability, and impulsiveness (Matthews & Krantz, 1976). Horn, Plomin, and Rosenman (1976) found further support for the heritability of certain personality traits associated with the Type A behavior pattern. In a study of 99 pairs of fraternal adult male twins, Horn *et al.* (1976) found that such personality factors as conversational poise, compulsiveness, and social ease, as measured by the California Psychological Inventory, were related to heritability. The sociability factors accounted for 28% of the variance of the genetic items in this study, which suggested a possible genetic factor in the development of the trait of sociability.

## Gender and Physiological Reactivity

Another approach to determine the role of biological predisposition in the development of Type A behavior has been to examine sex differences in psychophysiological reactivity. As discussed in a previous section, differences in physiological responding between Type A and Type B men have been reported. Until recently, the majority of studies supporting the general hypothesis that Type A individuals show excessive sympathetic arousal under challenging conditions have used male subjects. Comparatively little consistent research has emerged evaluating the psychophysiological response differences between Type A and Type B females. An early study by Rosenman and Friedman (1961) demonstrated that women selected solely on the basis of Type A behavior had higher levels of serum cholesterol and diastolic hypertension. Several more recent studies have not found physiological reactivity differences between female Type A's and Type B's (Frankenhaeuser, Lundberg, & Forsman, 1980; Lott & Gatchel, 1978; Manuck, Craft, & Gold, 1978). It appears that the Type A behavior pattern may be expressed differently in females than males. Frankenhaeuser *et al.* (1980), for instance, found that both male and female Type A subjects chose to work faster at a self-paced reaction time task than did Type B's, but did not show more physiological arousal. However, males of both types excreted more epinephrine and reported exerting a greater effort during the task than did females. In another study, MacDougall *et al.* (1981) compared the cardiovascular responses of Type A and Type B college women to a variety of stressors. In contrast to the men studied earlier, no differences were found between the women in heart rate or systolic and diastolic blood pressure responses during either a cold pressor test or a choice reaction time task. The responses of Type A women, however, were greater for systolic blood pressure than the Type B women during the structured interview and history quiz, but no differences in heart rate or diastolic blood pressure responses were seen, which indicates a situation-specific reactivity not observable in males.

More recently, a number of important studies have attempted to investigate the relationship between coronary-prone behavior and physiological responses to stress in older and younger women (Lawler, Rixse, & Allen, 1983; Lawler, Schmied, Mitchell, & Rixse, 1984). Lawler *et al.* (1983) assessed the physiological responsivity to stress in 41 Type A and B women between the ages of 25 and 55. All participants were required to complete the JAS and a health questionnaire. The psychological stressors included a mental arithmetic test and a Raven's Progressive Matrices, the latter involving two conditions — experimenter-controlled pacing and subject-controlled pacing. Throughout the experiment, physiological measures (heart rate, blood pressure, skin conductance) were monitored during each rest and task sequence. Based on the JAS, 90% of the executive-level women scored at the 65th percentile and above, thus identifying themselves as strong Type A's, whereas the unemployed or housewife group were identified as A's and B's. Differences were also found for employed Type A's, unemployed Type A's, and unemployed Type B's on mean physiological measures of heart rate, second-by-second heart rate, and systolic and diastolic blood pressure. The employed Type A women had a higher heart rate, the Type B women had the greatest phasic heart rate deceleration. When Type A and B women were directly compared within the unemployed group, Type A women showed a greater heart rate reactivity and greater systolic responses on all tasks. In this respect, the Type A women's hyperreactivity was similar to that in men. In an attempt to replicate these findings in a population of young college women, aged 18 to 25, Lawler *et al.* (1984) used the same psychological stressors, in addition to the JAS and a structured interview. The participants in this study consisted of 20 women who were matriculated in female-dominated majors and 17 women who were pursuing degrees in male-dominated or non-traditional fields for women. Lawler *et al.* (1984) found no physiological differences (heart rate or blood pressure) between Type A and Type B women on resting levels or on phasic response to the tasks. These findings, taken as a whole, suggest that age and associated experience in the work environment may play a role in the way women react to psychological stressors. With increased experience, a tendency toward hyperreactivity may occur.

A further explanation for the inconsistency of these findings may lie in the complex interplay of gender, Type A behavior, and family history of cardiovascular disease in influencing physiological reactivity. In order to assess the influence of these interacting variables on cardiovascular reactivity and its relationship to CHD, Lane, White, and Williams (1984) recruited 29 healthy female undergraduate students who were then classified into Type A's and Type B's on the scores obtained from the JAS. Five physiological recordings were taken throughout the Resting–Baseline and Task periods of the experiment and included heart rate, forearm blood flow, respiration, systolic blood pressure, and diastolic blood pressure. The experimental task consisted of a challenging mental arithmetic task involving the subtraction of 13 from a four-digit number and the subsequent subtraction of 13 from each new answer, with five trials being recorded over a six-minute period. Instructions emphasizing the speed and accuracy of subtraction, as well as the importance of continued striving during the entire task period, were given to the subjects. In addition, a bottle of champagne was offered as an incentive for the highest number of correct subtractions made.

When compared to the results of an earlier study that used an identical task with a similar reward in young male subjects (Williams, Lane, et al. 1982), the findings of Lane et al. (1984) indicate the existence of gender differences in physiological stress reactivity. Lane et al. (1984) found that, in contrast to the male subjects of the earlier study, female Type A subjects were on the whole *not* hyperresponsive (compared to Type B subjects) during the mental arithmetic task. Although the female subjects responded to the task with elevations in heart rate, blood pressure, and forearm blood flow, they did not show the greater degree of skeletal muscle vasodilation Type A males had during the mental arithmetic task. This finding may possibly be accounted for by Frankenhaeuser's observations regarding sex differences in cardiovascular responding (Frankenhaeuser, Dunne, & Lundberg, 1976; Frankenhaeuser, von Wright, Collins, von Wright, Sedvall, & Swahn, 1978; Frankenhaeuser, Dunne, & Forsman, 1980), in that males typically excrete more epiniphrine than females do during the stress response. One may speculate that because the skeletal-muscle vasodilation observed in males is probably being mediated by increased plasma epinephrine, differences in response seen in males and females may be accounted for by sex differences in epinephrine release.

Additional findings from the Lane et al. (1984) study regarding interactions of Type A's and Type B's with a *family history* of hypertension provide a further possible explanation for the lack of task-related cardiovascular hyperresponsivity in female Type A's as compared with Type A males. Lane *et al*. (1984) found that although female Type A's were not hyperresponsive as a group, a subset of those with a positive family history of hypertension were, in fact, hyperresponsive and were more so compared to Type B females with a positive family history. This study indicates that two new dimensions — gender and family history — should be further investigated in terms of their interactive role with Type A behavior in modulating the cardiovascular and neuroendocrine hyperresponsivity.

### Family Models

The notion that parents may serve as models for Type A behavior for their children has also been investigated as a possible factor contributing to the development of Type A behavior. Implicit in this notion is the assumption that parents and children should be similar on the Type A dimension. Some authors have shown that Type A behavior may be more prevalent in children of parents with higher education levels and occupational status. Butensky *et al*. (1976), for example, found that children and teenagers from suburban, middle-class homes displayed more Type A behavior than age- and sex-matched controls from rural working-class homes. Viewed from a social learning perspective, adult modeling and conditioning processes have been found that significantly affect competitive aggressive behavior in offspring (Bandura, Ross, & Ross, 1963; Bandura & Walters, 1959; McClelland, 1961; McKinley, 1964), thus explaining the potential influence of such behaviors when modeled by middle-class parents. It is not surprising, therefore, that behavior patterns resembling the Type A behavior pattern, albeit modest, have been found in children of both sexes over 11 years old (Bortner, Rosenman, & Friedman, 1970; Matthews & Krantz, 1976). The role of family models and their interaction with other mechanisms involved in the development of Type A behavior should be further explored.

### Other Learning Processes

Differential reinforcement of specific components of the Type A behavior pattern (achievement motivation, aggression, time-urgency) may also be implicated in the development of the coronary-prone behavior pattern. Matthews (1978) has hypothesized, for instance, that approval and disapproval contingent on improved performance in a child who is predisposed to a heightened response to "loss of control" or "disapproval" and who tends toward social comparison may help to explain the development of Type A behavior in children. Matthews supported her hypothesis with data from Type A college students who reported experiencing guilt in the absence of parental approval and who indicated that their parents were more strict than the parents of Type B students. Moreover, direct observations of mothers of extreme Type A children revealed that mothers tend to reinforce their children differentially (ages 4–10), that is, they disapproved of poor performance and encouraged their children to try harder following a good performance, to a greater degree than did mothers of extreme Type B children. Matthews (1978) also found that Type A mothers tended to evaluate their child's performance as positive less frequently than did Type B mothers. Two subsequent studies designed to evaluate the effects of extrafamilial approval on competitiveness and impatience revealed that positive performance evaluations and frequent urging to improve subsequent performance significantly increased competitive-striving behaviors, although impatience was not affected. In general terms, these findings suggest that the combination of frequent extrafamilial approval and intrafamilial contingent approval and disapproval may underlie the development of certain components of the Type A behavior pattern.

Another explanation for the development and maintenance of the Type A behavior pattern may be derived from the positive outcomes associated, both socially and economically, with such a behavior pattern, particularly in Western cultures. Chesney and Rosenman (1980), for example, provided evidence that suggested that Type A behavior is associated with socioeconomic status in both sexes and with occupational status, income, and rapid achievement in middle-class males. Although only modest, these associations justify the further investigation of the role of actual or expected rewards in maintaining the Type A pattern. Longitudinal research on fluctuations in the Type A pattern over time and on the respective role of economic and social factors would enhance our understanding of the maintenance of this pattern.

## TYPE A-CORONARY HEART DISEASE: THE PHYSIOLOGICAL TRANSDUCTION PROCESS

If there is a relationship between the Type A behavior pattern and CHD, one must ask how Type A behavior leads to the development of CHD. That is, what is the physiological process through which Type A behavior sets the stage or contributes to the development of CHD? It is important, when considering physiological mechanisms, to consider the various stages and clinical events of CHD because mechanisms that may produce or exacerbate the atherosclerotic process may be quite different from those involved in sudden cardiac death or MI. Thus, any consideration of the possible role Type A behavior may play in the physiological development of CHD must consider the pathogenesis of atherosclerosis and the effects of Type A behavior on various complications of coronary atherosclerosis, including MI, angina pectoris, and sudden arrhythmic death.

Does the behavior pattern play an etiological role in atherosclerosis? Currently, there is no evidence that Type A behavior contributes directly or indirectly to the primary event or the formation of atheromata. It would be quite difficult, however, to demonstrate such a role definitively. This specific question cannot currently be addressed adequately in humans, but the use of animal models in which the process of atherogenesis could be accelerated under controlled conditions is one viable methodological approach to studying the problem.

A major focus for research on physiological mechanisms is the relationship between catecholamines and CHD. As discussed earlier, it has been shown that Type A's tend to have a heightened sympathetic reactivity, in contrast to Type B's. Recent work has indicated that regulation of the circulation and lipid mobilization, platelet aggregation, and other processes potentially related to atherogenesis can be influenced by catecholamines. It has been found that norepinephrine, or its metabolites, in both urine and plasma are increased in individuals classified as Type A and, interestingly, in ambulatory persons with CHD. Type A individuals tend to be more reactive than Type B in response to environmental challenges and stressors but resting levels apparently do not differentiate the Type A from the Type B subject. Although there is evidence that sympathetic reactivity may influence cholesterol metabolism (accountants had increased serum cholesterol levels as the April 15 tax deadline approached), such findings are only correlates of stress and Type A behavior and may have little to do with the development of CHD. Clearly, more research is needed to identify the pathophysiological links between Type A and CHD.

The Type A behavior pattern, with its associated sympathetic reactivity to challenge, could contribute to the exacerbation of coronary atherosclerotic complications (sudden arrhythmic death, angina and MI). Some studies have suggested that stress and high catecholamine levels can trigger complicated arrhythmic activity, angina, and MI. It is possible that increased sympathetic activity can exert an effect on CHD through environmentally induced changes in cardiovascular functioning via circulating catecholamines. That is, the response to stress, which is characteristically defined as an increased cardiac output and/or peripheral resistance, could impose an additional work load on the cardiac muscle such that the blood supply to the heart via diseased coronary arteries is insufficient for the metabolic needs of the heart, resulting in anginal pains or MI. Similarly, this sympathetic arousal could exacerbate the occurrence of abnormal rhythms in the heart of an individual with documented atherosclerosis.

## TYPE A AND THE WORK ENVIRONMENT

Chesney and Rosenman (1980) have studied the interaction of Type A behavior and the work environment. This research is based upon a conceptualization of job stress proposed by French, Rogers, and Cobb (1974), the *person–environment fit theory.* The theory hypothesizes that an incompatibility, or "poor fit," between job demand, worker's skills and abilities, and/or difficulty in the job fulfilling a worker's personal needs results in occupational stress. According to this theory, the lack of fit results in job stress, psychological distress (depression, anxiety, job dissatisfaction), and/or negative health outcomes (e.g., CHD). The person–environment fit theory empahsizes aspects of the job environment and personal characteristics or personality and their dynamic interaction.

Given the findings of heightened physiological reactivity in specific situations (i.e., challenge) in Type A's, consideration of the nature of the work environment (challenge/no challenge) is particularly important. Chesney and Rosenman (1980) attempted to test the complicated person–environment fit theory as it related to Type A behavior. These investigators studied 145 male managers, classified as A or B by the SI. The subjects were requested to monitor work load and work pressure weekly. A symptom checklist was also completed on five occasions to measure anxiety. Although no differences were observed on anxiety between the A's and B's, when job environment characteristics (work load and pressure) were considered, work load and pressure were found to be correlated with anxiety for Type A's only. Further analysis with a subsample (76 subjects) revealed that a Type A individual perceives the work environment (Work Environment Scale, WES) as one in which he was in control, in contrast to a Type B individual. Chesney *et al.* hypothesized that an *extremely* controlled environment would present a threat or challenge to the Type A manager, who if placed in such an environment, would experience greater distress (i.e., poor person–environment fit) than in a work environment that he could control. Chesney tested this hypothesis by classifying A's and B's into three groups, based upon WES "control" subscale scores: (1) low externally controlled environment group; (2) middle group; and (3) high externally controlled environment group. The results indicated that the Type A's in the high externally controlled environment group experienced higher Trait Anxiety than A's in the low externally controlled environment. In contrast, *lower* Trait Anxiety was observed in the high externally controlled environment for Type B's.

Chesney and Rosenman (1980) argued that these findings support the hypothesis that Type A's who characteristically need to be in control become distressed when forced to interact with an environment that is *excessively* controlled, whereas Type B's experience anxiety when confronted with an environment characterized by minimal structure and minimal external control. This work is an important example of research that examines the laboratory and clinically observed characteristics of Type A individuals within the actual work environment to test the validity of the various constructs of challenge and control.

Figure 10-2 presents a framework (model) relating Type A behavior to the work environment. The model was proposed by two British psychologists, Davidson and Cooper (1980). The model identifies five major categories: (1) susceptible Type A individual; (2) work environment; (3) control conflict; (4) maladaptive coping behavior; and (5) symptoms. Davidson and Cooper (1980) reviewed the research on these five factors.

Research related to the "susceptible Type A individual" indicates the following: (1) time-urgency and ambition decrease with age (beyond 36–55 years); (2) high-stress occupations (e.g., air traffic controller) do *not* necessarily facilitate increased Type A behavior among employees;

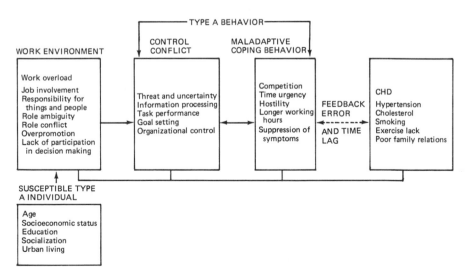

**FIGURE 10-2.** Type A behavior and work environment. From "Type A Coronary-Prone Behavior in the Work Environment" by M. J. Davidson and C. L. Cooper, 1980, *Journal of Occupational Medicine, 22,* 376. Copyright 1980 by American Occupational Medical Association. Reprinted by permission.

(3) higher Type A scores are associated with higher occupational status (e.g., professional/technical); and (4) although Type A behavior is more prevalent among males than females, there is a tendency for women in the work force to be Type A, and Type A in women is related to higher occupational status.

In regard to the *work environment:* (1) correlations exist between work load and anxiety in Type A individuals with varying occupations (e.g., university computer worker, male accountants, managers); (2) Type A workers tend to indicate dissatisfaction with subordinates, feel misunderstood by supervisors, and are more inclined to wish to work alone when under threat; (3) no significant relationship between Type A and job satisfaction has been reported, although Type A and company growth rate are related; (4) job involvement is correlated with Type A behavior; and (5) it is assumed that Type A individuals self-select into occupations that involve increased exposure to stressors, although no data support this assumption.

Type A managers tended to feel more in control than Type B managers and became distressed if challenged by external control at work. This finding illustrates the *control conflict* component in the model.

*Maladaptive coping behaviors* that have been investigated in the laboratory and work setting include time-urgency and suppression of symptoms. This research indicates that (1) time pressures are felt by Type A's in the work environment, primarily because they underestimate the time needed to complete a task; (2) pressured Type A's elicit hostility on meeting Type A co-workers who appear to be uninfluenced by time; and (3) laboratory research suggests that Type A's tend to suppress symptoms and feelings of fatigue. The symptom suppression, according to Cummings and Cooper (1979), is a manifestation of maladaptive coping. They use cybernetic theory to suggest that adaptive coping is a function of the individual's ability to isolate the existence of environmental strain through the use of information feedback. The magnitude of such feedback (feedback gain) affects the extent to which strain-reducing behaviors (stress-reduction strategies) are judged to be effective by the individual. Ineffective or maladaptive coping occurs when there is *feedback error*—when feedback information regarding strain is either *distorted* or *delayed* (time of feedback)—which, in turn, delays the adaptive coping process. According to this concept, feedback error is likely when an employee experiences work overload. Davidson and Cooper (1980) have added the concept of distorted or delayed feedback into the Type A work environment model and hypothesize that "the feedback error proposition adequately explains the link between coping behavior and symptom outcome in Type A individuals" (p. 380). They hypothesize that the Type A individual is *less* perceptive in the identification of environmental stressors and that the tendency to suppress symptoms leads to time lags in terms of identifying the existence of cardiovascular disease risk factors and problems in identifying signs and sources of strain.

The final component of the model shown in Figure 10-2 is *symptoms*. These symptoms are presumably further enhanced by the processes of feedback error and time lag. Symptoms include CHD, hypertension, elevated cholesterol and norepinephrine levels, lack of exercise, and poor family relations. The symptoms, other than family problems, have been discussed in other contexts in this book. Type A behavior is associated with family alienation, poor family health, decreased marital satisfaction, and marital breakdown. For example, some research has demonstrated that higher levels of Type A behavior in male prison administrators were associated with lower marital satisfaction and poor physical and psychological state of wives, including greater feelings of social isolation. This latter finding (social isolation) may be an artifact of the sample structure (spouses of prison administrators tend to be more susceptible to feelings of social isolation and alienation). The Davidson and Cooper (1980) framework illustrates certain key factors that should be considered when attempting to understand the Type A behavior pattern in the work environment a setting that commonly evokes much Type A behavior.

## THE ECOLOGICAL APPROACH

Margolis, McLeroy, Runyan, and Kaplan (1983) have outlined an *ecological approach* to the study of Type A behavior that provides a broad-based integrative framework for understanding the behavior pattern. The approach argues that focusing on individual characteristics of the Type A behavior pattern is limiting and, in order to elaborate the nature of Type A behavior and its relationship to health and illness, it is necessary to consider multiple levels of human experience. These ecological approach levels include (1) intrapersonal, (2) interpersonal, (3) institutional, and (4) cultural.

The interpersonal level includes the psychological processes underlying the behavior pattern, as discussed earlier in this chapter. Margolis *et al.* identify intense achievement striving and attributional processes as major factors at this level. They hypothesize that (1) individuals with Type A behavior possess higher performance standards than others and (2) Type A's tend to make attributions to effort rather than ability and to expect that future outcomes are a consequence of this heightened effort, not ability. According to this ecological approach, the intrapersonal factors, or "internal environment," are expressed within a set of environments of increasing complexity. This ecological approach to understanding Type A is shown in Table 10-5. The approach identifies the specific environments and highlights certain hypothesized factors that contribute to the development and expression of Type A behavior. Although these contributing factors require further elaboration and empirical support, such a perspective is useful for summarizing factors related to Type A.

The earlier discussion on Type A in the work environment is an example of an ecological approach. In considering the role of the environment, we include interpersonal and institutional components as proposed in the ecological approach.

This type of ecological analysis may also help identify areas for future preventive efforts. It may be necessary to direct effective prevention at multiple levels, including intrapersonal, interpersonal, institutional, and, perhaps, cultural, in order for primary prevention efforts to have an enduring effect. The prevention programs, to date, have been primarily directed at the intrapersonal level. Prevention of the complex Type A behavior pattern, if indeed such prevention appears warranted (at least at the primary prevention level), will require much thought. We

### TABLE 10-5
Ecological Levels of Analysis of Type A Behavior

| Environment | Contributing factors |
| --- | --- |
| Intrapersonal | Unrealistic social comparison processes |
| | Attributional dimensions of locus of control in which high achievement orientation is combined with unstable (effort rather than ability), internal (rather than external), and specific (rather than global) attributions |
| Interpersonal | High expectations by salient others (achievement striving) |
| | Unclear performance feedback |
| | Rewards for aggressive, competitive behavior |
| | Diffuse, heterogeneous, dispersed social networks |
| Institutional | Reward systems which foster aggressiveness |
| | Limited controllability of success or failure |
| | Numerous role demands |
| | Numerous time demands |
| Cultural | Individualistic orientation toward causality combined with devaluation of individuals |
| | Time orientation |
| | Cultural complexity |
| | Rapid rates of cultural change |

Note. From "Type A Behavior: An Ecological Approach" by L. H. Margolis, K. R. McLeroy, C. W. Runyan, and B. H. Kaplan, 1983, *Journal of Behavioral Medicine, 6,* 256. Copyright 1983 by Plenum Publishing Corporation. Reprinted by permission.

will now review current attempts (somewhat limited, given the ecological perspective) to modify the Type A behavior pattern.

## MODIFYING THE TYPE A BEHAVIOR PATTERN

This section will review the issues that confront interventions in Type A behavior; it will be structured according to the guidelines provided in Roskies (1980). Illustrative examples of current research relevant to prevention of the coronary-prone behavior pattern, as well as to intervention with postmyocardial infarct patients, will be provided.

A major issue of concern is the choice of target behaviors for modification (Roskies, 1980). For instance, is it more beneficial to attempt a global approach to changing life-style in Type A individuals or to focus on a specific behavior (hostility, time-urgency) that is related to a hypothesized mechanism by which Type A behavior leads to coronary CHD? The problem with the former approach is that not all the constellation of characteristics descriptive of the Type A behavior pattern seem to be predictive of CHD. Jenkins, Rosenman, and Zyzanski (1974), for example, found that the speed and impatience of the JAS were not adequate predictors of CHD. A global intervention, although it has the potential of eliminating certain Type A characteristics, may not necessarily alter the individual's risk for CHD. Moreover, this approach may be detrimental to the adaptive qualities of the Type A behavior pattern in some individuals. Mettlin (1976), for example, has indicated that Type A behavior may play an integral role in career success, despite findings by Friedman and Rosenman (1974) that Type A behavior may not be necessary for professional success. However, in support of Mettlin's contention, several independent studies have found that Type A behavior is positively correlated with socioeconomic status as defined by education and occupation (Zyzanski, 1978). The absence of research examining the impact of modifying various characteristics of Type A behavior on immediate and long-term productivity, professional advancement, and accomplishments indicates that caution should be taken when implementing global life-style changes, particularly in individuals with no history of CHD, as these may adversely affect career planning.

An alternative approach to modifying the Type A behavior pattern is to examine the mechanisms by which it leads to an increase in atheriosclerosis and eventually to an increased risk of CHD (Williams, Friedman, Glass, Herd, & Schneiderman, 1977), as discussed in a previous section. Type A individuals, for instance, have been distinguished from Type B persons by their psychological and physiological hyperresponsivity to challenge. A series of studies have reported that Type A individuals, in comparison to Type B, have higher autonomic and neuroen-docrine responses under challenge and slower recovery rates (Dem-broski, MacDougall, & Shields, 1977; Frankenhaeuser, 1977; Friedman, Byers, Diamant, & Rosenman, 1975; Glass, 1977). These findings are considered important in the light of the postulated relationship between sympathetic arousal, with its associated endocrine activity, and the de-velopment of atheriosclerosis (Davis, 1974; Gilmore, 1974; Obrist, 1976; Williams, 1975). Since, as discussed, hostility is an emotion that has been found in Type A individuals under challenge (Glass, 1977; Glass, Snyder, & Hollis, 1974), and since high levels of hostility are positively associated with degree of coronary atherosclerosis (Williams, 1978) and risk of heart disease (Matthews, 1977), it is quite possible that persons with the coronary-prone behavior may either be more responsive to cues eliciting anger or tend to label any arousal they experience as anger. Further, it may be that anger generates a somatic response pattern that may be more damaging than response patterns produced by other emo-tions. Following such a conceptualization, treatment would then be tar-geted at managing the individual's reactivity to anger. An approach along these lines would provide several advantages in that the Type A individual could be taught to change the frequency, intensity, and dura-tion of his or her stress responses (reducing his or her risk of CHD) without necessarily requiring the individual to change his or her exter-nal environment radically. The economy of such an approach, in terms of time, would appeal to a wide range of individuals.

Based on the assumptions that Type A individuals respond to chal-lenge with excessive sympathetic arousal and dramatically increase their pace and aggressiveness whenever they experience anxiety associated with threatened loss of control over their environment, Roskies and Avard (1982) developed a multimodal treatment approach to intervene in this process. A combination of progressive muscular relaxation, ra-tional emotive therapy, communication skills training, problem-solving skills training, and stress inoculation was suggested by Roskies and Avard (1982) to be helpful in controlling coronary-prone behavior in managers. The goal of the treatment program developed by Roskies and Avard is to help the participants of the program to become problem-rather than technique-oriented. Instead of applying the techniques ster-eotypically, the participants are encouraged to adapt to the demands of specific situations by flexibly combining techniques or even parts of techniques. The order of presentation of techniques is considered to be important in such a program and is designed to facilitate the construc-tion of an integrated repertoire.

Progressive muscular relaxation (PMR) is presented as the first tech-nique because of the ease with which it may be practiced, as well as the immediacy of its benefits. The goal here is for the participant to learn to monitor and reduce tension. Second, rational emotive therapy (RET) is presented to practice control of such negative emotions as anger, anxiety, guilt, and depression. As does PMR, RET brings about an immediate increase in a sense of well-being. Third, communication and problem-solving skills designed to reduce the stress associated with interpersonal conflict and decision making, are taught. Communications skills training helps the individuals send and receive messages that are clear and better formulated, that is, they focus on the problem rather than attack the other person or question the relationship itself. Problem-solving skills training is provided as an aid for resolving more efficiently some of the problems of daily living. This technique includes defining the problem, brain-storming all possible solutions, appraising the positive and negative features of each alternative, choosing a course of action, making a plan for executing it, and establishing when and how the result of this course of action will be evaluated. Finally, stress inoculation is implemented, with the goal of increasing the participant's awareness of and enhancing current labeling of physical and cognitive cues of stress. During the course of practicing stress-inoculation procedures, the participant is instructed to monitor feelings of time pressure throughout the week, and record the circumstances under which they occurred and the types of emotional and physical reactions they evoked. Following this step, the participant is taught procedures to change the situations and/or the reactions. For example, if the individual is pressured by time, distress can be reduced by engaging in active relaxation and making reassuring and positively reinforcing self-statements.

In an early study assessing the effectiveness of teaching Type A individuals alternative strategies for managing their stress responses, Roskies, Spevack, Surkis, Cohen, and Gilman (1978) compared a group psychotherapy intervention with a behavioral group intervention. Participants in this study included 29 healthy (no CHD), male, Type A volunteer subjects, between 39 and 57 years of age, who were randomly assigned to either a psychotherapy or a behavioral therapy group.

The psychotherapy treatment, which consisted of modifying the need of Type A individuals for mastery and control over their environment was conducted by psychoanalytically trained therapists. The behavioral treatment, however, concentrated on teaching the Type A individuals a sequence of relaxation techniques to modify their behavior in response to stress. Following the 14-week course of therapy, individuals in both treatment groups showed significant pre-post treatment reductions in mean systolic blood pressure, serum cholesterol levels, self-reported time pressure, and number of psychological symptoms. No significant differences were found on either mean diastolic blood pressure or serum triglycerides.

The results of this study should be viewed with caution because there was not an adequate control group. Nonetheless, the reduction in serum cholesterol and self-report changes reported by Roskies *et al.* suggested that Type A behavior and CHD risk may be amenable to change. These findings were, in fact, confirmed in a later report (Roskies, Kearny, Spevack, Surkis, Cohen, & Gilman, 1979), which showed good maintenance of treatment effects (decrease in serum cholesterol levels) after a six-month follow-up, particularly in the behavior therapy group.

Another approach to modifying the coronary-prone behavior pattern is that of Suinn (1980). The development of this program, known as cardiac stress management training (CSMT), was prompted by questions about the type of reinforcers maintaining Type A behavior, the type of alternative behaviors considered to be desirable, and the method of achieving such behaviors. Suinn conceptualizes the maintaining factors of Type A behavior to be primarily cultural in origin. Western society generally admires and rewards Type A behavior; thus, many individuals learn that they will be reinforced for engaging in timeless, aggressive, "workaholic"-type behaviors. Type A individuals tend to internalize these values and impose these stresses upon themselves. The internal stress, in turn, creates its own reward for hard work in the form of negatively reinforcing reduction of anxiety, thus furthering the maintenance of the Type A behavior pattern. In Suinn's view, the only way that Type A individuals can retain productivity, and control an uncertain world, is through Type A behavior. They cannot consider less stressful methods of achieving, since those methods, for them, have not yet been associated with reward.

Cardiac stress management training basically consists of two procedures: anxiety management training (AMT) and visuomotor behavior rehearsal (VMBR). In AMT, individuals are trained to identify physical cues of arousal to stress and taught to use relaxation techniques to reduce their stress response. In VMBR, individuals are instructed in a covert rehearsal procedure designed to help them utilize alternative behaviors incompatible with the Type A pattern in those situations that typically elicit Type A responses (e.g., imagine taking a coffee break during a peak work period). In Suinn's view, the advantage of CSMT is that it provides the patient with behavior patterns that allow him or her to retain their productivity, while reducing the risks of CHD of the previous Type A pattern.

In order to evaluate the effectiveness of CSMT in a non-clinical population, Suinn and Bloom (1978) administered the JAS to a small group (12 male and 2 female) before and after the six treatment sessions. Subjects were randomly assigned to either a nontreatment control group or to a treatment group, which received six sessions of CSMT. Compared to the control, significant reductions on the State and Trait Anxiety scales of the STAI (Spielberger, Gorsuch, & Lushene, 1970) and on the JAS Speed and Impatience and Hard-Driving subscales were found in the treatment group following intervention. Further, no significant change was found following treatment on the JAS Type A scale, an important finding, since only the Type A scale on the JAS has been found to be predictive of CHD (Jenkins et al., 1974). Although reductions in blood pressure were noted, these were not significant and do not support the findings of Roskies et al. (1978). In addition, no significant changes in serum lipid levels were found — contrary to findings in an earlier study by Suinn (1975) with postcoronary patients.

Increasing attention has recently been paid to the potential beneficial effects of physical fitness programs as a preventive approach to CHD, and a number of large-scale epidemiological studies have associated habitual physical activity with reduced incidence of CHD (Morris, Chave, Adam, Sircy, Epstein, & Sheehan, 1973; Paffenbarger & Hale, 1975). In a more recent study, Blumenthal, Williams, Williams, and Wallace (1980) evaluated the role of a systematic exercise program in the modification of the Type A behavior pattern in a group of healthy, middle-aged adults. The sample consisted of 46 subjects, classified as either Type A or Type B on the basis of their scores on the JAS. The exercise program consisted of three supervised sessions per week over a period of 10 consecutive weeks. Each session required the subjects to engage in a series of stretching exercises for 10 minutes followed by 30 to 45 minutes of continuous walking or jogging (equivalent to approximately three miles). Throughout the first week of training, almost all subjects were walking only, whereas by the final week, over one-half the subjects were jogging continuously for 30 minutes and approximately 30% of the group were doing at least some jogging. Exercise intensity was prescribed to produce elevations of heart rate equal to 70% to 85% of the maximal heart rate achieved on each person's initial treadmill test, and subjects were shown how to determine their own heart rate by carotid or radial artery palpation. In addition, subjects were encouraged to limit their dietary intake of total calories, salt, cholesterol, and saturated fats.

Measures of physiological variables (blood pressure, serum lipids, body weight, plasminogen-activator release, and treadmill performance) and psychological variables (scores on the JAS) were obtained before and after the exercise program. Blumenthal et al. (1980) found that, in comparison to Type B subjects, Type A subjects were able to successfully reduce the physiological cardiovascular risk factors, in addition to lowering their scores on the JAS. Despite the absence in this study of an adequate control group, which made it difficult to specify the mechanisms by which the Type A scores were modified, the beneficial effects of physical fitness programs on reduction of coronary risk factors, found in Blumenthal et al.'s study, do merit further investigation.

The notion that beta-adrenergic hyperreactivity may be implicated as a physiological mechanism underlying Type A behavior and a mediating factor in the development of CHD has recently been investigated by several authors (Krantz, Durel, Davia, Schaffer, Arabian, Dembroski, & MacDougall, 1982; Schmieder, Friedrich, Neus, Rudel, & von Eiff, 1984). Krantz et al. (1982), for instance, employed a correlational design to compare the behavioral and psychophysiological characteristics of coronary patients who were either medicated or not medicated with the beta-adrenergic blocking drug propranolol. Eighty-two men and six women underwent a structured Type A interview (SI) and a history quiz (stressor) while their heart rate and blood pressure were monitored. Data were analyzed controlling for age, sex, extent of coronary artery disease, and history of angina. The findings of the study indicated that patients taking propranolol were significantly lower in intensity of Type A behavior than patients not taking propranolol. Patients taking propranolol also showed lesser rate–pressure responses (a correlate of myocardial oxygen demand) to the interview (Figure 10-3). No differences in blood pressure responses were found. A component analysis of Type A characteristics revealed that the propranolol patients scored lower on such factors as speech stylistics (i.e., loud/explosive, rapid/accelerated, potential for hostility), but there were no differences between the groups in terms of the content of responses to the SI and the scores on the JAS. These findings were not demonstrated when patients received diuretics, nitrates, or other CNS active drugs, which illustrated the specificity of the beta blocker.

Krantz et al.'s study, (1982), which demonstrated the effect of propranolol on the Type A behavior pattern, is important in that it highlights the possible role of biological substrates in Type A behavior. One interpretation of the findings offered by Krantz and his colleagues has been that Type A behavior pattern is an interaction between cognitive and physiological components. Such variables as speech stylistics, which responded to propranolol medication, may reflect physiological processes. On the other hand, such variables as "content" (related to the SI) and scores on the JAS, which were not affected by beta-adrenergic blockade, may be more closely associated with cognitive-perceptual or psychological factors. The interaction of these cognitive and physiological variables may result, therefore, in coronary-prone behavior mediated

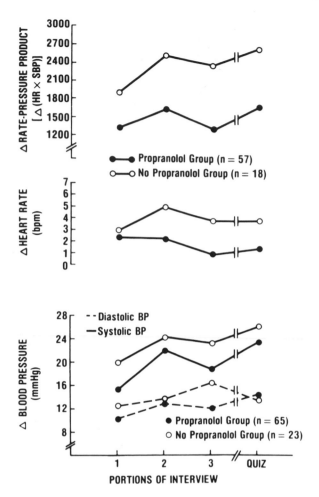

**FIGURE 10-3.** Changes in cardiovascular reactivity in propranolol and no propranolol patients, showing changes in heart rate, blood pressure, and rate-pressure product in propranolol and no propranolol patients during the structured interview and quiz. From "Propranolol Medication among Coronary Patients: Relationship to Type A Behavior and Cardiovascular Response" by D. S. Krantz, L. A. Durel, J. E. Davia, R. T. Schaeffer, J. M. Arabian, T. M. Dembroski, and J. M. MacDougall, 1982, *Journal of Human Stress, 8,* 9. Copyright 1982 by Heldref Publications. Reprinted by permission.

by a feedback system from peripheral sympathetic responses. The individual's response to or perception of these peripheral cardiovascular responses would then reinforce energetic Type A stylistics. Thus, by selectively decreasing peripheral sympathetic activity, beta-blockers may play a role in reducing the intensity of Type A behavior.

A more recent study by Schmieder *et al.* (1984) provides further support for the potentially beneficial effects of beta-blockers on cardiovascular reactivity and Type A behavior pattern. Schmieder *et al.* (1984) tested the effect of beta-blockers on Type A behavior pattern and cardiovascular reactivity in a sample of 19 white, male hypertensive patients. Patients were randomly assigned to two treatment groups, one receiving beta-blockers, the other (control group) receiving diuretics. Each patient underwent the German version of the SI before therapy and, at a minimum of a few weeks after normalization of clinical resting, casual blood pressure. No differences in age, blood pressure at rest, cardiovascular reactivity, and Type A were noted between the two groups before therapy. Following therapy, however, the patients treated with beta-blockers showed significant changes in Type A speech characteristics (loud/excessive, rapid/accelerated, response latency) toward Type B, regardless of where they had been on the Type A scale. Further, the patients treated with beta-blockers showed diminished reactivity in systolic blood pressure, diastolic blood pressure, and heart rate in response to the second SI, compared to those patients treated with diuretics (Fig. 10-4). It may be concluded from this study that beta-blockers may indeed be a useful way of altering the coronary-prone behavior pattern and its underlying psychophysiology as well as serving as a prophylactic in the prevention of CHD. It would be of interest to investigate the role of other techniques in reducing sympathetic overreactivity; these include relaxation training, stress inoculation, and combinations of drug and biobehavioral interventions.

Work on modifying the Type A behavior pattern and reducing the risk factors associated with CHD has also been undertaken with postmyocardial infarction patients. The first large-scale, long-term attempt to test the feasibility of altering a Type A life-style and to evaluate the effectiveness of such an alteration on the incidence of CHD has been reported in an impressive study by Friedman, Thoresen, *et al.* (1984), in which 862 postmyocardial infarction patients participated. Patients in this study met the following criteria: they had ostensibly suffered one or more documented MIs within the last six months, were 64 years old or under, had either never smoked or had quit for six months or longer, and had never been treated for diabetes. The patients were randomly assigned to either a control group (*Section 1*) and were given only cardiological counseling regarding diet, exercise, and general information concerning the possible medical and surgical procedures employed in the treatment of postinfarction patients, or to an experimental group (*Section 2*), who were given the same cardiological counseling plus Type A behavioral counseling. All participants received, on entry, a focused cardiovascular examination including ECG, serum cholesterol, and urine analysis. Blood samples for serum cholesterol analysis were ob-

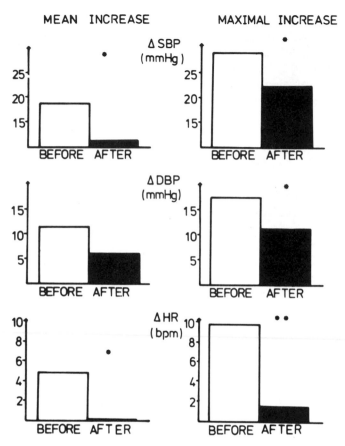

**FIGURE 10-4.** Increase in blood pressure and heart rate during Type A interview before and after treatment with beta-blockers. The left column shows the mean increase of BP and HR, the right column the maximal increase of BP and HR. * = $p < .05$; ** $p = < .01$. From "The Influence of Beta Blockers on Cardiovascular Reactivity and Type A Behavior Pattern in Hypertensives" by R. Schmieder, G. Friedrich, H. Rüdell, and A. W. von Eiff, 1984, *Psychosomatic Medicine, 45* (5), 420. Copyright 1984 by Elsevier Science Co., Inc. Reprinted by permission.

tained biannually, in addition to an interval medical history, physical examination, and ECG examination, which were repeated at $1\frac{1}{2}$ and 3 years after entry.

The evaluation of changes in Type A behavior was conducted via three types of questionnaires and a videotaped structured interview (VSI). The questionnaires consisted of (1) a participant questionnaire composed of 88 items assessing the presence of specific Type A habits under specific situations; (2) a spouse questionnaire to be filled out by spouses of Section 2 participants, with the aim of confirming the information obtained from self-report; and (3) a monitor questionnaire to be filled out by a colleague at work. In the case of Section 1 participants, spouse and monitor questionnaires were not utilized, as this may have increased these participants' awareness and possible self-correction of Type A behavior. The questionnaires were completed on entry and then at yearly intervals. Finally, the VSI (a 15-minute test to detect and score any of the 38 psychomotor, physiological, behavioral, and biographical manifestations presently considered diagnostic by Friedman, Thoresen, et al., 1982, of Type A behavior) was administered and scored by an experienced Type A interviewer who was not participating in the study and was kept blind to the section status of the participants both at entry and at subsequent interviews.

The cardiological counseling by cardiologists given participants consisted of 24 group sessions for 90 minutes in the 3-year period. During these sessions, patients received information regarding (1) the pathogenesis of MI; (2) the alteration of standard coronary risk factors (e.g., hypertension, hypercholesterolemia, excess cigarette smoking), excluding the Type A behavior pattern; (3) recent advances in the surgical and drug management of CHD; and (4) the avoidance of certain daily activities (heavy meals rich in fat, overexertion, excess caffeine or alcohol) believed to precipitate cardiac events.

The behavioral counseling, described by Powell, Friedman, Thoresen, Gill, and Ulmer (1984) (Table 10-6), was given by a psychiatrist or psychologist to the Section 2 cardiac treatment/Type A patients, who also were given cardiological counseling. The behavioral counseling sessions were based on the cognitive social learning model of behavior developed by Bandura (1977). Sessions were designed to teach patients how to identify manifestations of the Type A behavior pattern (e.g., polyphasic activity, vehement arguments about petty issues, hypersensitivity to criticism, reliving anger about the past, interrupting others), first in other individuals and then in themselves. Patients were taught to recognize excessive physiological, cognitive, and behavioral responses to stressful situations and to develop mastery in physical and mental relaxation as incompatible responses to stress. In addition, as treatment progressed, topics that surrounded the patients' typical beliefs about themselves (e.g., unrealistic appraisals of personal qualities, overemphasis on achievements as a way of measuring self-worth), their attitudes toward others (e.g., suspicion, vindictiveness, hostility, competition), and their global beliefs about life (e.g., the role of the Type A behavior pattern in achieving occupational success, the optimum balance between quantitative and qualitative appreciation) were discussed. The treatment package emphasized the importance of the group process

**TABLE 10-6**
Comprehensive Intervention Program for Modifying the Type A Behavior
Pattern in Postmyocardial Infarct Patients

---

Cardiac Counseling
  Provision of information
  Pathogens of myocardial infarct
  Alteration of standard coronary risk factors
  Current advances in the surgical and drug management of coronary heart disease
  Avoidance of certain daily activities suspected of precipitating recurrent cardiac
    events
Behavioral Counseling
  Identification of overt manifestations of Type A behavior pattern
  Increasing patients' awareness of the cognitive, physiological, and behavioral
    components of their stress response
  Instruction in cognitive and muscular relaxation procedures
  Behavioral rehearsal
  Cognitive restructuring

---

Note. From "Can the Type A Behavior Pattern Be Altered after Myocardial Infarction? A Second Year
Report from the Recurrent Coronary Prevention Project" by L. H. Powell, M. Friedman, C. E. Thor-
esen, J. J. Gill, and D. K. Ulmer, 1984, *Psychosomatic Medicine, 46*(4). Copyright 1984 by Elsevier Science
Co., Inc. Adapted by permission.

in facilitating and promoting change, as well as in getting away from
adversarial peer relationships.

The results reported by Friedman *et al.* (1984) are encouraging. Type
A behavior was significantly reduced in 43.8% of the 592 patients who
received Type A behavior counseling, in addition to cardiological counseling (Section 2). Of this sample, 17.6% evidenced *marked* reductions in
Type A behavior, whereas the remaining 26.2% showed an *overall* reduction following three years of treatment. Those participants in Section 2
who *actually* continued to receive counseling for at least three years
showed even greater reductions in Type A behavior with 31.7% of the
sample in the *markedly* reduced category and 47.3% of the sample in the
*overall* reduction category. These reductions in Type A behavior were
significantly greater than those observed in participants who received
only group cardiological counseling (marked reduction, 7.2%; overall
reduction, 41.7%).

Other findings reported in this study showed that significantly
fewer Section 2 participants suffered angina at the end of the third year,
compared to Section 1 participants, although at entry this difference did
not exist. Further, the mean serum cholesterol levels of both Section 1
and 2 participants dropped significantly from entry levels at the end of
the first year and were maintained at this lower level for the remaining
two years. Finally, the cumulative 3-year cardiac rate was found to be

7.2% in patients who had been assigned to the cardiological group and Type A behavioral counseling in comparison to the higher recurrence rate of 13% observed in patients receiving only cardiological counseling (Figure 10-5). The Friedman *et al.* (1984) study is a good example of a large-scale pioneering effort in positively altering Type A behavior and reducing the risk of CHD in individuals with postmyocardial infarction. Future research in this area should evaluate the nature of the treatment components most effective in maintaining long-term treatment gains and in preventing another MI.

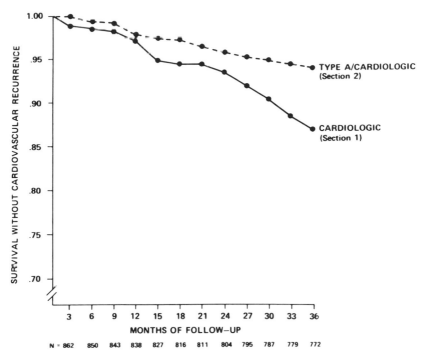

**FIGURE 10-5.** Effects of Type A/cardiological intervention versus cardiological intervention only on survival without cardiac recurrence. Illustration of the cumulative "survival without cardiac recurrence" curves for Type A/cardiological and cardiological sections employing the "intention-to-treat" principle. *N* indicates the total number of participants followed at the beginning of each time point. A participant is censored (i.e., removed from further calculations) upon cardiovascular recurrence or inability to trace. The Section 2 curve is significantly different from that of Section 1 (chi-square = 7.8, *p* < .01). From "Alteration of Type A Behavior and Reduction in Cardiac Recurrences in Postmyocardial Infarction Patients" by M. Friedman, C. E. Thoresen, J. J. Gill, L. H. Powell, D. Ulmer, L. Thompson, V. A. Price, D. D. Rabin, W. S. Breall, T. Dixon, R. Levy, and E. Bourg, 1984 *American Heart Journal, 108* (2), 244. Copyright 1984 by C. V. Mosby Co. Reprinted by permission.

In conclusion, several issues remain to be addressed on coronary-prone behavior pattern intervention. In order to measure the changes in various Type A dimensions or in other risk factors considered to be precursors of CHD (e.g., psychophysiological reactivity and lipid and hormone levels), multiple-outcome measures will help evaluate the respective contribution of such multimodal intervention methods as stress management, cognitive restructuring, exercise, and drug therapy. Other variables that will require further attention in the context of Type A and CHD research are the careful matching of subject characteristics (age, sex, coping skills), selecting targets for intervention (e.g, changing completely from Type A to Type B, reduction in magnitude of Type A behaviors), choosing methods of intervention (e.g., single-method strategy versus multimodal strategies), and inclusion of appropriate control groups (e.g., minimal treatment control). Finally, the long-term goal of intervention programs for Type A behavior should be to evaluate the mechanisms contributing to the *maintenance* of therapeutic effects in the prevention of recurrent MI.

## SUMMARY

The past three decades have witnessed the sharp rise in incidence of coronary heart disease (CHD), which has been described as the primary cause of premature death in the United States. This chapter attempted to illustrate the various contributions of the subdisciplines of psychology (e.g., developmental, clinical, social, psychophysiological) in furthering our understanding of the psychobiological mechanisms implicated in the development of coronary heart disease and in the reduction of risk factors associated with it.

An overview of etiological considerations, including a definition of CHD and specification of risk factors, was first presented. This overview was then followed by a detailed discussion of the "coronary-prone behavior pattern," or the Type A behavior pattern, as it relates to the development and maintenance of CHD. Given the importance of the Type A behavior pattern as the first well-defined *psychological* or *behavioral* risk factor in the history of risk factor research in health and illness, particular consideration was given in the chapter to defining the Type A behavior pattern and providing a historical perspective, describing the pattern and the methods of measuring and identifying it, reviewing research on the validation of the Type A construct, and reviewing the psychophysiological research, which attempts to examine the possible physiological mechanism accounting for the Type A–CHD relationship.

Developmental aspects of Type A behavior and factors in the work environment contributing to the development of Type A behavior pattern were also discussed.

Finally, the chapter reviewed various strategies used in modifying the Type A behavior pattern. Particular emphasis was placed on prevention research representing efforts to modify Type A and its subsequent potential negative health consequences and on reviewing intervention studies with patients displaying the Type A behavior pattern with CHD (e.g., postmyocardial infarction patients).

## REFERENCES

Arlow, J. A. (1945). Identification mechanisms in coronary occlusion. *Psychosomatic Medicine, 7*, 195–210.

Bandura, A. (1977). *Social learning theory*. Englewood Cliffs, NJ: Prentice-Hall.

Bandura, A., & Walters, R. H. (1959). *Adolescent aggression*. New York: Roland.

Bandura, A., Ross, D., & Ross, S. A. (1961). Transmission of aggression through initiation of aggressive models. *Journal of Abnormal Social Psychology, 63*, 575–582.

Barefoot, J. C., Dahlstrom W. G., & Williams, R. B. Jr. (1983). Hostility, CHD incidence, and total mortality: A 25-year follow-up study of 255 physicians. *Psychosomatic Medicine, 45*(1), 59–63.

Blumenthal, J. A., Williams, R. S., Williams, R. B., & Wallace, A. G. (1980). Effects of exercise on the Type A (coronary-prone) behavior pattern. *Psychosomatic Medicine, 42*, 289–296.

Bortner, R. W., Rosenman, R. H., & Friedman, M. (1970). Familial similarity in pattern A behavior: Fathers and sons. *Journal of Chronic Disease, 23*, 39–43.

Brehm, J. (1966). A theory of psychological reactance. New York: Academic Press.

Brunson, B. I., & Matthews, K. A. (1981). The type A coronary-prone behavior pattern and reactions to uncontrollable stress: An analysis of performance strategies, affect, and attributions during failure. *Journal of Personality and Social Psychology, 40*(5), 906–918.

Butensky, A., Forelli, V., Heebner, D., & Waldron, I. (1976). Elements of the coronary-prone behavior pattern in children and teenagers. *Journal of Psychosomatic Research, 20*, 439–444.

Carver, C. S. (1980). Perceived coercion, resistance to persuasion, and the Type A behavior pattern. *Journal of Research in Personality, 19*, 467–481.

Chesney, M. A., & Rosenman, R. H. (1980). Type A behavior in the work setting. In C. L. Cooper & R. Payne (Eds.), *Current concerns in occupational stress*. London: Wiley.

Chesney, M. A., Black, G. W., Chadwick, J. H., & Rosenman, R. H. (1981). Psychological correlates of the Type A behavior pattern. *Journal of Behavioral Medicine, 4*, 217–229.

Chesney, M. A., Eagleston, J. R., & Rosenman, R. H. (1981). Type A behavior: Assessment and intervention. In C. K. Prokop & L. A. Bradley (Eds.), *Medical psychology: Contributions to behavioral medicine*. New York: Academic Press.

Cooper, T., Detre, T., & Weiss, S. M. (1981). Coronary prone behavior and coronary heart disease: A critical review. *Circulation, 63*, 1199–1215.

Cummings, T. G., & Cooper, C. L. (1979). A cybernetic framework for studying occupational stress. *Human Relations, 32*, 395–418.

Davidson, M. J., & Cooper, C. L. (1980). Type A coronary-prone behavior in the work environment. *Journal of Occupational Medicine, 22,* 375–383.

Davis, R. (1974). Stress and hemostatic mechanisms. In R. S. Eliot (Ed.), *Stress and the heart* (pp. 97–122). New York: Futura.

Dembroski, T. M., & MacDougall, J. M. (1978). Stress effects on affiliation preferences among subjects possessing the type A coronary-prone behavior pattern. *Journal of Personality and Social Psychology, 36*(1), 23–33.

Dembroski, T., MacDougall, J. M., & Shields, J. L. (1977). Physiologic reactions to social challenge in persons evidencing the Type A coronary-prone behavior pattern. *Journal of Human Stress, 3*(3), 2–9.

Dembroski, T. M., MacDougall, J. M., Shields, J. L., Petitto, J., & Lushene, R. (1978). Components of the Type A coronary-prone behavior pattern and cardiovascular responses to psychomotor performance challenge. *Journal of Behavioral Medicine, 1,* 159–176.

Dembroski, T. M., MacDougall, J. M., Herd, A. J., & Shields, J. L. (1979). Effect of level of challenge on pressor and the heart rate response in Type A and Type B subjects. *Journal of Applied Social Psychology, 9,* 209–228.

Diamond, E. L. (1983). The role of anger and hostility in essential hypertension and coronary heart disease. *Psychological Bulletin, 92*(2), 410–433.

Diamond, E. L., Schneiderman, N., Schwartz, D., Smith, J. C., Vorp, R., & Pasin, R. D. (1984). Harassment, hostility, and type A as determinants of cardiovascular reactivity during competition. *Journal of Behavioral Medicine, 7*(2), 171–189.

Dongier, M. (1974). Psychosomatic aspects in myocardial infarction in comparison with angina pectoris. *Psychotherapeutics and Psychosomatics, 23,* 123–131.

Fontana, A., & Dovidio, J. F. (1984). The relationship between stressful life events and school-related performances of Type A and Type B adolescents. *Journal of Human Stress, 10*(1), 50–55.

Frankenhaeuser, M., Dunne, E., & Lundberg, U. (1976). Sex differences in sympathetic-adrenal medullary reactions induced by different stressors. *Psychopharmacology, 47*(1), 1–5.

Frankenhaeuser, M., von Wright, M. R., Collins, A., von Wright, J., Sedvall, G., & Swahn, C. G. (1978). Sex differences in psychoneuroendocrine reactions to examination stress. *Psychosomatic Medicine, 47*(4), 334–343.

Frankenhaeuser, M., Lundberg, U., & Forsman, L. (1980). Dissociation between sympathetic-adrenal and pituitary-adrenal responses to an achievement situation characterized by high controllability: Comparison between Type A and B males and females. *Biological Psychology, 10,* 79–91.

French, J. R. P., Rogers, W., & Cobb, S. (1974). Adjustment as person–environment fit. In G. V. Coelko, D. A. Hamburg, & J. E. Adams (Eds.), *Coping and adaptation.* New York: Basic Books.

Friedman, M., & Rosenman, R. H. (1959). Association of specific overt behavior pattern with blood and cardiovascular findings: Blood cholesterol level, blood clotting time, incidence of arcus senilis and clinical coronary artery disease. *Journal of the American Medical Association, 169,* 1286–1296.

Friedman, M., & Rosenman, R. H. (1974). *Type A behavior and your heart.* New York: Fawcett Books.

Friedman, M., Byers, S., Diamant, J., & Rosenman, R. H. (1975). Plasma catecholamine response of coronary-prone subjects (Type A) to a specific challenge. *Metabolism, 24,* 205–210.

Friedman, M., Thoresen, C. E., Gill, J. J., Ulmer, D., Thompson, L., Powell, L., Price, V. A., Elek, S. R., Rabin, D. D., Breall, W. S., Piaget, G., Dixon, T., Bourg, E., Levy, R.

A., & Tasto, D. L. (1982). Feasibility of altering type A behavior pattern after myocardial infarction. Recurrent Coronary Prevention Project Study: Methods, baseline results and preliminary findings. *Circulation, 66*(1), 83–92.

Friedman, M., Thoresen, C. E., Gill, J. J., Powell, L. H., Ulmer, D., Thompson, L., Price, V. A., Rabin, D. D., Breall, W. S., Dixon, T., Levy, R., & Bourg, E. (1984). Alteration of type A behavior and reduction in cardiac recurrences in postmyocardial infarction patients. *American Heart Journal, 108*(2), 237–248.

Gilmore, J. P. (1974) Physiology of Stress. In R. S. Eliot (Ed.), *Stress and the heart* (pp. 69–90). New York: Futura.

Glass, D. C. (1977). *Behavior patterns, stress, and coronary disease.* Hilldale, NJ: Erlbaum.

Glass, D. C., Snyder, M. L., & Hollis, J. F. (1974). Time-urgency and the Type A coronary-prone behavior pattern. *Journal of Applied Social Psychology, 4*, 125–140.

Glass, D. C., Krakoff, L. R., Contrada, R., Hilton, W. F., Kehoe, K., Manucci, E. G., Collings, C., Snow, B., & Elting, E. (1980). Effect of harassment and competition upon cardiovascular and catecholamine responses in Type A and B individuals. *Psychophysiology, 17*, 453–463.

Haynes, S. G., Levine, S., Scotch, N., Feinleib, M., & Kannel, W. B. (1978). The relationship of psychosocial factors to coronary heart disease in the Framingham study. I. Methods and risk factors. *American Journal of Epidemiology, 107*(5), 362–383.

Haynes, S. G., Feinleib, M., & Kannel, W. B. (1980). The relationship of psychosocial factors to coronary heart disease in the Framingham study. III. Eight-year incidence of coronary heart disease. *American Journal of Epidemiology, 111*(1), 37–58.

Horn, J. M., Plomin, R., & Rosenman, R. (1976). Heritability of personality traits in adult male twins. *Behavior Genetics, 6*(1), 17–30.

Jenkins, C. D. (1966). Components of the coronary-prone behavior pattern: Their relation to silent myocardial infarction and blood lipids. *Journal of Chronic Diseases, 19*, 599–609.

Jenkins, C. D. (1971). Psychologic and social precursors of coronary disease. *New England Journal of Medicine, 284*, 244–255, 307–317.

Jenkins, C. D. (1978). Behavioral risk factors in coronary artery disease. *Annual Review of Medicine, 29*, 543–562.

Jenkins, C. D., Rosenman, R. H., & Friedman, M. (1967). Development of an objective psychological test for the determination of the coronary-prone behavior pattern in employed men. *Journal of Chronic Diseases, 20*, 371–379.

Jenkins, C. D., Rosenman, R. H., & Zyzanski, S. J. (1974). Prediction of clinical coronary heart disease by a test for the coronary-prone behavior pattern. *New England Journal of Medicine, 290*, 1271–1275.

Julian, D. G. (1978). *Cardiology* (3rd ed.). London: Cassell.

Keys, A., Aravanis, C., Blackburn, H., van Buchem, F. G. P., Buzina, R., Djordjevic, B. X., Fidanza, F., Karvonen, M. J., Nenotti, A., Puddu, V., & Taylor, H. L. (1972). Probability of middle-aged men developing coronary heart disease in five years. *Circulation, 45*, 815–828.

Krantz, D. S., Durel, L. A., Davia, J. E., Schaeffer, R. T., Arabian, J. M., Dembroski, T. M., & MacDougall, J. M. (1982). Propranolol medication among coronary patients: Relationship to type A behavior and cardiovascular response. *Journal of Human Stress, 8*, 4–12.

Lane, J. D., White, A. D., & Williams, R. B. Jr. (1984). Cardiovascular effects of mental arithmetic in Type A and Type B females. *Psychophysiology, 21*(1), 39–46.

Lawler, K., Allen, M., Critcher, E., & Standard, B. (1981). The relationship of physiological responses to the coronary-prone behavior pattern in children. *Journal of Behavioral Medicine, 4*, 203–216.

Lawler, K. A., Rixse, A., & Allen, M. T. (1983). Type A behavior and psychophysiological responses in adult women. *Psychophysiology, 20*(3), 343–350.

Lawler, K. A., Schmied, L., Mitchell, V. P., & Rixse, A. (1984). Type A behavior and physiological responsivity in young women. *Journal of Psychosomatic Research, 28*(3), 197–204.

Lott, G. G., & Gatchel, R. J. (1978). A multi-response analysis of learned heart rate control. *Psychophysiology, 15,* 576.

Lovallo, W. R., & Pishkin, V. (1980). Type A behavior, self-involvement, autonomic activity, and the traits of neuroticism and extroversion. *Psychosomatic Medicine, 42,* 329–334.

MacDougall, J. M., Dembroski, T. M., & Krantz, D. S. (1981). Effects of types of challenge on pressor and heart rate responses in type A and B women. *Psychophysiology, 18*(1), 1–9.

Manuck, S. B., Craft, S. A., & Gold, K. J. (1978). Coronary-prone behavior pattern and cardiovascular response. *Psychophysiology, 15,* 403–411.

Margolis, L. H., McLeroy, K. R., Runyan, C. W., & Kaplan, B. H. (1983). Type A behavior: An ecological approach. *Journal of Behavioral Medicine, 6,* 245–258.

Matthews, K. A. (1977). Caregiver–child interactions and type A coronary-prone behavior pattern. *Child Development, 48,* 1752–1756.

Matthews, K. A. (1978). Assessment and developmental antecedents of pattern A behavior in children. In T. M. Dembroski, S. M. Weiss, J. L. Shields, S. G. Haynes, & M. Feinleib (Eds.), *Coronary-prone behavior.* New York: Springer-Verlag.

Matthews, K. A. (1982). Psychological perspectives on the type A behavior pattern. *Psychological Bulletin, 91*(2), 293–323.

Matthews, K. A., & Angulo, J. (1980). Measurement of the type A behavior pattern in children: Assessment of children's competitiveness, impatience–anger, and aggression. *Child Development, 51*(2), 466–475.

Matthews, K. A., & Krantz, D. S. (1976). Resemblances of twins and their parents in pattern A behavior. *Psychosomatic Medicine, 38*(2), 140–144.

Matthews, K. A., & Siegel, J. M. (1982). The Type A behavior pattern in children and adolescents: Assessment, development, and associated coronary risk. In A. R. Baum & J. E. Singer (Eds.), *Handbook of Health and Medical Psychology* (Vol. 2). Hillsdale, NJ: Erlbaum.

Matthews, K. A., Glass, D. C., Rosenman, R. H., & Bortner, R. W. (1977). Competitive drive, Pattern A, and coronary heart disease: A further analysis of some data from the Western Collaborative Group Study. *Journal of Chronic Diseases, 30,* 489–498.

McClelland, D. (1961). *The achieving society.* New York: Free Press.

McKinley, D. G. (1964). *Social class and family life.* New York: Free Press.

Menninger, K. A., & Menninger, W. C. (1936). Psychoanalytic observations in cardiac disorders. *American Heart Journal, 11,* 10–21.

Mettlin, C.(1976). Occupational careers and the prevention of coronary-prone behavior. *Social Science and Medicine, 10,* 367–372.

Morris, J. N., Chave, S. P., Adam, C., Sircy, C., Epstein, L., & Sheehan, D. J. (1973). Vigorous exercise in leisure time and the incidence of coronary heart disease. *Lancet, 1,* 333–339.

Murray, J. L., Bruhn, J. G., & Bunce, H. (1983). Assessment of Type A behavior in preschoolers. *Journal of Human Stress, 9,* 32–39.

Obrist, P. A. (1976). The cardiovascular-behavioral interaction — as it appears today. *Psychophysiology, 13*(2), 95–107.

Osler, W. (1892). *Lectures on angina and allied states.* New York: Appleton.

Paffenbarger, R. S., & Hale, W. E. (1975). Work activity and coronary heart mortality. *New England Journal of Medicine, 292*(11), 545–550.

Powell, L. H., Friedman, M., Thoresen, C. E., Gill, J. J., & Ulmer, D. K. (1984). Can the Type A behavior pattern be altered after myocardial infarction? A second year report from the recurrent prevention project. *Psychosomatic Medicine, 46*(4), 293–313.

Rahe, R. H., Hervig, L., & Rosenman, R. H. (1978). Heritability of Type A behavior. *Psychosomatic Medicine, 40,* 478–486.

Rosenman, R. H., & Friedman, M. (1961). Association of a specific overt behavior pattern in females with blood and cardiovascular findings. *Circulation, 24,* 1173–1184.

Rosenman, R. H., Rahe, R. H., Borhani, N. O., & Feinleib, M. (1976, November). Heritability of personality and behavior. Proceedings of the First International Congress of Twin Studies, Rome, Italy. *Acta Geneticae Medicae et Gemellologiciae (Rome) 25,* 221–224.

Roskies, E. (1980). Considerations in developing a treatment program for the coronary-prone (Type A) behavior pattern. In P. O. Davidson, & S. M. Davidson (Eds.), *Behavioral Medicine: Changing health life-styles.* New York: Brunner/Mazel.

Roskies, E., & Avard, J. (1982). Teaching healthy managers to control their coronary prone (Type A) behavior. In K. R. Blankstein & J. Polivy (Eds.), *Self-control and self-modification of emotional behavior.* New York: Plenum Press.

Roskies, E., Spevack, M., Surkis, A., Cohen, C., & Gilman, S. (1978). Changing the coronary-prone (Type A) behavior pattern in a non-clinical population. *Journal of Behavioral Medicine, 1,* 201–216.

Roskies, E., Kearney, H., Spevack, M., Surkis, A., Cohen, C., & Gilman, S. (1979). Generalizability and durability of treatment effects in a intervention program for coronary-prone managers. *Journal of Behavioral Medicine, 2,* 195–208.

Scherwitz, L., Berton, K., & Leventhal, H. (1978). Type A behavior, self-involvement, and cardiovascular response. *Psychosomatic Medicine, 40,* 593–609.

Schmieder, R., Friedrich, G., Neus, H., Rüdel, H., & von Eiff, A. W. (1984). The influence of beta blockers on cardiovascular reactivity and Type A behavior pattern in hypertensives. *Psychosomatic Medicine, 45*(5), 417–423.

Shekelle, R. M., Gale, M., Ostfeld, A. M., & Paul, O. (1983). Hostility, risk of coronary heart disease, and mortality. *Psychosomatic Medicine, 45,* 109–114.

Siegel, J. M. (1984). Anger and cardiovascular risk in adolescents. *Health Psychology, 3*(4), 293–313.

Siegel, J. M., & Leitch, C. J. (1981). Behavioral factors and blood pressure in adolescence: The Tacoma Study. *American Journal of Epidemiology, 113*(2), 171–181.

Spielberger, C. D., Gorsuch, R. L., & Lushene, R. (1970). *State–trait anxiety inventory.* Palo Alto, CA: Consulting Psychologists Press.

Suinn, R. M. (1975). The cardiac stress management program for Type A patients. *Cardiac Rehabilitation, 5*(4), 13–15.

Suinn, R. M. (1980). Pattern A behaviors and heart disease: Intervention approaches. In J. M. Ferguson, & C. B. Taylor (Eds.), *The comprehensive handbook of behavioral medicine* (Vol. 1). Jamaica, NY: Spectrum Publications.

Suinn, R. M., & Bloom, L. J. (1978). Anxiety management training for Pattern A behavior. *Journal of Behavioral Medicine, 1,* 25–36.

Theorell, T., Lind, E., & Floderus, B. (1975). The relationship of disturbing life changes and emotions to the early development of myocardial infarction and other serious illnesses. *International Journal of Epidemiology, 4,* 281–293.

Williams, R. B. (1975). Physiological mechanisms underlying the association between psychosocial factors and coronary disease. In W. D. Gentry & R. B. Williams (Eds.), *Psychological aspects of myocardial infarction and coronary care* (pp. 37–50). St. Louis: Mosby.

Williams, R. B. (1978, April). *Arousal, relaxation, and biofeedback.* Paper presented at the Symposium on Concepts of Stress/Stress Management, Houston.

Williams, R. B., Friedman, M., Glass, D. C., Herd, J. A., & Schneiderman, N. (1977). Summary statement: Mechanisms linking behavioral and pathophysiological processes. In T. Dembroski (Ed.), *Proceedings of the Forum on Coronary-Prone Behavior* (Publication No. NIH78–1451, pp. 157–169). Washington, DC: Department of Health, Education and Welfare.

Williams, R. B., Haney, T. L., Lee, K. L., Hong Kong, Y., Blumenthal, J. A., & Whalen, R. E. (1980). Type A behavior, hostility, and coronary atherosclerosis. *Psychosomatic Medicine, 42,* 539–549.

Williams, R. B., Lane, J. D., Kuhn, C. M., Melosh, W., White, A. D., & Schanberg, S. M. (1982). Type A behavior and elevated physiological and neuroendocrine responses to cognitive tasks. *Science, 218,* 483–485.

Zyzanski, S. J. (1978). Associations of the coronary-prone behavior pattern. In T. M. Dembroski, S. M. Weiss, J. L. Shields, S. G. Haynes, & M. Feinleib (Eds.), *Coronary-prone behavior.* New York: Springer-Verlag.

# CHAPTER 11

# SMOKING

## SMOKING BEHAVIOR

### Significance of the Problem

Historically, the development of smoking behavior may be traced back to the fifteenth century; this developmental pathway is summarized in Table 11-1. The increase in recent years in the number of reviews on the theoretical aspects of why people smoke and the effectiveness of current interventions to eliminate as well as to prevent smoking behavior (Frederiksen & Simon, 1979; Hunt & Matarazzo, 1981, Leventhal & Cleary, 1980; Lichtenstein, 1982) reflects the significance of this health risk factor. Given the accumulation of research studies on the effects of cigarette smoking, a strong statement can be made regarding the negative effects of smoking on health, particularly with regard to heart disease, cancer, emphysema, peptic ulcers, and chronic bronchitis (USPHS, 1983). There is also clear evidence that excessive smoking has deleterious health effects on nonsmokers (USPHS, 1975). The presence of smoke in a closed environment can produce a variety of problems for the nonsmoker, ranging from mild irritation to allergic reaction and cardiovascular

**TABLE 11-1**

Historical Development of Smoking Behavior

| Important dates | Major trends | |
|---|---|---|
| 1492: 12 October. Columbus first encounters tobacco and later records the incident in his journal. | Pre-history to 15th century: the use of tobacco smoke, probably initially for religious and ritual purposes, but later also for pleasure, plays an important role in Mayan civilization and ultimately spreads throughout central and north America. | 1828: Posselt and Reiman isolate the "active ingredient" in tobacco and call it "nicotine." |
| | | 1840–70: the development of new strains of plant and new methods of curing result in a milder and mellower tobacco. |
| 1519: tobacco leaves brought to Europe. | 16th century: tobacco cultivation and the medicinal use of the leaf becomes widespread in Europe, although the recreational use of tobacco is at first largely confined to American colonists, sailors, and inhabitants of the maritime ports. | 1848: fall of one of the last bastions against tobacco; smoking is allowed on the streets of Berlin. |
| 1543: tobacco recommended for its healing properties. | | 1854–56: Europeans introduced to the cigarette by the Crimean War. |
| 1556: tobacco seeds arrive in France. 1570: tobacco plant named Nicotiana after Jean Nicot, French ambassador to Portugal, who enthused about tobacco's medicinal uses and introduced the leaves to France. | | 1881: the cigarette-making machine patented in the U.S.; with a speed of 200 cigarettes per minute (now over 5000) each machine produces as much in a day as 500 workers, and heralds the era of mass production. 1914–18: The Great War spreads cigarette smoking. |
| | | 20th century: the cigarette conquers the world. |

| Events | Commentary |
|---|---|
| 1585–86: English colonists in Virginia take to smoking tobacco and bring the habit to England. Sir Walter Raleigh, a devotee, does much to popularize smoking for pleasure. | |
| 1604: the tobaccophobe James I's "Counterblaste to Tobacco" inveighs against the habit. | |
| 1660: snuff introduced to England from France by courtiers of Charles II. | |
| 17th century: the ascendancy of the pipe<br>1. Pipe smoking spreads from England to Holland and then throughout Europe, helped by the marauding armies of the Thirty Years War.<br>2. Smoking reaches Russia via the Baltic ports and the Near East through the Venetians; the habit proliferates in the Far East where it was introduced by Spanish and Portuguese sailors and merchants.<br>3. Harsh persecution in Turkey, Persia, Russia and Japan fails to check the habit.<br>4. the tobacco trade plays a major part in developing the English North-American colonies; the need for ships to carry leaf to Europe aids the devel- | |
| Post-1918: the rise of the female smoker.<br>1929: the introduction of du Maurier—Britain's first filter cigarette. | 1. The low cost and convenience of the cigarette, combined with increasing prosperity, the growth of leisure and the democratization of society, provide unprecedentedly favourable conditions for a massive growth in consumption.<br>2. The use of mellower tobacco encourages the inhalation of smoke. |
| 1937: for the first time, cancer is produced in laboratory animals by cigarette tar.<br>1938: Raymond Pearl of Johns Hopkins University produces statistics showing nonsmokers live longer than smokers.<br>1950–56: Doll and Hill and others assemble evidence linking cigarette smoking with cancer of the lung; known carcinogens identified in cigarette smoke. | 3. Detailed epidemiological studies in the 1950s and 1960s confirm the increased health risks associated with cigarette smoking.<br>4. Governments introduce health-education campaigns and legislation designed to reduce the prevalence of smoking, while cigarette manufacturers become interested in the concept of developing a "safer" cigarette. |
| 1962: first report on smoking and health by the Royal College of Physicians. | 5. Great growth in the proportion of the total market taken by filter cigarettes, accompanied by a general downward trend in tar deliveries. This trend is especially pro- |

(continued)

**TABLE 11-1** *(Continued)*

| Important dates | Major trends | | |
|---|---|---|---|
| | opment of England's maritime power and revenue from tobacco subsidizes military adventure on land.<br>5. Tobacco is used as a currency, to buy wives in Virginia, slaves and land in Africa. | 1964: U.S. Surgeon General's report on smoking and health.<br>1965: UK ban on cigarette advertising on television. A health warning appears on cigarette packets sold in the U.S.<br>1970: radio and TV advertising of cigarettes banned in U.S. | nounced in the U.S. and West Germany.<br>6. In the developed world, the proportion of the population smoking tends to fall and the total consumption of cigarettes plateaus. Perhaps because of this, tobacco companies engage in "aggressive" marketing in the Third World where consumption rises, governments are slow to take action, and cigarettes remain high in tar and nicotine. |
| | 18th century: during which a good part of the world fell to "snuffing" and the pipe circumnavigated the globe. | | |
| 1820s: introduction of the flue-curing of tobacco. | 19th century: the age of the cigar and the tobacco quid. | 1971: the health warning appears in the UK.<br>1973: publication by the UK government of tar and nicotine "league tables"; low-tar "milder" brands of cigarette introduced.<br>1977: the introduction and rapid commercial failure of cigarettes containing tobacco substitutes. | |

*Note.* From *Smoking: Psychology and Pharmacology* (pp. 14–17) by H. Aston and R. Stepney. Copyright 1982 by Tavistock Publications. Reprinted by permission.

stress. Smoking during pregnancy significantly increases the likelihood of deleterious effects on the fetus, including stillbirths, higher infant mortality, prematurity, and decreased birthweight (USPHS, 1975). Because of the powerful negative impact of cigarette smoking on health, efforts to achieve a better understanding of smoking behavior and to improve methods of treatment are continually being made. Table 11-2 summarizes some of the findings on smoking as slow-motion suicide. However, it is impossible to provide an equally strong statement as to why people smoke and as to the effectiveness of current treatment strategies, even though a considerable amount of research has been done in these areas. A critical review of the more current theories on the establishment and maintenance of smoking behavior and smoking cessation interventions will be presented. Smoking prevention efforts will also be discussed.

## TABLE 11-2
Cigarette Smoking: Slow-Motion Suicide

1. Cigarette smoking is the largest preventable cause to death in the United States
2. Cigarette smoking is causally related each year to
    80,000 deaths from lung cancer
    22,000 deaths from other cancer
    up to 225,000 deaths from cardiovascular disease
    more than 19,000 deaths from pulmonary disease
3. Overall, cigarette smokers experience a 70% greater coronary heart disease death rate than do nonsmokers
4. Cigarette smoking is a major independent risk factor for CHD, it acts synergistically with other risk factors (particularly hypertension and elevated serum cholesterol), to greatly increase the risk of CHD
5. Women who use oral contraceptives and who smoke increase their risk of myocardial infarction tenfold, compared to women who neither use oral contraceptives nor smoke
6. Cigarette smoking has been found to significantly elevate the risk of sudden death. Overall, smokers experience two to four times greater risk than nonsmokers
7. There is an association between cigarette smoking and cerebrovascular disease
8. Cigarette smoking is the strongest risk factor predisposing to atherosclerotic peripheral arterial disease
9. Death from rupture of an atherosclerotic abdominal aneurysm is more common in cigarette smokers than in nonsmokers
10. Annual cost of smoking-related health damage (in medical care absenteeism, accidents, and decreased work productivity) is estimated at $27 billion

*Note.* From *The Health Consequences of Smoking* by U.S. Public Health Service, 1975, 1983. Reprinted by permission of the U.S. Government Printing Office.

## ESTABLISHMENT AND MAINTENANCE OF SMOKING BEHAVIOR

There are several approaches to explaining why people smoke. Many approaches focus on one particular process or mechanism as the main cause of cigarette smoking, such as nicotine addiction or social learning. Recent dissatisfaction with these simplistic models has produced a number of theories that attempt to integrate several factors, that is, nicotine addiction, social learning, operant and classical conditioning, and developmental phases (new smoker to chronic, heavy smoker). Lichtenstein and Brown (1980), for example, have described four stages in the development and maintenance of smoking behavior and these are presented in Table 11-3. Psychosocial factors appear to play a more important role in the *initiation* phase of the smoking habit, whereas a combination of the pharmacological effects of nicotine along with psychosocial and cognitive factors seem to be crucial in the *maintenance* phase. Smoking cessation appears to be largely determined by both psychosocial factors and the degree of physical dependence on nicotine. Finally, a combination of psychosocial and physiological factors (e.g., social pressures, withdrawal symptoms) tend to be implicated in the resumption of smoking behavior. A brief review of the biological, psychological/behavioral, and psychobiological theories of smoking behavior will be presented, with the psychobiological model representing the most comprehensive approach.

**TABLE 11-3**
Stages in the Development and Maintenance of the Smoking Habit

| Starting: psychosocial | Continuing: physiological and psychosocial | Stopping: psychosocial | Resuming: psychosocial and physiological |
|---|---|---|---|
| Availability | Nicotine | Health | Withdrawal |
| Curiosity | Immediate positive | Expense | symptoms |
| Rebelliousness | consequences | Social support | Stress and |
| Anticipation of | Signals (cues) in | Self-mastery | frustration |
| adulthood | environs | Aesthetics | Social pressure |
| Social confidence | Avoiding negative | Example to others | Alcohol |
| Social pressure/ | effects | | consumption |
| modeling: Peers, | (withdrawal) | | Abstinence vio- |
| siblings, parents, | | | lation effect |
| and media | | | |

*Note.* From "Smoking Cessation Methods: Review and Recommendations: by E. Lichtenstein and R. A. Brown in *The Addictive Behaviors: Treatment of Alcoholism, Drug Abuse, Smoking, and Obesity* edited by W. R. Miller. Copyright 1980 by Pergamon Press, Inc. Reprinted by permission.

## Biological Theories

An individual who smokes a pack a day takes more than 50,000 puffs per year. Each puff delivers to the lungs and bloodstream a variety of chemicals that may be the reinforcing pharmacological agents involved in smoking behavior. Out of these many chemicals, nicotine is thought to be the most important in smoking; however, tar and carbon monoxide have also been considered (Jarvik, 1979).

When a cigarette is smoked, nicotine is rapidly extracted. After entering the pulmonary circulation it is pumped to the aorta where it stimulates the aorta and carotid chemoreceptors. At this point, reflex stimulation of the respiration and cardiovascular centers in the brainstem may occur. During one circulation, one-fourth of the nicotine passes through the brain capilliaries. The blood–brain barrier is highly permeable to nicotine, which passes quickly into the brain. In the brain, nicotine stimulates nicotine receptors and releases biogenic amines, which stimulate a variety of hypothalamic and pituitary hormones. The other three-fourths of the inhaled nicotine is delivered to the rest of the body, where it activates other nicotine receptors. Nicotine releases epinephrine from the adrenal gland, which is associated with sympathetic arousal. Nicotine increases free fatty acid levels. Although nicotine appears to be the prime candidate for the reinforcing pharmacological effects of cigarettes, the evidence is circumstantial (Jarvik, 1979). Cigarette smokers prefer cigarettes with nicotine. However, smokers will continue to smoke cigarettes even after receiving nicotine intravenously.

Given that nicotine appears to have a reinforcing biochemical effect, biological theories focus on nicotine addiction as the primary etiological and maintaining factor in cigarette smoking. *Nicotine regulation models* conceptualize smoking behavior as an escape response to nicotine withdrawal in an addictive cycle (Jarvik, 1977). The characteristic symptoms of nicotine withdrawal are irritability, anxiety, inability to concentrate, disturbance of arousal, and intensified craving (Shiffman, 1979). This biological approach hypothesizes an internal regulatory mechanism that detects the level of nicotine and maintains it within certain limits by regulating the frequency of smoking. Smoking occurs when the level of nicotine in the body falls below a *set point*, thus suggesting that sustaining the level of nicotine acts as a mechanism for maintaining smoking behavior. A biological mechanism (often referred to as a "nicostat") senses the lowered nicotine level and provides the motivation for directed behavior, that is, smoking the cigarette. Smoking the cigarette increases the nicotine in the blood, which is, in turn, reinforcing.

In the past, little attention has been paid to the effects of nicotine deprivation and withdrawal symptoms. These physiological factors are more commonly recognized now, but most behavioral scientists maintain that smoking does not occur in a psychosocial vacuum and that psychosocial factors are equally important. Some of the problems associated with the nicotine regulation model include a failure of the model to explain (1) how changes in plasma nicotine levels are related to craving and smoking behavior, (2) the high relapse rates seen in cigarette smokers even after nicotine levels have remained at zero for long periods of time, (3) smoking responsiveness to emotional states that change rapidly, (4) why individuals have difficulty quitting smoking when under stress, and (5) the apparently long developmental history of smoking (Leventhal & Cleary, 1980). More information is needed on the physiological effects of nicotine. These include the biochemistry of nicotine, specific arousal mechanisms, and the differences in individuals' sensitivity to nicotine so that the relative importance of nicotine addiction in the establishment and maintenance of smoking can be understood.

### Psychological/Behavioral Theories

Three theories of smoking that are representative of the various types of approaches generated from a psychological/behavioral perspective will be discussed. These include an affect reduction model, a social learning model, and a habit and associative learning model.

Tomkins (1966, 1968) presented an *affect reduction model*, suggesting that smoking is used to regulate emotional states. Smoking produces positive emotional reactions and minimizes negative emotional reactions in a variety of situations. The research strategy used to investigate this model is primarily based on self-report questionnaires and factor analyses of the results of the questionnaires. Based on his work, Tomkins proposed four "general types" of smoking. These general types are based on the smoker's use of cigarettes to control the affective experience. The four general types of smoking are (1) positive affect smoking to obtain pleasure; (2) negative affect smoking to obtain relief from unpleasantness; (3) habitual smoking, which occurs automatically without reference to affect; and (4) craving, as seen in the seriously addicted smoker who exhibits craving behavior whenever he or she is prevented from smoking. There is some evidence that confirms the reliability of individuals' reports for smoking and of the conditions that stimulate smoking. Leventhal and Avis (1976) and Ikard and Tomkins (1973), after dividing subjects into those with high and those with low scores on particular scales, assessed the smoking behavior of the subjects in different situations. When given cigarettes adulterated with vinegar, those subjects high on the pleasure-taste factor showed a significant decrease in number of cigarettes smoked, compared to those low on this factor.

Habit smokers significantly reduced their smoking when asked to monitor each cigarette smoked, whereas pleasure-taste smokers did not. Subjects who use smoking as a means of reducing anxiety smoked more after viewing a fear film. Although these studies support earlier findings (Schwartz & Dubitzky, 1968), the relationship between self-report and behavior is not perfect. Also, the report that smoking reduces tension, the phenomenon often referred to as Nesbitt's paradox, is not accounted for. Nesbitt's paradox refers to evidence that people who report that smoking produces relaxation often demonstrate autonomic arousal, which is inconsistent with a state of relaxation (Schachter, 1973).

The research on the affect reduction model initially raised a great deal of interest in the role of psychological variables other than personality in the establishment and maintenance of smoking. In general, the reported research used inadequate experimental designs to explain relatively few phenomena associated with cigarette smoking. Other components of the affect reduction model have been incorporated into more complex models, such as the multiple-regulation model, to be discussed in a later section.

The *social learning approach* to smoking has not been presented as a formal, integrated model. Rather, the approach has been one of creating and evaluating various smoking cessation interventions, based on the principles of social learning. A social learning approach to the establishment and maintenance of cigarette smoking as suggested by Pomerleau (1980) will be discussed.

A social learning explanation can be thought of as an extension of operant-conditioning principles to situations that involve interpersonal activity. It also incorporates the concepts of imitation, social reinforcement, and symbolic, vicarious, and self-regulatory processes (Bandura, 1977). Within this approach, a habit is believed to be acquired under conditions of social reinforcement, usually through peer pressure. Smoking cigarettes is initially aversive behavior, but after sufficient practice, habituation or tolerance occurs. After habituation occurs, smoking behavior begins to provide adequate positive reinforcement in itself, so that social reinforcement is not a necessary maintaining factor. Smoking also generalizes to other situations via operant conditioning.

The individual gradually learns that certain external and internal cues now control smoking behavior and act as discriminative stimuli for situations that are punishing, neutral, or reinforcing. Situations associated with smoking, such as an empty cigarette pack, may serve as a conditioned stimulus, which will elicit covert responses, such as physical changes perceived as craving, that increase the likelihood of smoking. The same situation may serve as a discriminative stimulus that sets the occasion for the reinforcement of smoking. Also, stimuli that prepare one for the act of smoking can serve as a secondary reinforcer for behaviors preceding them, as well as discriminative stimuli for behaviors following them. For example, the sight of a cigarette can reinforce the act of opening a full cigarette pack and the sight of a cigarette can also serve as a discriminative stimulus for lighting the cigarette. In essence, the smoking ritual forms a linked chain of responses. These responses are initially established through social reinforcement and are maintained by internal and external cues.

Internal events, such as emotion, influence smoking. Smoking behavior is thought to be in part an avoidance/escape response to such negative emotional events as the experience of anger. This escape response is a potential coping response, and although it initially provides relief, it has long-term negative health consequences. However, when the reinforcement effects become powerful, the response may generalize to other negative emotional states, such as anxiety and sadness. Given the various possible mechanisms described above, smoking can be seen as providing both positive and negative reinforcement over a wide array of internal and external events. This view is reflected in the multicomponent treatment approach advocated by a social learning model.

A critical evaluation of social learning theory as applied to smoking cannot be made, since there is currently insufficient longitudinal evidence to support this relationship. Indirect support, through evaluation of multifactor procedures, has made it difficult to pinpoint and evaluate the factors involved in treatment success (Hunt & Matarazzo, 1982).

Hunt and Matarazzo (1970, 1982) apply their discussion of *habit* and *associative learning* to explaining smoking behavior (Hunt, Matarazzo, Weiss, & Gentry, 1979). Initially, they defined habit as a "stable behavior pattern overlearned to the point of becoming automatic and marked by decreasing awareness and increasing dependence on secondary rather than primary reinforcement." More recently, they defined *habit* as a "stable behavior pattern marked by automaticity, decreasing awareness, and a partial independence of reinforcement." This newer definition attempts to place more emphasis on the explanatory power of the immediate and automatic aspects of such habitual behavior, as well as its relative independence of reinforcement. Few studies have examined the concept of habit as defined above. This type of automatic behavior may appear to occur spontaneously and independently of reinforcement, and oftentimes in apparent opposition to reinforcement contingencies. A habit is established in the following manner. A behavior is initially acquired via commonly recognized reinforcement processes. In time, these processes are short-circuited as the behavior becomes a function of associative learning and thus becomes automatized.

In essence, reinforcement is the primary process in the acquisition of a new behavior, whereas associative learning is seen as important in maintenance. Furthermore, operant principles and associative learning are not independent, but rather are interactive. Although Hunt and Matarazzo (1982) discuss treatment implications for smoking, the basic hypothesis they make about habit and associative learning has not been researched.

## Psychobiological Models

Psychobiological models integrate and emphasize physiological factors associated with cigarette smoking, as well as behavioral, psychological, and emotional factors. Two theories that represent this approach are the opponent-process model and the multiple-regulation model.

The *opponent-process model of acquired motivation* attempts to explain the process of addiction in general (Solomon, 1977, 1980; Solomon & Corbit, 1973, 1974). This model has been used to explain cigarette smoking; however, research evidence to support the model has mainly come from laboratory studies with animals (Ternes, 1977).

The opponent-process model postulates central nervous system (CNS) mechanisms that operate homeostatically to reduce significant departures from affective equilibrium. The affective departure may be either positive or negative. Return to homeostatic balance is brought about by activation of an opponent process. Thus, if the initial change is a positive increase in affect, then a negative process would be initiated, via CNS mechanisms, to counteract the change. Unconditioned stimuli (UCS) or primary reinforcers, for instance, can produce this initial imbalance.

The UCS, an affect-arousing stimulus, can elicit primary affective processes (UCRs). These UCRs are called *a-processes*. The a-process may reflect a positive, pleasant, or negative affect, depending on the UCS that elicits it. For example, drinking several glasses of wine may produce relaxation and good feelings in a particular person. However, the elicitation of the a-process triggers a second response, called the *b-process*. The b-process is always an opposite affective response. To continue with the example of a person who had several glasses of wine, the b-process would be associated with a headache and stomach upset or a hangover the next morning. Furthermore, the a-process is closely associated with the UCS and does not show much habituation. The b-process is slower in response than the a-process and is also slower to peak or return to baseline following the termination of the UCS. In our example, then, two things can be predicted: The person will experience the pleasure of drinking wine more rapidly and for a shorter time than the negative affect associated with a hangover, which will take longer to experience and will last for a longer time.

Given the nature of these two processes, a biphasic pattern of affective or hedonic tone can be predicted. Initially a > b, and the affective state is predicted by the a-process. When the UCS is terminated, then a < b, and the affective state correspond to b-processes. The a and b processes are nonassociative. They are not based on conditioning or learning; however, the processes may be conditioned by stimuli other than the initial UCS.

This simple model becomes more complex when it is realized that the growth of the b-process can be affected by the intensity, duration, and frequency of and interval between the UCS presentations. The b-processes are strengthened by increases in intensity, frequency, and duration of the UCS and decreases in the interval between UCS presentations. The b-processes are weakened through reduction or discontinuation of the UCS.

The opponent-process model can be applied to the establishment and maintenance of cigarette smoking in the following general way. To begin with, cigarettes must contain substances (UCS) that evoke the a-process and provide pleasure during their initial use. Aversive affective responses may occur on the first few occasions of smoking, but these negative affects are offset by other reinforcers, such as peer pressure. As cigarette smoking continues, the opposing b-process becomes stronger. In time, the pleasurable A state weakens and the aversive B state and associated withdrawal symptoms intensify. The best way for the smoker to reduce the B state is to smoke more and thus produce the A state. The addictive cycle is now established—smoking is positively reinforced by providing pleasure and negatively reinforced by terminating the withdrawal symptoms of the b-process. As tolerance to the UCS in the cycle occurs, the person will smoke more and more, which will only strengthen the underlying b-process. Also, stimuli associated with the a-process, such as a full pack of cigarettes or the sight of an ashtray, may elicit a brief conditioned response similar to the pleasure associated with the a-process. Stimuli associated with the cessation of smoking, such as an empty pack of cigarettes and "no smoking" signs, may elicit a conditioned response similar to the negative b-process. To make matters worse, the brief, conditioned A state elicited by the conditioned stimuli will be followed by conditioned b-processes, which in turn, intensify the desire for a cigarette.

Some evidence does point to the fact that nicotine may possess some intrinsically rewarding actions, which, in turn, lead to tolerance. Deprivation of nicotine, then, may elicit withdrawal symptoms similar to those observed in drug addiction. Based on such observations, Stepney (1980) provided a description of cigarette smoking in terms of an addictive behavior, as illustrated in Figure 11-1. Stepney hypothesizes that the main motivation behind the continuation of smoking behavior, once it is established, is to alleviate the withdrawal symptoms that accompany the fall in tissue nicotine levels as the effect of each cigarette wears off.

Affective experiences predicted by the opponent-process model have been reported by former smokers (Pomerleau, 1980). For instance, smokers have reported that an initial brief acquisition phase occurred during which smoking itself was not that pleasurable, but was reinforced by external events, such as peer approval. Smoking became pleasurable for a while (a-process > b-process); however, in time, more cigarettes were smoked and the pleasure of smoking became minimal in comparison to the discomfort of not smoking (a-process < b-process). Smokers who quit for a period of time and then began smoking again report that the first few cigarettes smoked seemed very pleasurable (a-process > b-process).

The opponent–process model does provide a psychobiological framework as it attempts to integrate concepts from both social learning

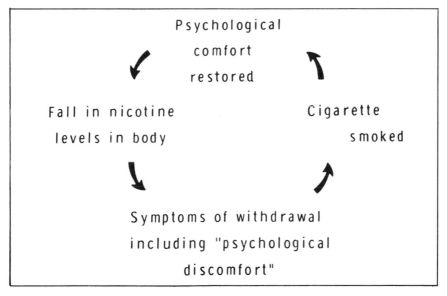

**FIGURE 11-1.** Mechanisms mediating smoking behavior: The addiction model. From "Smoking Behaviour: A Psychology of the Cigarette Habit" by R. Stepney, 1980, *British Journal of Diseases of the Chest, 74,* 64. Copyright 1980 by Baillière Tindall. Reprinted by permission.

and biological models. It does predict both affective and physiological responses that may be assessed and evaluated. Some supporting evidence from animal experiments and research in the area of opiate addiction has been found for the opponent-process model (Pomerleau, 1980). The model, although quite convincing in its ability to explain phenomena associated with smoking, has yet to be empirically tested as a model for smoking in humans.

Leventhal and Cleary (1980) present a *multiple-regulation model*, which attempts to integrate the psychological and biological factors associated with smoking. The theory is placed within a developmental context as it describes the stages of smoking. The four stages discussed are preparation, initiation, "becoming a smoker," and maintenance. The first stage preparation includes all the factors that may lead a person to pick up a cigarette and smoke it. Many researchers believe that social pressure is probably a prime initiator of experimentation with cigarettes, particularly for children and adolescents. Smoking cigarettes is seen as mature, rebellious, and sexually attractive (Leventhal, 1973). Grade-school students view smokers as foolish, tough, often in trouble, lazy, easygoing, and so forth (Bland, Bewley, & Day, 1975). Although these students do not view themselves as possessing these characteristics, they may be attracted to this ideal of a smoker, since these characteristics reflect an individual who is independent, tough, and expresses impulses freely (Leventhal & Cleary, 1980). Other preparatory factors include smoking by family members which appears to reduce the barrier to peer pressure to smoke and increases the opportunity for obtaining cigarettes to smoke. Some children may have different preparatory sets. For example, children who experience a lack of social acceptance may smoke to become part of the gang. Young adults who begin smoking may believe that smoking will improve their ability to cope with stress, as is often seen in college and medical students (Smith, 1970). Whatever the specific cognitive set toward smoking cigarettes, the important issue to be recognized is that attitudes and beliefs about smoking, modeling of authority or admired figures, and peer pressure are some of the psychosocial factors that motivate the individual to experiment with cigarettes initially. Understanding these psychosocial factors is important in the prevention of smoking.

Initiation of smoking is marked by the actual smoking of one's first cigarette. During this second stage of smoking one's first few cigarettes, many people decide not to continue with their experimentation. Over 80% of youngsters report trying at least one cigarette (Palmer, 1970), yet students in grade school through high school who are regular smokers rarely exceed 50% of those who attempt smoking. One may speculate as to why some people do not proceed past the second stage of smoking, although no conclusive answers have as yet been found to this question. Certainly, having a better understanding of what the factors are that inhibit smoking behavior at this point would also be useful in designing prevention programs for individuals at risk for developing long-term smoking behavior (i.e., people who experiment with cigarettes). For those individuals who do not quit at this point, the development of tolerance to the physiological effects of smoking occurs. The initial data suggest that it takes about two years and possibly longer for smoking to become consistent and frequent (Leventhal & Cleary, 1980). During the "becoming a smoker" stage, biological factors appear to play a critical role. However, social, cognitive, and behavioral factors may further enhance the process. The fourth stage, maintenance, begins when smoking is an integral part of self-regulation in many different situations. Leventhal and Cleary emphasize the importance of both biological and psychological factors at this level.

After describing the four stages of smoking, Leventhal and Cleary (1980) provide a detailed discussion of the underlying assumptions of the multiple-regulation model. The model is an elaboration of similar models by Tomkins and Solomon and Corbit and attempts to account for the problems found with Schacter's model of nicotine regulation.

Essentially, six assumptions are made. The first and most critical assumption is that *emotional regulation* rather than nicotine regulation is involved in smoking. Fluctuations from emotional or hedonic homeostasis or general optimal levels stimulate smoking behavior. Leventhal and Cleary believe that although heavy dependent smokers regulate nicotine intake, they do so not because of the drop in nicotine level *per se*, but rather because of the negative emotional state associated with the sensation of craving. The craving sensation becomes linked to drops in nicotine level in two possible ways. First, craving can be caused by a drop in nicotine level itself. In this case, the phenomenon that occurs is predicted by the opponent-process model. Craving would be associated with the negative, opponent B-state. The more one smokes to reduce craving, the greater the underlying b-processes become. This results in an increased intensity of craving. External stimulation can provide the second source of craving. For example, smoking is used in various anxiety-provoking situations. In time, these situations may elicit the negative emotions that become conditioned to decreased levels in plasma nicotine.

The second assumption is that several emotional processes may be operating simultaneously. These may be multiple external situations that provoke affective responses as well as multiple internal (opponent-processes) sources of affect. For example, an individual can feel the pain from an intense physical workout followed by a positive opponent affect and a positive affect from smoking followed by a negative affect. The third assumption is that these affective states can combine algebraically at any given point in time. Thus, the positive or the negative opponent process can be combined with a negative or positive affect from a variety of situations, therefore facilitating conditioning. The fourth assumption is that changes in plasma nicotine level generate a variety of bodily sensations that can be conditioned to the emotional states experienced. These first four assumptions attempt to develop the concept of craving to include more than the direct effects of changes in nicotine plasma level. In essence, these assumptions state that the externally induced or opponent negative emotional reactions to these sensations (resulting from changes in nicotine plasma level) can be conditioned and reflect what smokers experience as craving.

The fifth assumption is that smoking can be used as a coping skill. The multiple regulation model indicates that smoking enhances relaxation and helps to control negative affect, such as fear, anger, and tension. The sixth and final assumption states that there exists an "emotional memory" for the events outlined above. Thus, the smoking experience will be strongly associated with memories of smoking to cope with aversive events. Schematic emotional memories would combine image-like representations of situations with impressions of motoric and physiological reactions in these situations, for example, the subjective emotions experienced in the situation and the autonomic, expressive, motor, and instrumental behaviors performed in the setting. This concept is somewhat similar to aspects of the bioinformational theory discussed in Chapter 4. Schemata of this sort will sustain the conditioning of a range of memories experienced as craving to nicotine levels in a variety of situations (Leventhal & Cleary, 1980, p. 393). It is the schema that provides the mechanism for tying together all the events discussed thus far (external stimulus cues, internal stimulus cues, subjective emotional experience, and expressive motor and autonomic reactions associated with the emotional response to smoking). The appearance of any of these elements can produce the other elements. The complexity of the model and the allowance for idiosyncratic combinations of events make it feasible to account for different "types" of smokers. Thus, depending on the elements of the schema, smokers will call themselves a particular type of smoker: social, addicted, habitual, and so forth. According to Leventhal and Cleary, the breaking up of these conditioned emotional schemata will eliminate the conditioned experience of craving and increase the likelihood that the person will stop smoking. This model represents the most comprehensive psychobiological model of smoking to date. The complexity of the model calls for innovative systematic research to test the specific assumptions proposed.

## TREATMENT APPROACHES

There is widespread interest in developing smoking cessation programs. Types of techniques designed to enhance smoking cessation range from self-help manuals to community projects. Treatment strategies can be classified in a variety of ways. This section will discuss clinical or individual approaches, followed by community or large-scale efforts. Besides a description of the smoking interventions, research evaluating the different approaches will be discussed. The final portion of the discussion of smoking cessation strategies will focus on the problems associated with research in this difficult area.

Research has primarily focused on the evaluation of smoking cessation strategies rather than on the issue of why people smoke. Based on a critical review of the smoking treatment literature, Leventhal and Cleary (1980) draw four interesting conclusions. First, there appears to be a significant decrease in smoking behavior during the treatment phase, regardless of whether the outcome variable is quitting or significant reduction. Second, there is a relatively high drop-out rate of those in treatment, up to 50% of the initial sample. Third, those who quit smoking generally return to smoking. And fourth, different therapies do not seem to differ significantly in terms of their effectiveness. These general findings suggest that smoking cessation programs work well at helping people stop smoking, but have few long-term effects.

### Clinical or Individual Approaches

Behavioral interventions, cognitive modification, hypnosis, and physician intervention are the most researched and widely implemented smoking cessation programs. *Behavioral interventions* include stimulus control, reinforcement of nonsmoking, affect or tension reduction techniques, aversion techniques, and multicomponent programs. Stimulus control techniques are based on operant principles, with the goal of determining and controlling environmental stimuli that elicit smoking behavior. Since smoking usually takes place in a wide variety of settings, the number and extensiveness of controlling cues or discriminative stimuli make it difficult for the smoker not to smoke. Treatment generally involves the gradual elimination of smoking by instructing the smoker to choose either a few particular locations or times to smoke. In time, as smoking becomes restricted to a few well-controlled environments, not smoking should become easier in other situations, since those cues eliciting the smoking response loose their saliency. Eventually, the smoker is expected to abstain from smoking in all situations. Results from studies evaluating stimulus control techniques indicate that most smokers will reduce their smoking but tend to plateau at 10 to 12 cigarettes a day. It has been suggested that the reinforcement value of these few cigarettes becomes so great that the individual finds it extremely difficult to refrain from smoking. In general, stimulus control procedures do not provide significant initial or long-term effects in reduction of smoking, as compared to other active or placebo treatments. Drop-out rates are also very high (Glasgow & Bernstein, 1981; Shapiro, Tursky, Schwartz, & Schnidman, 1971).

Reinforcement of nonsmoking attempts to modify smoking behaviors indirectly by reinforcing nonsmoking behaviors, particularly those incompatable with smoking. Most often money is used as the reward for specified periods of nonsmoking. Recent research indicates that positive reinforcement strategies tend to have good initial results. Thus, this approach seems effective in helping the smoker make initial changes (Bernstein & Glasgow, 1979). However as with other smoking cessation strategies, the long-term effects are questionable.

The use of affect or tension reduction techniques in smoking control is based on the assumption that cigarette smoking is more likely to occur in anxiety-provoking situations and that cigarette smoking is then a coping technique to reduce stress. Tension reduction techniques are aimed at eliminating the distress and anxiety that stimulate smoking. Common techniques used are relaxation training and systematic desensitization. Relaxation is used as a counter response to anxiety-producing situations. If anxiety is relieved through relaxation, then the desire for a cigarette should also be reduced. Systematic desensitization also uses muscular relaxation, but combines it with images of various smoking situations. Imagined situations are arranged in a hierarchical fashion in terms of difficulty of abstention. The goal is to be able to feel relaxed in situations in which one would have the most difficult time not smoking. Results of studies of tension reduction techniques have not been promising in this area; they have either failed to demonstrate greater effectiveness over other approaches or have reported unimpressive success rates (Frederiksen & Simon, 1979).

Aversion therapy was a commonly used and studied behavioral intervention for smoking. Electric shock, aversive taste stimuli, and smoke are the aversive stimuli used. The general strategy is to pair the aversive stimuli with actual or imagined smoking. An advantage of electric shock is that it allows for specific and precise application in pairing the conditioned stimulus (smoking) and unconditioned stimulus (shock). It may also be used in the natural environment, such as a cigarette case that shocks the person when a cigarette is withdrawn. Controlled evaluations of electric shock have shown the procedure not to be that effective, with studies reporting faradic shock as being equally effective to control conditions and lacking in significant long-term success rates. An interesting study utilizing a multiple baseline component analysis design to evaluate an electric aversion procedure employed many daily sessions and intense levels of shock (Dericco, Brigham, & Garlington, 1977). Eighty percent of the subjects reported abstinence from smoking at a 6-month follow-up. It has also been suggested that the procedure may be more effective if the shock is paired with preparatory events, such as thinking about taking a cigarette out of the case. Shock then may be paired with the urge to smoke (Berecz, 1976). Criticisms of faradic shock include the lack of generalization in humans (i.e., they can readily discriminate when shock is not present), ethics of the use of electric shock to modify behavior, and the fact that stimuli more commonly associated with cigarette smoking, (e.g., smoke) may produce better results.

Very few studies have used aversive taste stimuli. The poor results reported by those investigators who have evaluated such procedures most likely generated little enthusiasm for further exploration of this procedure. An example of the procedure used can be found in a study by Whitman (1972) who used a tablet that produced a bitter and burning sensation in the mouth. No significant differences were found between the treatment group and a waiting-list control group at a six-month follow-up.

The use of smoking itself as the aversive stimulus has been more widely studied and appears to be a promising procedure. The basic procedure is to expose or require the smoker to inhale large quantities of smoke and would entail, for instance, blowing warm smoky air as the person smokes, instructing the individual to chain smoke or requiring him or her to take more puffs at a faster than normal rate. This last example has been termed *rapid smoking*, and of all the aversive approaches, it appears to have the greatest impact on smoking cessation. Two issues have been raised in regard to rapid smoking. The first is that rapid smoking appears most effective when paired with a particular therapeutic setting. The setting must be one in which the subject is given warm, strong social support and positive expectancy. Also, the intervention must be individually tailored; thus, one may have to vary the number of sessions and trials per session, depending on the particular individual one is treating. Because of the need for this type of setting, it is questionable whether the effects of rapid smoking are due to a straightforward aversive conditioning or punishment process. The second issue concerns some initial findings that rapid smoking is not a safe procedure, since it produces various, potentially dangerous, physiological side effects. One study found that rapid smoking led to a significant increase in heart rate, blood pressure, carboxy hemoglobin levels, and even cardiac abnormalities (Horan, Hackett, Nicholas, Linberg, Stone, &

Lukoski, 1977). However, other studies completed at the same time reported no adverse effects (Miller, Schilling, Logan, & Johnson, 1977). Sachs, Hall, and Hall (1978) point out that the risk–benefit ratio of rapid smoking is favorable. Thus, it is more logical for the smoker to risk highly improbable negative effects from rapid smoking than to refrain from treatment and be exposed to the much greater risk of premature death secondary to heart disease and cancer. Most researchers continue to agree that patients who suffer from pulmonary or cardiovascular disease and individuals over 55 should not engage in rapid smoking. Physician approval is also essential for all patients (Lichtenstein & Glasgow, 1977). In general, the rapid smoking procedure provides the best results of all the behavioral smoking cessation interventions discussed thus far. If the procedure is combined with a supportive therapeutic environment, expected results would indicate that 30 to 44% of all subjects who entered treatment would be abstinent two to six years after treatment (Danaher, 1977a, Lichtenstein & Penner, 1977). Short-term abstinence rates for this procedure are at least 50% (Lichtenstein & Brown, 1980).

Multicomponent procedures are often a structured treatment package including some of the behavioral procedures described thus far. Multicomponent programs may also include self-monitoring procedures, such as keeping a record of cigarette intake. Initially, reports of multicomponent programs were encouraging, with some demonstrating an abstinence rate approaching 60% to 70% at 6-month follow-up (Delahunt & Curran, 1976; Lando, 1977). Other studies, however, indicate that some multicomponent programs have demonstrated that they were no more effective than a single component approach and are sometimes even less effective than the component parts themselves (Barbarin, 1978; Danaher, 1977b). The overall effects of a multicomponent approach, however, warrant further investigation to delineate which components work best together and in what format.

For those who adopt a psychobiological model for smoking, a multicomponent program would be one treatment approach consistent with the emphasis on the importance of both physiological and behavioral factors in the etiology, maintenance, and cessation of smoking behavior. A multicomponent program may include procedures that would modify physiological as well as psychological factors. For example, nicotine fading could be combined with a contingency management procedure or aversive therapy. A nicotine fading procedure requires the patient to switch to cigarettes with a progressively lower tar and nicotine content until he or she is ready to quit completely. Foxx and Brown (1979) have reported interesting results for subjects who self-monitored their smoking behavior and employed nicotine fading. At an 18-month follow-up,

40% of the smokers remained abstinent, whereas the remaining 60% reported smoking cigarettes lower in nicotine and tar content than their baseline brands.

Arguments leveled against nicotine fading include concerns that more cigarettes per day would be smoked, the smoker may inhale more deeply and thus increase exposure to harmful gases, or reduction in tar and nicotine may create greater exposure to carbon monoxide, thus making consumption of these lower tar and nicotine cigarettes quite hazardous (Hammond, Garfinkel, Seidman, & Lew, 1976). In general, studies investigating these issues have found that most often changing to low tar and nicotine cigarettes does not produce the above changes in behavior or lead to adverse health effects (Forbes, Robinson, Hanley, & Coulburn, 1976; Schachter, 1977, 1978). However, because of the limited amount of data, research is needed to delineate the relationship between reduction in tar and nicotine intake, exposure to carbon monoxide, and the potential for associated health risks.

The underlying assumption of *covert modification procedures* in the treatment of smoking is that such internal cues as self-statements, urges, and visual images are discriminative stimuli for smoking behavior. It is thought that these cognitive processes occur before, during, and after smoking (Frederiksen & Simon, 1979). The goal of cognitive modification is to change those internal cues to ones that would promote behavior incompatable with smoking. Several strategies have been evaluated. Frederiksen and Simon (1979) suggest the following four categories: "(1) increased anti-smoking or pro-smoking self-statements, (2) overt or covert reinforcement for such self-statements, (3) presentation of covert aversive stimulation following smoking urges or images, and (4) overt aversive stimulation contingent upon smoking urges or images" (p. 507). The fourth strategy has been discussed in the section on aversion therapy. Outcome studies investigating these various procedures have failed to demonstrate that they are superior to behavioral interventions and there is little evidence that these strategies have significant long-term effectiveness as compared to placebo controls (Glasgow & Bernstein, 1981). Although cognitive modification procedures do not show more impressive results than many of the behavioral interventions discussed, some positive changes have been reported. Based on available research, it has been emphasized that covert antecedents of smoking should not be ignored and that a multicomponent program for smoking cessation should include modification of these internal cues.

*Hypnosis* is a smoking cessation procedure that has been used for over 30 years. Many studies, mostly uncontrolled reports, have been reported and suggest that hypnosis is a useful procedure. Other studies, however, indicate poor results. Reviews on the evaluation of hypnosis as a smoking cessation strategy report treatment success ranging from no change to 94% (von Dedenroth, 1968). The lack of experimental control, a failure to specify and control hypnotic procedures adequately, the lack of long-term follow-up, and the use of other supportive procedures have made it impossible to provide valid statements regarding the effectiveness of hypnosis on smoking cessation (Hunt & Matarazzo, 1982).

*Physician Intervention.* Many people seek medical treatment or have physical checkups and will therefore have contact with a physician. It has been thought that physician intervention could have a powerful impact on smoking cessation for those patients. Many physicians will instruct their patients to stop smoking. This intervention may include a brief comment on the part of the physician on smoking-related health risks or an intervention that lasts several minutes. Sometimes a patient will be given literature consisting of serious advice and suggestions to quit smoking. Given the minimal procedure utilized and the time in contact with the physician, it is surprising that studies evaluating physician intervention for smoking provide any positive results at all. For instance, studies using single group designs report results ranging from 17 to 38% patients remaining abstinent after 6 months or longer (Handel, 1973). A review of studies that used control groups also indicates a wide range of effectiveness with 33 to 90% remaining abstinent at 6-month follow-up. However, most studies had no proper experimental controls. Despite the relatively few studies reporting the effectiveness of physician intervention, the findings currently available are promising in that this type of smoking cessation intervention appears to be at least as effective as all the approaches we have discussed thus far. Physician intervention may also be less expensive and time-consuming than behavioral, cognitive, or hypnotic procedures. It would seem beneficial to continue research in this area in order to determine how the effects of physician intervention could be enhanced. One way, for instance, might be to explore the manner in which the physician gives suggestions to quit smoking. Should the physician use a threatening, demanding approach or a supportive, educational one? Should literature be provided to the patient accompanied by a physician's warning and what types of information should be included in the literature?

## Community or Large-Scale Clinical Projects

This section will focus on types of programs and studies that attempt to reach large groups of individuals. Often the target population consists of individuals at "high risk" for coronary heart disease (CHD) or respiratory disease. The types of studies/programs that will be discussed are clinical studies focusing on individuals at risk and community studies.

In *large-scale clinical interventions*, individuals are referred either to an intervention group for smoking cessation or to their usual source of medical care. Although some of these studies have focused only on smoking behavior, others have included interventions aimed at reducing or eliminating other risk factors, such as hypertension. The actual treatments used in the interventions are often ones that have been discussed in the previous section, particularly behavioral, cognitive, and multicomponent treatment programs.

Table 11-3 lists intervention, follow-up, and cessation results for five major controlled clinical trials that were included in the 1983 report of the Surgeon General, *Consequences of Smoking*. The multiple risk factor intervention trial (MRFIT) will be described, since it exemplifies a large-scale clinical study. The MRFIT was a randomized clinical prevention trial followed for an average of seven years. This program was designed to test the effects of a multifactor intervention program on CHD. The risk factors of interest were cigarette smoking, hypertension, and elevation of serum cholesterol levels. A sample of 12,866 men, between the ages of 35 to 57 who were considered to be at risk, were selected from 22 clinical centers and randomly assigned to one of two groups. The controlled condition identified as the usual care (UC) condition received their usual health care in the community. The UC group subjects returned for annual assessments of risk factor levels, physical examination status, and laboratory studies. In addition, their morbidity status was assessed with the evaluation of the examination sent to the subjects' usual source of medical care. The second group was the special intervention (SI) group. The SI group was treated for hypertension, cigarette smoking, and elevated blood cholesterol levels. Treatment for smoking began at the third screening visit. During this visit, the subject met with a physician who described the effects of smoking on the respiratory and cardiovascular systems. The physician strongly advised the patient to stop smoking. The smoker then met with a "smoking specialist," who discussed the smoking intervention program. Of the subjects, 96% agreed to participate in an intensive intervention that would meet in group form and 6% agreed to be seen individually. Group treatments consisted of about 10 members per group who met for 10 sessions. The treatment focused on interventions for all three risk factors. Subjects were encouraged to bring family and friends to these meetings. The smoking intervention program presented during these group meetings was a multicomponent one. The program included educational, cognitive, and behavioral approaches to cigarette smoking cessation. In order to provide comparable treatment among the 10 groups, common protocols and educational materials were used. Following the intensive group program phase, individual counseling was provided. An intervention team, often headed by a behavioral specialist, included a nutritionist, nurses, physicians, and health counselors who planned and carried out the individualized program. Depending on the status of the smoker, the individual program for those who had quit smoking focused on maintenance of smoking cessation; those who had not quit smoking were placed in an extended intervention program. The extended intervention program was individualized for maximum treatment effects; thus, subjects in these programs did not always receive the same treatment. The goal at this phase of the trial was an optimal treatment effect. All subjects in the SI group were assessed on a yearly basis in the same way as the UC group.

In addition to measures of self-report of smoking, serum thiocyanate (SCN) and carbon monoxide levels (CO) were also evaluated. The SCN and CO levels were used as a validity check for self-report of smoking. The results (Table 11-4) appear impressive, given the 6-year follow-up period: 43% of the SI smokers reported smoking cessation and 25% of the UC reported smoking cessation. (When the rates were adjusted for SCN levels, the difference between the two groups was statistically significant.)

A comparison of the five large-scale studies indicated in the table lead to some interesting and promising conclusions. First, these studies are quite impressive for their utilization of randomized control and treatment groups, long-term follow-up of three years or longer, and standardized points of follow-up (USPHS, 1983). Second, the results indicate that for all trials, except the Goteborg study, significant differences between the control and treatment groups were obtained at the three-year follow-ups. Data from these findings revealed that the control groups showed a steady increase in cessation as the study progressed (MRFIT, London Civil Service Study). The MRFIT data, however, indicate that a significantly smaller percent of control group smokers who reported cessation were long-term stoppers, as compared with the intervention group. Third, when the types of intervention used were examined, in general, success of smoking intervention programs appears to be related to the amount of intervention provided (USPHS, 1983).

Despite the sophistication of the MRFIT study in controlling for such problems as using SCN levels as a validity check on self-report, the majority of studies on smoking cessation appear to have several methodological flaws. Some of the problems with such studies include the lack of adequate comparison groups, classification differences, lack of follow-up data, different methods used in reporting data, variable treatment criteria used across studies, and lack of information and precautions needed to interpret outcomes adequately (USPHS, 1983). These problems will be described in more detail in the next section, since such methodological pitfalls apply to most smoking cessation studies in general.

*Community investigations* involve the randomization of *entire populations* to an intervention or a nonintervention group. Studies may involve the random allocation of factory sites to intervention or regular care. Alternatively, entire geographical areas may be studied. Table 11-5 indicates three community investigations reviewed by the Surgeon General (USPHS, 1983).

Community investigators generally employ the use of mass media, which may include information and warning about the danger of smoking to one's health and advice on how to stop smoking. Sometimes a mass media approach is compared to a more intense, individualized clinical program. Often subjects who are found to be at very high risk for CHD or respiratory disorder will be given individualized treatment, in addition to the mass media intervention.

The Belgian Heart Disease Prevention Project will be described as an example of a community investigation. The Belgian trial examined an intervention in the work environment for the reduction of risk factors associated with heart disease. Thirty Belgium industries were paired and, for each pair, one work unit was randomly assigned to an intervention condition and the other to a control condition. The subjects were between the ages of 40 to 59, and 83.7% of the 19,390 possible male workers agreed to be screened. The final number of subjects consisted of 7,398 men in the intervention group and 8,821 men in the control group. Of the control group subjects, 10% from each work site were randomly selected and given an examination similar to that given the intervention group. The other 90% had resting electrocardiograms performed. Those subjects in the intervention group who were in the top 21% of the risk score distribution were placed in the individualized treatment program ($N = 1,601$), which included twice-yearly counseling and a physical examination by two project physicians. The subjects assigned to the intervention condition received information from the mass media. The mass media approach included such interventions as posters, groups, films, and demonstrations, and subjects received a report of their results along with printed advice for change. All families of the subjects and physicians regularly received information on the subject's risk factors.

Subjects' reports of smoking rates were not validated with objective assessment. At a 2-year follow-up, a 5% random sample in the intervention group was compared with a 10% random sample of the control group. The results indicated no differences in reported smoking cessation, since only 12.5% of subjects from both groups said that they had

**TABLE 11-4**

Intervention, Follow-Up, and Cessation Results for Five Major Controlled Clinical Trials

| Clinical trial | Intervention | Control group contact | Follow-up | Reported cessation rates/(objective measures) | | |
|---|---|---|---|---|---|---|
| | | | | Treated | Control | Time |
| London Civil Servants Smoking Trial | Letter inviting patient to meet with MD Initial 15-min session Three more 15-min visits (with MD) in 10 weeks 6-mo visit Additional help if needed | Not told of high risk status or trial participation | Physical exams & smoking & medical Hx questionnaire at 1, 3, & 9 yrs for both groups Missed visit rates<br>IG NC Year<br>19% 19 1<br>30% 30% 3<br>17% — 9 | 51%* (cigs) 31% (all smoking) 36% (cigs) 46% (cigs) (no objective measures used) | 10% (cigs) 14% (cigs) — | 1 yr 3 yrs 9 yrs |
| Göteborg (Sweden) Study | Smokers ≥ 15 g tobacco/day invited to antismoking clinic Five biweekly small group sessions 2d session: patients given nicotine chewing gum Follow-up letters at 3, 5, 12 mo | Baseline smoking & medical Hx questionnaire sent to all patients in one CG 2% random sample of one CG screened | Physical exams & smoking & medical Hx questionnaire at 4 yrs for all IG males & all males in one CG No missed visit rates noted | 31%* (no objective measures used) | 26% | 4 yrs |
| Oslo (Norway) Study | Initial 15- to 20-min session with MD Group session for men with wives "5-day smoking" | Yearly examination | IG: Physical exam & assessment every 6 mos CG: same as above each year | 29% (cigs) 31% (cigs) 18% (all tobacco) (measured SCN at end, but | 13% (cigs) 18% (cigs) 1% (all tobacco) | 3 yrs 5 yrs |

| Study | Methods | Intervention | Follow-up / Missed visit rates | Cessation rates | |
|---|---|---|---|---|---|
| | | "cessation program" halfway through for those who continue to smoke<br>6-mo exam & contact for smoking intervention | Missed visit rate: 1% at 5 yrs for males still living | rates not reported | |
| Multiple Risk Factor Intervention Trial (MRFIT) | Three screening visits<br>Yearly exam & assessments<br>Results sent to MD | Session with MD at 3d screen<br>Ten group intervention sessions for all risk factors<br>Maintenance protocol if stopped smoking cigarettes<br>Extended intervention protocol if still smoking<br>Follow-up at least every 4 mo | SI: every 4 mo for at least 6 yrs<br>UC: yearly exam & assessment for at least 6 yrs<br><br>Missed visit rates<br>   SI   UC   Year<br>4.5%  5.2%  1<br><10%  <10%  6 | 40%** (29% SCN adjusted) — 13% (11% SCN adjusted) | 1 yr |
| | | | | 40%** (35% SCN adjusted) — 16% (15% SCN adjusted) | 3 yrs |
| | | | | 43%** (42% SCN adjusted) — 26% (24% SCN adjusted) | 6 yrs |
| Stanford Three Community Study | Baseline survey (physical + interview)<br>1-, 2-, & 3-yr surveys repeated: 40-min contact<br>Medical results sent to MD | Media: TV, radio, posters, mail, phone, newspapers<br>Face-to-face intervention: group sessions 10 wks, then biweekly, yr 1<br>Continued intervention for yrs 2 & 3 | Surveys (physical + interviews) yrs 1, 2, & 3<br>High nonattendance rate each yr<br>Highest rate for WII group | Year 3<br>WII: 32% cessation**<br>W-RC: 0% cessation<br>GMO: 11.3% cessation (nonattenders excluded)<br>TC: 14.9% cessation (nonattenders excluded)<br>(SCN measured, but not used to adjust cessation rates) | |

*Note.* From *The Health Consequences of Smoking: Cardiovascular Disease* (pp. 250–251) by U.S. Public Health Service, 1983. Reprinted by permission of the U.S. Government Printing Office.

*P ≤ 0.05; **P ≤ 0.01; ***Not significant.

IG: Intervention Group; CG: Control Group; SI: Special Intervention group; UC: Usual Care group; WII: Watsonville Intensive Intervention group; W-RC: Watsonville media-only group; GMO: Gilroy media-only group; TC: Tracy Control Group.

## TABLE 11-5
### Intervention, Follow-Up, and Cessation Results for Three Community Prevention Trials

| Community trial | Intervention | Control group contact | Follow-up | Reported cessation rates/ (objective measures) | | |
|---|---|---|---|---|---|---|
| | | | | Treated | Control | Time |
| WHO European Collaborative Trial: United Kingdom | Mass media intervention for all factory workers Antismoking clinics for all smokers High-risk smokers (top 10% to 15% risk) offered individual treatment (four 15-min sessions in year 1 with company physician) | Random 10% sample invited for screening The rest of control males not told of their participation in the trial | Random 5% IG examined yearly All survivors examined at end of trial Same random 10% CG screened, reexamined at 2 years | 12%* (high risk smokers) 9% (all smokers) 7% (non- high-risk smokers) (no objective measures used) | (no change) | 5 yrs |
| WHO European Collaborative Trial: Belgium | Mass media intervention for all factory workers High-risk smokers (top 21% risk) offered counseling and examination by project physicians twice a year | Random 10% invited for screening Other 90% had resting ECG only | Random 5% IG examined yearly All survivors examined at end of trial | 18.7%** (high risk smokers) 12.5% (all smokers) (no objective measures used) | 12.2% (high risk smokers) 12.6% (all smokers) | 2 yrs |
| North Karelia (Finland) Project | Comprensive "community action" program against risk factors All forms of media used Special groups set up as needed | 6.6% random sample examined at baseline and 5 years | Random 6.6% of each community surveyed and examined in 1977 Results compared to assess RF change | 17%*** (male smokers) (SCN drawn for random subsamples) (Correlations reported, but adjustments not made) | 15% (male smokers) | 5 yrs |

Note. From The Health Consequences of Smoking: Cardiovascular Disease by U.S. Public Health Service, 1983. Reprinted by permission of the U.S. Government Printing Office.
*$P \leq 0.01$; **$P \leq 0.05$; ***Not significant.

quit smoking. The study also compared the results of the high-risk subjects in the intervention group with the results of the high-risk subjects selected from the 10% random sample of the control groups. The results of the comparison at the two-year follow-up indicated a significant reduction for the high-risk intervention subjects, with 18.7% reporting smoking cessation, as compared to 12.2% of the control group high-risk subjects.

In general, the community investigation demonstrated that a mass media approach to smoking cessation had a minor impact on the population studied. Leventhal and Cleary (1980) point out four reasons why a mass media approach may be less effective than a clinical approach in changing beliefs and behaviors. First, exposure to the message is uncontrollable in the field, whereas in face-to-face interventions, information is directly given to the subject, thus increasing its impact. Second, media messages are symbolic and abstract, and generally do not focus on concrete experiences of interest to the individual. Third, information or messages chosen to be delivered via mass communication are often based on hunches of what should be effective. Few studies have thus far evaluated the individual's actual interest in and response to media messages regarding health risk prevention or reduction. Finally, the subject may be in a variety of situations, when receiving the message. The context of the situation—home, school, work, or among friends—may have a dramatic impact, either negative or positive, on the subject's attention to and evaluation of that message.

A final issue with regard to the community investigation is the problem associated with the design of these studies. The methodological flaws are similar to those noted in large-scale clinical trials and include the lack of objective data to verify self-report measures, an absence of cohort analyses and the almost exclusive reliance on cross-sectional analysis, a lack of specification of outcome criteria, and no evaluation on the relative effectiveness of the various components of treatment programs.

## General Problems in Smoking Cessation Interventions

Two areas appear particularly problematic in the smoking cessation literature. First, is the problem of assessment. Is self-report a reliable measure of smoking behavior and does the number of cigarettes smoked, even if accurately reported, truly reflect the impact of smoking on one's physiology and eventual health status? Second, a review of the literature indicates that success rates reported from both clinical and large-scale interventions are disappointingly low and that recidivism is very high.

In terms of problems in assessment, it has been argued that an optimal assessment procedure would involve both self-monitoring of the number of cigarettes smoked per day and two physiological measures (Brownwell, 1982). The two most commonly used physiological measures include carbon monoxide (CO) and thiocyanate (TCN) (Pechacek & McAlister, 1980). Carbon monoxide levels are influenced by many other factors other than smoking, such as ambiant CO mostly from automobile exhaust. Carbon monoxide also has a short half-life from two to six hours. Elevated CO levels appear to be associated with increased risk of CHD, and once CHD has been diagnosed, survival rates are notably reduced (USDHEW, 1979).

Carbon monoxide levels are assessed by measuring the CO concentration in air samples. Despite the presence of sources other than smoking that may influence CO levels, in addition to the short CO half-life, CO levels do provide a relatively valid physiological measure that may be considered along with self-report data (Frederiksen & Martin, 1979).

Thiocyanate levels are another potential physiological variable that may be evaluated. Thiocyanate is the body's end product of the detoxification of cyanide compounds. Thiocyanate can be measured in urine, blood, or saliva. The advantages of TCN are that it distinguishes smokers from nonsmokers, correlates moderately with smoking rate, has a longer half-life (10–14 days) than CO levels, and cannot be confounded by nonsmoking sources (Prue, Martin, & Hume, 1980).

It is highly recommended that future investigations consider the use of physiological measures. Physiological measures can validate the accuracy of self-report, and the discrimination power of CO and TCN can be significantly increased when both these measures are used (Brownell, 1982).

Another issue related to self-report is that the rate of smoking itself does not always accurately reflect the dose of CO, tar, and nicotine the body receives (Frederiksen, Martin, & Webster, 1979). Other important factors that should be considered along with the rate of smoking are the substance or quality of the cigarette and the *topography* of smoking. Substance may be assessed by observing the brand of cigarette smoked. Measurement of the topography of smoking, however, is not quite so clear cut. Topography may vary in terms of puff frequency, duration, volume, intensity, and distribution; interpuff interval; amount of tobacco used; and smoking duration. The impact of varying smoking topography is illustrated in the following example. A smoker has been instructed to smoke fewer and less harmful cigarettes. However, the smoker may begin taking more puffs per cigarette and may draw more heavily on the cigarette. Such changes in smoking, while reducing the number of cigarettes smoked per day, have no effect on the smoker's health status. Future investigations will need to address the problems associated with changes in smoking topography, so that intervention may be designed to deal directly with such problems. Also, the assessment of smoking patterns at an individual level requires closer examination.

The issue of low success rates and problems with maintenance of treatment gains cannot be ignored. Hunt and Matarazzo (1982) point out the amazingly high current output of research studies on smoking and smoking cessation and the likelihood of continued interest in this area, despite the apparent low success rate often reported. One motivating factor in this area of research may be the recent awareness that many of the intervention studies reported thus far are not based on any comprehensive model of smoking and that the intervention procedures often used are based on hunches that they may have an effect on smoking. More investigators are beginning to conclude that a successful intervention procedure should include components that would affect physiological, behavioral, cognitive, and affective factors. The point here is that most interventions to date have not been derived from a psycho-biological model, but rather focused on one narrow area, such as changing environmental cues for smoking or briefly producing an aversive response to smoking. Recent attempts to address this issue have utilized multicomponent programs. Results from many of these studies support a psychobiological approach, suggesting that some multicomponent programs appear to be more effective than a single-factor approach. However, other multi-component programs have shown negligible success rates, and some report even less success than a single component program. These conflicting findings may be a result of either the unsystematic choice of components or the lack of consideration given to individual differences. For instance, a chronic heavy smoker may need a different combination of techniques than a light, primarily social smoker. One solution to the problem of low success rates may be to focus on a systematic evaluation of multicomponent programs, based on a psychobiological model of smoking, much like the model presented by Leventhal and Cleary, (1980).

Maintenance effects is the final problem to be considered. In the past, improving maintenance has been studied by extending treatment procedures into follow-up periods. These booster sessions have not met with success. Brownell (1982) suggests that in accordance with the framework of phases of smoking, maintenance issues should be considered a different type of problem than issues relating to initial cessation and treatment. Accordingly, different procedures may have to be utilized at different phases and would probably include more than a basic behavioral package.

Hall (1980) proposed a model that emphasizes the interactive role of coping strategies and commitment in maintaining change in addictive disorders. The model of preventing relapse includes both behavioral and cognitive components. More specifically, it highlights three areas of concern. First, both knowledge and performance of relapse skills are needed. Second, continued commitment is needed to motivate performance of coping skills. Third, commitment to maintenance is a function of perceived costs and benefits of the problem behavior and change attempts (see Chapter 8). Factors thought to be important in determining cost/benefit perceptions are the severity of withdrawal symptoms, feedback on the intermediate effects of change attempts, and difficulties in performing change strategies. Based on this model of preventing relapse, a model specific to prevention of smoking relapse has recently been evaluated (Hall, Rugg, Tunstall, & Jones, 1984). The model assumes that coping skills training must address the issue of withdrawal symptoms, as well as situational factors related to relapse. In the treatment program evaluated by Hall *et al.*, cognitive relaxation was used to decrease the anxiety and irritability often associated with withdrawal symptoms and skills training for high-risk relapse situations was offered. The cognitive relaxation training and skills training were individualized to maximize the effects for each subject. A second aspect of the study was to evaluate two levels of aversive smoking (6-second versus 30-second frequency of inhalation). Of the group, 123 subjects completed treatment and were assigned to one of four groups that included skills training with either 6-second aversive inhalation or 30-second aversive inhalation. The results of the study indicate that relapse-prevention skill training did prevent relapse among cigarette smokers who had quit. More subjects in the skill training prevention relapse were abstinent or smoked less at 6 and 52 weeks from the start of the study. It was also found that subjects in the skill training condition were more likely to report using coping skills. However, they did not differ from the discussion condition in perceived cost and benefit of change or of smoking, or in mood dysphoria or physical complaints.

Another example of recent work in the area of maintenance was reported by Shiffman (1984) in a study on coping with the temptation to smoke. The effectiveness of reported coping responses related to the temptation to smoke were analyzed. Seventy-five ex-smokers reported to a hotline when dealing with the temptation to smoke. The results of the study demonstrate that the number of coping responses used had no effect; however, combining cognitive and behavioral responses enhanced the effectiveness of the response. Table 11-6 lists the specific coping responses used and how frequently they were used, in addition to the effectiveness of a response. The use of willpower and self-punitive statements did not help the smoker cope with the temptation to smoke. If the results of the study prove to be valid, one may be able to

TABLE 11-6

Behavioral and Cognitive Coping Responses Used to Control Smoking Behavior[a]

| Coping response | Frequency (% of cases) | % not smoking | Relation to outcome | |
|---|---|---|---|---|
| | | | Effect compared to no response ($\phi$) | Effect compared to other responses ($\phi$) |
| Behavioral ($N = 228$) | | | | |
| Eating or drinking | 24.3 | 84.4 | .52 | .07 |
| Distracting activity | 12.1 | 89.3 | .48 | .10 |
| Escape | 3.4 | 100.0 | .37 | .12 |
| Delay | 4.3 | 70.0 | .23 | .09 |
| Physical activity | 8.6 | 80.0 | .37 | .02 |
| Relaxation | 5.2 | 83.3 | .33 | .01 |
| Other behavior | 10.8 | 75.0 | .33 | .08 |
| Any behavioral response | 55.6 | 81.7 | .51 | |
| Cognitive ($N = 221$) | | | | |
| Positive consequences—health | 1.0 | 88.9 | .37 | .11 |
| Negative consequences—health | 8.9 | 84.2 | .44 | .12 |
| Negative consequences—other | 11.2 | 84.0 | .46 | .11 |
| Willpower | 17.0 | 55.3 | .24 | −.20[c] |
| Distraction | 3.1 | 85.7 | .32 | .15 |
| Intent to delay | 3.1 | 100.00 | .32 | .08 |
| Self-punitive | 3.6 | 37.5 | .05[b] | −.18[c] |
| Other self-talk | 38.1 | 70.0 | .40 | .00 |
| Any cognitive response | 63.8 | 80.5 | .39 | |
| Any coping response | 71.5 | 70.3 | .47 | |

Note. From "Coping with Temptations to Smoke" by S. Shiffman, 1984, *Journal of Consulting and Clinical Psychology, 52,* 265. Copyright 1984 by the American Psychological Association. Reprinted by permission.
[a]Identification of specific behavioral and cognitive coping responses: frequency, survival rate, and effect compared to no coping and to other responses. Column 2 represents the percentage of subjects performing the coping response who did not smoke. The phi coefficients were computed from tables cross-tabulating whether or not the person smoked with performance of a specific coping response. In column 3, people performing the coping response are contrasted to those who did no coping. In column 4, they are contrasted to those who performed any other coping response. All phi coefficients in column 3 are significant and those in column 4 are nonsignificant unless otherwise noted.
[b]Phi coefficient nonsignificant.
[c]Phi coefficient significant.

draw the conclusion that, in most cases, the type of coping response used is not as important as the fact that a coping response is used at all. The implications for maintenance programs are that concern for an individualized maintenance program may not be necessary, and that relapse prevention should focus on teaching the individual a variety of cognitive and behavioral coping responses.

Schachter (1982), for instance, took a different approach to studying recidivism in ex-smokers. Rather than studying individuals undergoing active treatment, he investigated people who had quit smoking on their own. Schachter pointed out that many people choose to quit smoking on their own and are very successful with long-term abstinence. He proposes that if one includes the success of all the self-quitters, a more optimistic conclusion can be drawn for the cessation of smoking. He also noted that those people who are unable to quit on their own are a special "hard-core" group who are unwilling or unable to help themselves. This population is typically the one most frequently studied in smoking cessation research, and therefore the results of these studies are based on this self-selected group. Schachter completed a study in which he interviewed 161 individuals. Subjects were from one of two groups—employees of and students at the Psychology Department at Columbia University and a substantial portion of the entrepreneurial and working population of Amagansett, a small town in eastern Long Island, New York. Of the 161 people interviewed, 94 reported a history of smoking cigarettes. Interestingly, of the smokers who attempted cessation, 63.6% had been successful at the time of the interview! This represents a fairly large number compared to most treatment outcome studies. The average person had maintained abstinence from cigarettes for 7.4 years. He found that of the heavy smokers, 45.8% had more difficulties than light smokers in quitting, and reported such symptoms as fever, chills, sweating spells, and marked irritability; 25.4% had minor difficulties; and 28.8% reported no problems. Light smokers reported fewer problems in quitting than heavy smokers; however, they were not more successful. Schachter suggested that these findings indicate that quitting smoking for long periods of time may not be as problematic for many people as has been suggested from the treatment study results. Additional questions that need to be addressed are what differences, if any, exist between self-quitters and those who seek treatment, and whether these differences affect treatment outcome. Another concern in this area, if differences do exist, is whether therapy affects treatment outcome in a negative manner for some people.

Summarizing the area on maintenance, health psychologists are becoming more concerned with issues of maintenance and follow-up. Some conceptualize maintenance as a different process than treatment and, thus, one that should be studied separately and possibly require different types of intervention procedures. Presently, various behavioral and cognitive coping skills are under evaluation in order to determine their effect on maintenance.

## CURRENT ISSUES IN SMOKING

### Social Support

There has been recent interest in understanding the influences of social situations and interpersonal relationships on the etiology and treatment of smoking. The role that social influence plays in smoking may vary from individual to individual as well as phase the smoker is in; for instance, whether the smoker is developing or maintaining his or her smoking habit. As discussed in the section dealing with the phases of smoking, it was noted that peer pressure and family history, in addition to social views of smoking, have an apparent impact, at least for many smokers, on the initiation of smoking behavior. Once a person begins smoking regularly, smoking rate and topography are susceptible to social influences (Antonuccio & Lichtenstein, 1980). Finally, quitting smoking and remaining abstinent may also be related to peer and family pressure. A 5-year follow-up study of 599 participants who attended a smoking withdrawal clinic reported differences in maintenance effects between smokers whose spouses did not smoke (42% relapse) and smokers whose spouses did smoke (58% relapse) (West, Graham, Swanson, & Wilkinson, 1977). Other surveys report that smokers often relapse during social situations (Best, 1978; Marlatt & Gordon, 1979). Because of the potential impact of social influences on smoking behavior, it has been suggested that smoking cessation programs might include social influence as part of the intervention (Colletti & Brownell, 1983).

Two kinds of social support systems that may increase long-term smoking cessation have been described and studied. Those are continued contact by the therapist after the treatment phase and the use of a buddy system during and after therapy. What has been termed *continued contact* has ranged from having a secretary phone and ask the smoker questions about his or her smoking behavior to having smokers attend sessions for new subjects who are about to receive treatment. The studies on continued contact show mixed results (Colletti & Brownell, 1983). The biggest problem in comparing studies is the differing modes of providing continued social support. Studies on the *buddy system* approach, in which smokers are paired and instructed to call each other daily and report their progress, present similar mixed results. Thus, no conclusive evidence regarding the efficacy of either continued contact or the buddy system has yet been established.

Spouse involvement is another component of the social support approach used in smoking cessation. Lichtenstein and Stalgaitis (1980) report a study in which six smoking couples contracted for "reciprocal aversion." The couples were instructed that each time one spouse smoked a cigarette the other spouse would also have to smoke a cigarette. Five couples completed treatment, and four out of these five couples had at least one spouse who was abstinent at the six-month follow-up. The results are encouraging, although a replication study with a better-controlled design is needed, since the findings reported by Lichtenstein and Stalgaitis were based solely on self-report data, and a multiple-baseline design.

## Prevention

Given the disappointingly low success rate of treatment and maintenance, many experts in the smoking area are now turning to the concept of prevention. Smoking prevention programs may well prove to be more cost-effective and efficient than any attempts at helping people quit. Prevention studies have typically tended to include grade school and high school students as subjects. The majority of programs, however, have been geared to adolescents. It is believed that adolescents are at greater risk for developing smoking behavior than younger children. Adolescents experiencing the stressful transition to adulthood are greatly influenced by their peers (Hunt & Matarazzo, 1982). Smoking may be a symbol of belonging to the peer group and approaching adulthood, as well as a rebellion against parents and authority figures.

Most prevention programs take place at school; however, mass media may also be used, and includes posters, and radio and television commercials. The general framework of many of the prevention studies involves the test, treatment, and retest paradigm. Pre- and post-treatment assessment involves establishing the incidence of smoking. The positive effects of the prevention program are reflected by no changes or decreases in absolute number of smokers in the groups or no new smokers appearing. Evans and colleagues (Evans, 1976; Evans, Rozelle, Mittlemark, Hansen, Bane, & Havis, 1978; Evans, Rozelle, Maxwell, Raines, Dill, & Guthrie, in press) have provided examples of the typical smoking prevention program carried out in a school setting. For example, the effect of videotaped information combined with discussion was evaluated in a sample of 750 seventh-graders in schools in the Houston area (Evans *et al.*, 1978). The three treatment groups included a full treatment group, a feedback-only group, and a repeated-testing group.

Each group saw a series of four videotapes, each videotape being followed by the students answering questions and a group discussion. There were three post-test sessions at 1, 5, and 10 weeks for the experimental groups. The control group was tested only at pre-treatment and at the 10-week post-test. Results indicated that the smoking rates for the three treatment groups were similar, but lower than for the control group, with rates for the full treatment group, 10.0%; the feedback group, 8.6%; and the repeated testing group, 9.2%. In comparison, in the control groups, 18.3% continued to smoke.

Another example of the current trend in implementing large-scale smoking prevention programs may be drawn from the recent Oslo Youth Study conducted by Tell, Klepp, Vellar, and McAllister (1984). The study assessed the effectiveness of a two-year, school-based multicomponent smoking prevention program for 10- to 15-year-old students in Oslo, Norway. Participants were divided into three groups: "cohort 1" (students who were fifth-graders on entry to this study and who were in seventh grade at follow-up), "cohort 2" (students who were sixth-graders on entry to the study and in eighth grade at follow-up), and "cohort 3" (students who were seventh-graders on entry to the study and in ninth grade at follow-up). The reference group were students of similar age ranges in schools not participating in the study. The smoking prevention program for "cohort 1" is presented in Table 11-7. Cohorts 2 and 3 underwent similar programs, except sessions 4 and 5 were omitted. Tell *et al.* found that the smoking prevention program resulted in a significant reduction in the onset of smoking relative to a reference group. Based on reports of smoking behavior, the intervention group ($N=278$) experienced a smoking onset rate of 16.5%, the reference group ($N=208$) a smoking onset rate of 26.9%. In addition, intervention students were found to have a significantly larger increase in scores on a smoking knowledge index, reported a significantly larger increase in frequent exercise, and a significantly smaller increase in alcohol consumption. Other findings revealed that in both intervention and treatment groups, students who reported smoking at the follow-up survey had already displayed risk-taking tendencies at the time of the baseline survey two years earlier, regardless of whether they had smoked at baseline or not. Follow-up smokers also had more smoking friends and siblings at baseline and evidenced greater acceptability of smoking. It would appear from this project that school-based smoking education programs may be effective in the prevention of smoking onset in adolescents. This approach may well prove equally successful if implemented in other settings, such as the work environment.

In general, smoking prevention programs have more recently focused on social influence and peer pressure (Severson, 1984).

## TABLE 11-7
### Smoking Prevention Program Curriculum

| Session | Topic |
|---|---|
| 1. September, 1979 | Personal commitment, social pressures. Student leaders gave a general introduction to the program. Students made personal commitments to not start smoking (or to not become addicted smokers). Social pressures to start smoking, tobacco advertisement, parental smoking, and the development of nicotine addiction were discussed. |
| 2. September, 1979 | Pressure resistance training. Students prepared and acted out role-plays to learn pressure resistance skills. The role-plays symbolized everyday situations connected with pressures to start smoking. |
| 3. November, 1979 | Social pressures. Students' experiences with various kinds of smoking pressures were discussed. A film about a boy growing up and becoming an addicted smoker was shown and discussed. Arguments against smoking were summed up and made into a poster. |
| 4. March, 1980 | Coping with social anxiety. Situations causing social anxiety and the use of cigarettes and alcohol as a way of coping were discussed. Anxiety was raised by asking students to dance in front of the class (disco music was played). Self-image and boy–girl relationships were discussed; techniques used to cope with anxiety were practiced. |
| 5. May, 1980 | Presure resistance training. Student leaders talked about the harmful effects of smoking. Plays about life-style during summer vacation were prepared and acted out. |
| 6. October, 1980 | Smoking: Self-pollution and waste of resources. Prior to this session, smoking behavior was assessed. Smoking frequencies in each class were presented and changes (if any) during the intervention period were discussed. Students were informed about short-term consequences of smoking. Smoking as a form of self-pollution and tobacco growing as a waste of agricultural resources were discussed. |
| 7. November, 1980 | Passive smoking. A film focusing on second-hand exposure was shown and discussed. Parental smoking and peer pressure at youth clubs were also discussed. Students previously gathered written material from newspapers about smoking; these were presented and discussed. |
| 8. December, 1980 | Long-term effects of smoking, marketing of tobacco. Cancer and cardiovascular diseases related to cigarette smoking were discussed. Marketing of cigarettes in third-world countries was compared to the situation in Norway. |
| 9. January, 1981 | Social and health aspects of smoking. "The Smokewarning," a magazine for adolescents (National Council on Smoking and Health) was handed out and discussed. |
| 10. February, 1981 | "It is Your Choice." A film focusing on alcohol consumption among Norwegian adolescents was shown. Drinking pressure and the parallel with pressures to start cigarette smoking was discussed. |

Note. From "Preventing the Onset of Cigarette Smoking in Norwegian Adolescents: The Oslo Youth Study" by G. S. Tell, K. I. Klepp, O. D. Vellar, and A. McAllister, 1984, *Preventive Medicine, 13*, 261. Copyright 1984 by Academic Press, Inc. Reprinted by permission.

McAlister (1983) suggests that these prevention programs, which are based on peer leadership and psychological "inoculation," appear to have at least short-term positive effects. Many prevention programs, therefore, are going beyond teaching health consequences and providing skills for dealing with peer pressure to smoking cigarettes. Along with skills training, information on the social forces that encourage smoking onset and the negative short-term social and physiological consequences of smoking is needed. Successful prevention programs have been reported by a variety of researchers (Botuin & Eng, 1982; Evans *et al.*, 1978; Hurd, Johnson, Pechacek, Bast, Jacobs, & Luepker, 1980; Perry, Killen, Telch, Slinkard, & Donahar, 1980; Severson, Fallen, Nautel, Bislan, Ary, & Lichtenstein, 1981).

Hunt and Matarazzo (1982) have indicated the importance of implementing programs during the preventive phase of smoking behavior. Studies attempting to evaluate the different modes of presenting such programs are encouraging. Evans *et al.* (1981), for instance, used children of similar age to participate as role models in videotapes depicting social situations that may possibly exert pressure on children to smoke. Leventhal and Cleary (1980) are not as optimistic about the results of the prevention studies to date and suggest that the replication of such studies using more sophisticated methodology would be redundant. They do suggest that more basic research as to what type of information or change in the social context is needed, rather than more studies on marketing existing programs. They do acknowledge that prevention studies demonstrate that children's knowledge of smoking hazards become greater. However, they also indicate that prevention programs do not deal directly with the motivation to smoke, such as the child's need to be accepted; or the programs fail to sustain nonsmoking attitudes and beliefs.

An example of the ways society can sustain nonsmoking is provided in an interesting article that appeared in the Sunday edition of the New York Times (Klemesrud, 1984). The article, titled "If You Smoke, No Room at the Inn," describes the efforts of a 55-year-old motelier who opened a motel with a nonsmoking policy aimed at excluding smokers from such "Non-Smokers Inns." The nonsmoking policy of the motel is quite strict, as suggested in the following:

> Guests who showed evidence of being smokers were asked to pay $100 smoking deposits in advance. "You can normally tell a smoker, . . . You can see a pack of cigarettes in his pocket or stains on his fingers or you can smell the odor. A smoker has an odor that clings."
>
> The deposit is not returned, she said (referring to the manager) if butts and ashes are found during room inspections when guests check out. "We bring them in the office and show them the sample," she said. "But if there is only the smell of smoke in the room then we give the deposit back." (p. 64)

In conclusion, we agree that more basic research on identifying what types of behaviors and attitudes are more amenable to change within the social context of a school setting is needed; however, we also acknowledge that the prevention studies to date have been innovative and encouraging.

## SUMMARY

The significance of cigarette smoking as a health risk factor in the development of heart disease, cancer, emphysema, peptic ulcers, and chronic bronchitis cannot be ignored. The first section of this chapter reviewed the theoretical frameworks used to explain the establishment and maintenance of smoking behavior. Biological theories were discussed, with particular emphasis on the nicotine regulation model of cigarette smoking. Psychological/behavioral theories were then reviewed, and our focus was directed at research related to the affect reduction model, the social learning model, and the associative learning model of smoking behavior. This section of the chapter was concluded by a review of two psychobiological models of cigarette smoking—the opponent process model and the multiple regulation model.

Widespread interest in the development of smoking cessation programs has led to the development of numerous techniques to enhance smoking cessation. This chapter provided an illustrative review of various behavioral, cognitive, physician-oriented, community, and large-scale interventions utilized in smoking cessation programs. Finally, the chapter attempted to evaluate current issues in smoking, such as the role of social support, relapse prevention programs in smoking cessation maintenance, and prevention of smoking behavior.

## REFERENCES

Antonuccio, D. O., & Lichtenstein, E. (1980). Peer modeling influences on smoking behavior of heavy and light smokers. *Addictive Behavior, 5,* 299–306.

Ashton, H., & Stepney, R. (1982). *Smoking: Psychology and pharmacology.* London: Tavistock.

Bandura, A. (1977). *Social learning theory.* Englewood Cliffs, NJ: Prentice-Hall.

Barbarin, O. A. (1978). Comparison of symbolic and overt aversion in the self-control of smoking. *Journal of Consulting and Clinical Psychology, 46,* 1569–1571.

Berecz, J. (1976). Treatment of smoking with cognitive conditioning therapy: A self-administered aversion technique. *Behavior Therapy, 7,* 641–648.

Bernstein, D. A., & Glasgow, R. E. (1979). Smoking. In O. F. Pomerleau & J. P. Brady (Eds.), *Behavioral medicine: Theory and practice.* Baltimore, MD: Williams & Wilkins.

Best, J. A. (1978). Targeting and self-selection of smoking modification methods. *Proceedings of the international conference on smoking.* New York: American Cancer Society.

Bland, J. M., Bewley, B. R., & Day, I. (1975). Primary schoolboys: Image of self and smoker. *British Journal of Preventive and Social Medicine, 29,* 262–266.

Botuin, G. J., & Eng, A. (1982). The efficacy of a multicomponent approach to the prevention of cigarette smoking. *Preventive Medicine, 11,* 199–211.

Brownell, K. D. (1982). The addictive disorders. In C. M. Franks, G. T. Wilson, P. C. Kendall, & K. D. Brownell (Eds.), *Annual Review of Behavior Therapy and Practice.* New York: Guilford Press.

Colletti, G., & Brownell, K. D. (1983). The physical and emotional benefits of social support: Application to obesity, smoking and alcoholism. In Hersen, M., Eisler, R. M., & Miller, P. M. (Eds.), *Progress in behavior modification.* New York: Academic Press.

Danaher, B. G. (1977a). Research on rapid smoking: Interim summary and recommendations. *Addictive Behaviors, 2,* 151–156.

Danaher, B. G. (1977b). Rapid smoking and self-control in the modification of smoking behavior. *Journal of Consulting and Clinical Psychology, 45,* 1068–1075.

Delahunt, J., & Curran, J. P. (1976). The effectiveness of negative practice and self-control techniques in the reduction of smoking behavior. *Journal of Consulting and Clinical Psychology, 44,* 1002–1007.

Dericco, D. A., Brigham, T. A., & Garlington, W. K. (1977). Development and evaluation of treatment paradigms for the suppression of smoking behavior. *Journal of Applied Behavior Analysis, 10*(2), 173–181.

Evans, R. I. (1976). Smoking in children: Developing a social psychological strategy of deterrence. *Preventive Medicine, 5*(1), 122–127.

Evans, R. I., Rozelle, R. M., Mittlemark, M. B., Hansen, W. B., Bane, A. L., & Havis, J. (1978). Deterring the onset of smoking in children: Knowledge of immediate psychological effects and coping with peer pressure, media pressure, and parent modeling. *Journal of Applied Social Psychology, 8,* 126–135.

Evans, R. I., Rozelle, R. M., Maxwell, S. E., Raines, B. E., Dill, C. A., & Guthrie, T. J. (1981). Social modeling films to deter smoking in adolescents: Results of a three year field investigation. *Journal of Applied Psychology, 66,* 399–414.

Forbes, W. F., Robinson, J. C., Hanley, J. A., & Colburn, H. N. (1976). Studies on the nicotine exposure of individual smokers: I. Changes in mouth-level exposure to nicotine on switching to lower nicotine cigarettes. *International Journal of the Addictions, 11,* 933–950.

Foxx, R. M., & Brown, R. A. (1979). Nicotine fading and self-monitoring for cigarette abstinence or controlled smoking. *Journal of Applied Behavior Analysis, 12*(1), 111–125.

Frederiksen, L. W., & Martin, J. E. (1979). Carbon monoxide and smoking behavior. *Addictive Behaviors, 4*(1), 21–30.

Frederiksen, L. W., & Simon, S. J. (1979). Clinical modification of smoking behavior. In R. S. Davidson (Ed.), *Modification of pathological behavior* (pp. 477–555). New York: Gardner Press.

Frederiksen, L. W., Martin, J. E., & Webster, J. S. (1979). Assessment of smoking behavior. *Journal of Applied Behavior Analysis, 12,* 653–664.

Glasgow, R. E., & Bernstein, D. A. (1981). Behavioral treatment of smoking behavior. In C. K. Prokop & L. A. Bradley, (Eds.), *Medical psychology: Contributions to behavioral medicine.* New York: Academic Press.

Hall, S. M. (1980). Self-management and therapeutic maintenance: Theory and research. In P. Karoly & J. Steffan (Eds.), *Improving the long-term effects of psychotherapy* (pp. 263–300). New York: Gardner Press.

Hall, S. M., Rugg, D., Tunstall, C., & Jones, R. T. (1984). Preventing relapse to cigarette smoking by behavioral skill training. *Journal of Consulting and Clinical Psychology, 52*, 372–382.

Hammond, E. C., Garfenkel, L., Seidman, H. & Lew, E. A. (1976). *Some recent findings concerning cigarette smoking.* Unpublished manuscript, Department of Epidemiology and Statistical Research of the American Cancer Society, New York.

Handel, S. (1973). Change in smoking habits in a general practice. *Postgraduate Medical Journal, 49*, 679–681.

Horan, J. J., Hackett, G., Nicholas, W. C., Linberg, S. E., Stone, C. I., & Lukoski, H. C. (1977). Rapid smoking: A cautionary note. *Journal of Consulting and Clinical Psychology, 45*(3), 341–343.

Hunt, W. A., & Matarazzo, J. D. (1970). Habit mechanisms in smoking. In W. A. Hunt (Ed.), *Learning mechanisms in smoking* (pp. 65–106). Chicago, Aldine.

Hunt, W. A. & Matarazzo, J. D. (1982). Changing smoking behavior: A critique. In R. J. Gatchel, A. Baum, & J. E. Singer (Eds.), *Handbook of psychology and health: Vol. 1. Clinical psychology and behavioral medicine's overlapping disciplines* (pp. 171–209). Hillsdale, NJ: Erlbaum.

Hunt, W. A., & Matarazzo, J. D., Weiss, S. M., & Gentry, W. D. (1979). Associative learning, habit, and health behavior. *Journal of Behavioral Medicine, 2*, 111–124.

Hurd, P., Johnson, D., Pechacek, T., Bast, L., Jacobs, D., & Luepker, R. (1980). Prevention of cigarette smoking in seventh grade students. *Journal of Behavioral Medicine, 3*, 15–28.

Ikard, F. F., & Tomkins, S. (1973). The experience of affect as a determinant of smoking behavior: A series of validity studies. *Journal of Abnormal Psychology, 81*, 172–181.

Jarvik, M. E. (1977). Biological factors underlying the smoking habit. In M. Jarvik, J. Cullent, E. Gritz, T. Vogt, & L. West (Eds.), *Research on smoking behavior* (NIDA Research Monograph No. 17). Rockville, MD: National Institute on Drug Abuse.

Jarvik, M. E. (1979). Biological influences on cigarette smoking. In J. A. Califano (Ed.), *Smoking and health: A report of the Surgeon General.* Washington, DC: USDHEW.

Klemesrud, J, (1984, September). "If you smoke, no room at the inn." *New York Times*, p. 64.

Lando, H. A. (1977). Successful treatment of smokers with a broad-spectrum behavioral approach. *Journal of Consulting and Clinical Psychology, 45*(3), 361–366.

Leventhal, H. (1973). Changing attitudes and habits to reduce risk factors in chronic disease. *American Journal of Cardiology, 31*, 571–580.

Leventhal, H. & Avis, N. (1976). Pleasure, addiction, and habit: Factors in verbal report on factors in smoking behavior. *Journal of Abnormal Psychology, 85*, 478–488.

Leventhal, H., & Cleary, P. D. (1980). The smoking problem: A review of the research and theory in behavioral risk modification. *Psychological Bulletin, 88*, 370–405.

Lichtenstein, E. (1982). The smoking problem: A behavioral perspective. *Journal of Consulting and Clinical Psychology, 50*(6), 804–819.

Lichtenstein, E., & Brown, R. A. (1980). Smoking cessation methods: Review and recommendations. In W. R. Miller (Ed.), *The addictive behaviors: Treatment of alcoholism, drug abuse, smoking, and obesity.* Oxford: Pergamon Press.

Lichtenstein, E., & Glasgow, R. E. (1977). Rapid smoking: Side effects and safeguards. *Journal of Consulting and Clinical Psychology, 45*, 815–821.

Lichtenstein, E., & Penner, M. D. (1977). Long-term effects of rapid smoking treatment for dependent cigarette smokers. *Addictive Behavior, 2*, 109–112.

Lichtstein, K. L., & Stalgaitis, S. J. (1980). Treatment of cigarette smoking in couples by reciprocal aversion. *Behavior Therapy, 11*, 104–108.

Marlatt, G. A., & Gordon, J. R. (1979). Determinants of relapse: Implications for the maintenance of behavior change. In P. Davidson (Ed.), *Behavioral medicine: Changing health life styles.* New York: Brunner/Mazel.

McAlister, A. L. (1983). Social psychological approaches. In T. Glynn, C. Leukefeld, & J. Ludford (Eds.), *Preventing adolescent drug abuse: Intervention strategies.* (NIDA Research Monograph No. 47, D.H.H.S. Publication No. ADM 83-1280). Washington, DC: U.S. Government Printing Office.

Miller, L. C., Schilling, A. F., Logan, D. L., & Johnson, R. L. (1977). Potential hazards of rapid smoking as a technique for the modification of smoking behavior. *New England Journal of Medicine, 297*(11), 590–592.

Palmer, A. B. (1970). Some variables contributing to the onset of cigarette smoking among junior high school students. *Social Science and Medicine, 4,* 359–366.

Pechacek, T. F., & McAlister, A. L. (1980). Strategies for the modification of smoking behavior: Treatment and prevention. In J. M. Ferguson & C. B. Taylor (Eds.), *The comprehensive handbook of behavioral medicine,* (Vol. 3). New York: Spectrum.

Perry, C., Killen, J., Telch, M., Slinkard, L., & Danaher, B. (1980). Modifying smoking behavior of teenagers: A school-based intervention. *American Journal of Public Health, 70,* 722–725.

Pomerleau, O. F. (1980). Why people smoke: Current psychobiological models. In P. O. Davidson & S. M. Davidson (Eds.), *Behavioral medicine: Changing health life-styles* (pp. 94–115). New York: Brunner/Mazel.

Prue, D. M., Martin, J. E., & Hume, A. S. (1980). A critical evaluation of thiocyanate as a biochemical index of smoking exposure. *Behavior Therapy, 11,* 368–379.

Sachs, D. P., Hall, R. G., & Hall, S. M. (1978). Effects of rapid smoking. Physiologic evaluation of a smoking cessation therapy. *Annals of Internal Medicine, 88*(5), 639–641.

Schachter, S. (1973). Nesbitt's paradox. In W. C. Dunn, Jr. (Ed.), *Smoking behavior: Motives and incentives.* Washington, DC: Winston.

Schachter, S. (1977). Nicotine regulation in heavy and light smokers. *Journal of Experimental Psychology, 106,* 5–12.

Schachter, S. (1978). Pharmacological and psychological determinants of smoking. *Annals of Internal Medicine, 88,* 104–114.

Schachter, S. (1982). Recidivism and self-cure of smoking. *American Psychologist, 37,* 436–411.

Schwartz, J. L., & Dubitzky, M. (1968). Requisites for success in smoking withdrawal. In E. F. Borgatta & R. R. Evans (Eds.), *Smoking, health and behavior.* Chicago: Aldine.

Severson, H., Fallen, C., Nautel, C., Biglon, A., Ary, D., & Lichtenstein, E. (1981). Oregon Research Institute's smoking prevention program: Helping students resist peer pressure. *Oregon School Study Council Bulletin, 25,* 1–39.

Severson, H. H. (1984). Adolescent social drug use: School prevention program. *School Psychology Review, 13,* 150–161.

Shapiro, D., Tursky, B., Schwartz, G. E., & Schnidman, S. R. (1971). Smoking on cue: A behavioral approach to smoking reduction. *Journal of Health and Social Behavior, 12,* 108–113.

Shiffman, S. (1984). Coping with temptations to smoke. *Journal of Consulting and Clinical Psychology, 52,* 261–267.

Shiffman, S. M. (1979). The tobacco withdrawal syndrome. In *Cigarette smoking as a dependence process* (NIDA Research Monograph No. 23, DHEW Publication No. ADM-79-800). Washington, DC: U.S. Government Printing Office.

Smith, G. M. (1970). Personality and smoking: A review of the empirical literature. In W. A. Hunt (Ed.), *Learning mechanisms in smoking.* Chicago: Aldine.

Solomon, R. A. (1980). The opponent-process theory of acquired motivation: The costs of pleasure and the benefits of pain. *American Psychologist, 35,* 691–712.

Solomon, R. A., & Corbit, J. (1973). An opponent-process theory of motivation. II. Cigarette addiction. *Journal of Abnormal Psychology, 81,* 158–171.

Solomon, R. A., & Corbit, J. (1974). An opponent-process theory of motivation. I. Temporal dynamics of affect. *Psychological Review, 81,* 119–145.

Solomon, R. L. (1977). An opponent-process theory of acquired motivation: The affective dynamics of addiction. In J. Maser & M. Seligman (Eds.), *Psychotherapy: Experimental models.* San Francisco: W. H. Freeman.

Stepney, R. (1980). Smoking behavior: A psychology of the cigarette habit. *British Journal of Diseases of the Chest, 74,* 325–344.

Tell, G. S., Klepp, K. I., Vellar, O. D., & McAllister, A. (1984). Preventing the onset of cigarette smoking in Norwegian adolescents: The Oslo Youth Study. *Preventive Medicine, 13,* 256–275.

Ternes, J. (1977). An opponent-process theory of habitual behavior with special reference to smoking. In M. Jarvik, J. Cullen, E. Gritz, T. Vogt, & L. West (Eds.), *Research on smoking behavior* (NIDA Monograph No. 17). Rockville, MD: National Institute on Drug Abuse.

Tomkins, S. S. (1966). Psychological model for smoking behavior. *American Journal of Public Health, 56,* 17–20.

Tomkins, S. S. (1968). A modified model of smoking behavior. In E. F. Burgatta & R. R. Evons (Eds.), *Smoking, health and behavior.* Chicago: Aldine.

U. S. Department of Health, Education and Welfare. (1979). *Smoking and health: A report of the Surgeon General* (DHEW Publication No. PHS 79-50066). Washington, DC: U. S. Government Printing Office.

United States Public Health Service. (1975). *The health consequences of smoking.* Washington, DC: U. S. Department of Health, Education and Welfare.

United States Public Health Service. (1983). *The health consequences of smoking: Cardiovascular disease.* Washington, DC: U. S. Department of Health, Education and Welfare.

Von Dedenroth, T. E. A. (1968). The use of hypnosis in 1,000 cases of "tobaccomaniacs." *American Journal of Clinical Hypnosis, 10*(3), 194–197.

West, D. W., Graham, S., Swanson, M., & Wilkinson, G. (1977). Five-year follow-up of a smoking withdrawal clinic population. *American Journal of Public Health, 67*(6), 536–544.

Whitman, T. L. (1972). Aversive control of smoking behavior in a group context. *Behavior Research and Therapy, 10,* 97–104.

# CHAPTER 12

# PAIN

Pain is a prevalent and costly health problem. When pain persists beyond the "natural" course of an illness, extends beyond the typical time required for an injury to heal, or is associated with a progressive illness such as arthritis, the pain is designated chronic. It has been estimated that 86 million Americans suffer with some form of chronic pain (Bonica, 1979). Bonica estimates the cost of chronic pain in the United States at $60 billion annually. Such costs are related to hospitalization, outpatient treatment, medication, surgery, loss of work productivity, loss of in-

425

come, disability payments, and litigation settlements. The social impact of pain is also considerable.

Pain varies greatly in terms of duration, severity, quality, and the degree to which it interferes with adaptive functioning. There are several patterns of pain: pain may be acute, chronic-periodic, recurrent, chronic intractable-benign, or chronic-progressive (Turk, Meichenbaum, & Genest, 1983). This differentiation is important because the pattern of pain may provide helpful information in formulating hypotheses regarding mechanisms involved in the development, exacerbation, and maintenance of the pain problem, and the pain pattern also relates to intervention planning.

Interestingly, not all individuals suffering with chronic or recurrent pain find it impossible to cope with such persistent pain. Many individuals are able to accept and cope with such disorders as arthritis, migraine headache, and back pain without abuse of medication, invalidism, and overuse of the health care system. Others, however, develop a complex cluster of symptoms independent of the type of pathophysiology. These individuals display a constellation of problems, including personal and social difficulties as well as patterns of health care use that are quite consistent across pathologies. This cluster of problems has been called the *chronic pain syndrome* and will be discussed in detail in this chapter. First, we will focus on the phenomena of pain itself and review past and current theories with particular emphasis on the role of psychological factors in pain. Following this, we discuss clinical procedures used to evaluate or measure pain. Various pain control techniques commonly used in the management of pain are then presented and mechanisms proposed to explain these effects discussed. Finally, a review of recurrent headache is presented to illustrate a psychobiological approach to recurrent pain.

## THEORIES OF PAIN

Pain is certainly a common experience to us all. Yet as one sits and considers just what pain is, most of us find it difficult to define. Is it a sensation such as that experienced in vision or hearing? Is it an emotion? After all, for most of us pain is not pleasant, but rather quite aversive. Is it a reaction? Our response to burning our hand on the grill in the backyard while broiling hamburgers might suggest this. Just what is pain?

The ancient Greeks viewed pain as an essential component of the human spirit. The counterpart of pleasure. It was assumed that pain was the result of an imbalance among man's four vital fluids, an experience of the heart rather than a physical sensation. This view of pain as an emotion dominated Western thought for centuries until the French philosopher Decartes proposed the basis for a pain theory later identified as the specificity theory.

### Specificity Theory

Figure 12-1 illustrates the specificity theory of pain. In general, according to this theory, pain is communicated to the brain via an entirely independent sensing system devoted solely to pain. This primary sensory system is similar to that subserving vision and audition. Figure 12-1 diagramatically illustrates the pain-sensing pathway from the spinal cord to the brain. As our friend, Joe, is punched in the stomach, a signal of pain is triggered and sent to the brain along specific sensory pathways.

A major controversy regarding the specificity–nonspecificity view of pain relates to the multidimensional character of pain. Two components are typically involved in pain. One is the sensation and perception of pain, the second is the affective state or reaction to unpleasantness. The specificity position argues that the perception of tissue threat or

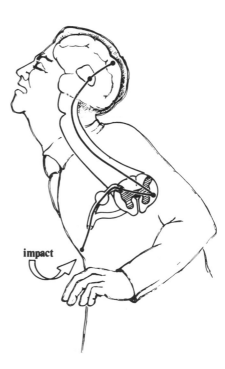

**FIGURE 12-1.** Conceptual view of specificity theory.

damage is pain and that such pain has a neural basis with *specific* anatomical and physiological characteristics. The affective state is simply a *reaction* to the primary pain sensation, that is, a consequence of pain. In contrast, the nonspecificity position argues that the affective component of pain (i.e., emotional concomitant and/or reaction) represents a major source of input influencing pain sensation, which requires input outside of the somatovisceral pain pathways. This distinction is not simply academic in that such a difference in views influences the manner in which pain is treated clinically. A middle range position is one that hypothesizes that a specificity-based view is appropriate for certain pain disorders and patients, whereas, for other pain disorders and patients, a nonspecificity view may be a more valid model for explaining the pain experience. The importance of careful clinical evaluation (medical and psychological) often helps determine potential modulators of pain in a given patient.

Let us review the basis behind the specificity view. Undifferentiated nerve endings are the receptors that transmit noxious stimuli. Certain receptors respond to only noxious mechanical stimuli or thermal stimuli, thus, they are *unimodal nociceptors.* There are also polymodal nociceptors, or receptors that respond to noxious stimuli as well as to chemical, mechanical, or thermal stimuli. Two active afferent fiber groups are involved in pain. The *A-delta fibers* are small myelinated fibers involved in sharp, pricking pain, the slower, unmyelinated *C fibers* are associated with a burning type of pain. Stimulation of peripheral nerves in man indicate that 100% of the unmyelinated C fibers respond to noxious stimuli. Putative receptor substances and neural transmitters have been identified in areas of the dorsal horn (marginal and gelatinosa layers) where pain fibers terminate, which suggests that such substances act on the receptors cells and affect the consequent pain experience (this is discussed in greater detail in a later section of this chapter).

The spinothalamic tracts (lateral and ventral) transmit pain impulses to the brain. Spinothalamic fibers connect with several levels of the reticular formation (plays a role in arousal and attention) as they ascend from the spinal cord. Projections of the spinothalamic tracts enter the thalamus (multiple thalamic nuclei) and cortex. The cerebral cortex, the periaqueductal gray matter in the brainstem, and the serotonin-releasing neurons in the raphe nucleus are involved in the descending modulation of pain signals and have a significant effect on neural transmission in the substantia gelatinosa of the dorsal horn, an area believed to play a major role in pain perception. Figure 12-2 illustrates the various pain transmission pathways.

Many medical techniques have been developed using the specificity assumption of pain as their base. Two such approaches include neu-

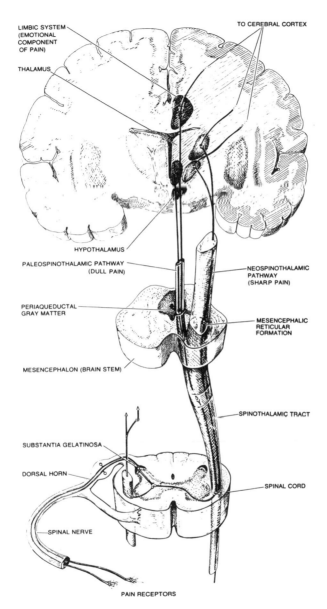

**FIGURE 12-2.** Pain pathways. From "Opiate Receptors and Internal Opiates" by S. H. Snyder, 1977, *Scientific American*, 236, 51. Copyright 1977 by W. H. Freeman. Reprinted by permission.

rosurgical procedures for pain control and nerve block techniques (Melzack & Wall, 1982). Figure 12-3 illustrates the anatomical sites and surgical techniques, and Figure 12-4 illustrates nerve block procedures used in pain control. From the figures, one can see that numerous potential pathways can be interrupted to block pain transmission. The various techniques include *cordotomy*—cutting a portion of the spinal cord, *neurectomy*—removing segments of sensory nerves, *tractotomy*— cutting a specific nerve tract within the spinal cord or brainstem. Figure 12-4 shows the various locations along the spinal cord at which nerves are often blocked and the area of pain most often affected by such local blocks. A nerve block involves injections of a substance, either a local anesthetic or an alcohol mixture, into the central nervous system (CNS) at critical sites in order to create a short-term (2–3 hours) or a fairly lengthy (3 months or longer) interruption of the pain pathways.

Unfortunately, in many cases, despite highly skilled surgery or nerve blocks, the pain may be eliminated for only a brief time (days or a few months), and, then, for some unknown reason, it reappears in full force. Why does this occur? Is it not logical that, if pain results from the transmission of pain messages along select pain pathways, damaging these pathways should prevent the pain messages from ever reaching

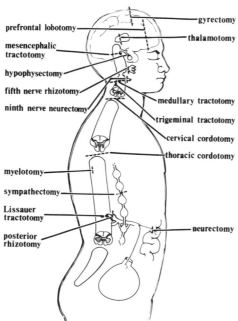

FIGURE 12-3. Neurosurgical procedures.

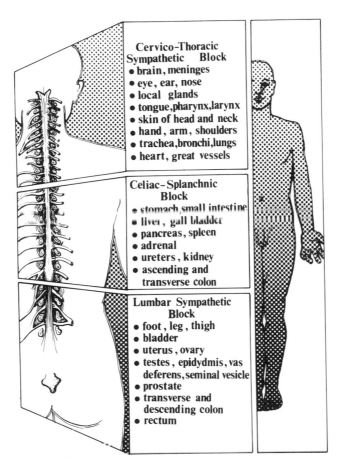

**FIGURE 12-4.** Nerve block procedures.

the brain? Before addressing this question, consider the following phenomena:

1. The football player who in the excitement of the game is unaware of the pain associated with a dislocated elbow experienced during a tackle in the first quarter.
2. Soldiers on the battlefield require much less analgesic medication than surgical patients in a hospital, despite the observation that tissue damage was much more severe in the soldiers.
3. Certain ethnic groups tend to report more pain to an identical pain stimulus than other groups. Italian, Greek, and Jewish women tend to report more pain than Irish-American women.

4. In remote Indian villages, an annual hook-swinging ceremony is undertaken in which two steel hooks are thrust into the lower back of the "celebrant." The celebrant is then placed on a special cart with an elevated pole from which he hangs as the cart is moved from village to village. The celebrant displays no sign of pain despite the assumed stimulation of pain-transmission routes. Figure 12-5 illustrates the position of the hooks and the crossbeam from where the celebrant is hung.

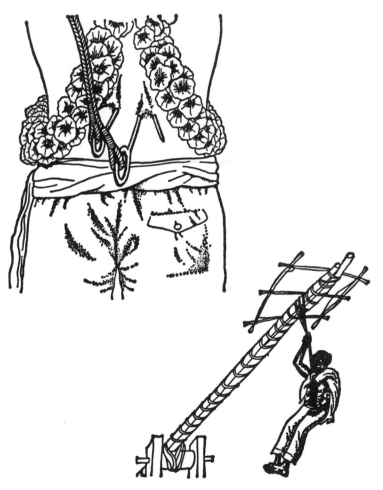

**FIGURE 12-5.** Hook swinging ceremony—"celebrant" experiences no pain. From "Living Prehistory in India" by D. D. Kosambi, 1967, *Scientific American, 216,* 110–111. Copyright 1967 by W. H. Freeman. Reprinted by permission.

How can such observations be explained by the specificity theory of pain? Indeed, laboratory and clinical research has demonstrated that a variety of psychological, cultural, and psychosocial factors influence the pain experience (Melzack & Wall, 1982).

## Gate Control Theory

The observations discussed above suggest that pain signals can be altered by a variety of psychological processes as they are transmitted within the nervous system. Pain is more than a simple transmission of sensory signals from a pain source ascending the spinal cord to the brain. Rather, it is the net result of a series of complex interactions of neurophysiological and neurochemical processes permitting such psychological processes as motivation, emotion, and cognition to modulate the pain experience. Melzack and Wall (1965) proposed a model that helps to explain the role of such psychological factors in CNS modulation of pain. This theory, the *gate control theory of pain*, has had a profound influence on the conceptualization and treatment of pain over the past two decades. It has been particularly important in stimulating interest in empirical research on psychological processes in pain and the use of psychological techniques in pain management. However, perhaps more importantly, it has emphasized the need for the use of an integrative psychobiological approach to theory and practice in the area of pain and pain control.

Figure 12-6 shows the gate control theory as it was first proposed by Melzack and Wall in 1965. Simply stated, the model assumes the following:

1. A spinal gate (SG) mechanism in the dorsal horn region of the spinal cord modulates the transmission of nerve impulses from afferent fibers to spinal cord transmission (T) cells. It is *assumed* that the substantia gelatinosa is the primary vehicle for gating.
2. The SG mechanism is influenced by the *relative* amount of activity in large-diameter (L) rapidly conducting and small-diameter (S) slowly conducting fibers. Activity in the large fibers tend to *inhibit* transmission, or close the gate; activity in the small fibers tend to *facilitate* transmission, or open the gate.
3. The SG mechanism is influenced by nerve impulses that *descend* from the brain.
4. A specialized system of large-diameter, rapidly conducting fibers (central control trigger) activates selective cognitive processes that then influence, via descending fibers, the modulating properties of the SG mechanism.

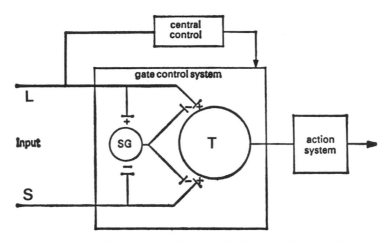

**FIGURE 12-6.** Gate control theory: Initial version. A schematic diagram of the gate control theory of pain (Mark I): L = the large diameter fibers; S = the small diameter fibers. The fibers project to the substantia gelatinosa (SG) and first central transmission (T) cells. The inhibitory effect exerted by SG on the afferent fiber terminals is increased by activity in L fibers and decreased by activity in S fibers. The central control trigger is represented by a line running from the large fiber system to the central control mechanisms; these mechanisms, in turn, project back to the gate control system. The T cells project to the action system. +, excitation; −, inhibition. From "Pain Mechanisms: A New Theory" by R. Melzack and P. D. Wall, 1965, *Science, 150,* 971. Copyright 1965 by the American Association for the Advancement of Science. Reprinted by permission.

5. When the output of the T cells exceed a critical level, the *action system* is triggered. This system represents those neural areas that form the basis for the complex, sequential patterns of behavior and experience characteristic of pain.

Figure 12-7 is a conceptual view of the gate control mechanism with gating in the spinal cord modulated by descending signals representing input from psychological processes. As the figure illustrates, the gate and the T cells trigger the complex reaction of facial grimace, crouching or bending, touching site of pain, and a variety of additional cognitive and behavioral reactions in reponse to the blow to the stomach.

The validity of the gate control theory has been widely debated over the past 15 years with the majority of critics arguing over the specific anatomical and neurophysiological mechanisms that can account for triggering the action system and the perceived pain. Questions regarding the exact function of the substantia gelatinosa within the gate model have been common. Recently, Melzack and Wall (1982) have revised the model, identifying changes in the original version necessitated by new knowledge in neurophysiology and neuroanatomy and the criticism of the earlier model. These changes are illustrated in Figure 12-8 and include the following:

1. The SG has multiple functions. It contains both excitatory (white circle) and inhibitory (black circle) links to the transmission (T) cells and descending inhibitory control from brainstem systems.

2. Because of the present uncertainty regarding the mechanisms of this inhibition, and in order to reduce misunderstanding as to whether this inhibition is a presynaptic mechanism, a bar has been placed at the end of the inhibitory link to indicate that its action may be presynaptic, postsynaptic, or both.

3. A separate input to the gate the descending inhibitory control was added to the model. This addition was necessitated by increased evidence of a significant brainstem inhibitory system influenced by sensory input after transmission through the gate (i.e., after T cell stimulation). As indicated in Figure 12-7, this system then projects back to the dorsal horn, providing the descending inhibition.

4. Based upon recent evidence for neuropeptide involvement in pain, observations that certain nerve fibers (particularly unmyeli-

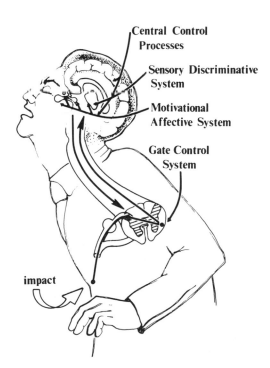

FIGURE 12-7. Conceptual view of gate control theory.

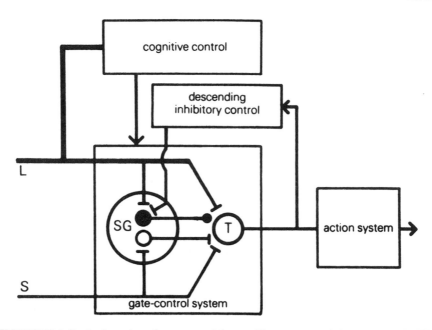

**FIGURE 12-8.** Revised version of gate control theory. The gate control theory: Mark II. The new model includes excitatory (open circle) and inhibitory (solid circle) links from the substantia gelatinosa (SG) to the transmission (T) cells as well as descending inhibitory control from brainstem systems. The round knob at the end of the inhibitory link implies that its action may be presynaptic, postsynaptic, or both. All connections are excitatory, except the inhibitory link from SG to T cell. From *The Challenge of Pain* by R. Melzack and P. D. Wall. Copyright 1982 by Basic Books, Inc. Reprinted by permission.

nated fibers) are rich in such peptides and that neuropeptide concentrations change slowly for several days following peripheral nerve injury, Melzack and Wall proposed a role for such peptides within the gate theory.

The SG also contains peptides (including enkephalins). The model proposes that following damage or poisoning of peripheral nerves, there is a slow change in the terminals of the fine fibers in the spinal cord and a concomitant disinhibition. In addition, an expansion of the receptive fields of the transmitting cells occurs. This establishes a condition resulting in a greater probability of activating the T cells and triggering the action system. The authors are suggesting that transmission to the CNS can be controlled by two mechanisms: (1) classic nerve impulses and (2) slow transport and release of neurochemicals that modify the structure and activity of the T cells. The conceptual model of gating and the assumptions underlying it continue to provide a useful heuristic tool in the area of pain research. Indeed, despite much controversy, a viable alternative has not yet been proposed.

In addition to the concept of pain gating, Melzack *et al.* conceptualized the pain experience as being comprised of three components: sensory-discriminative, motivational-affective, and cognitive-evaluative. The *sensory-discriminative component* is that system that transmits basic sensory information, such as location of pain in the body and the pain's sensory qualities, such as burning, aching, or piercing. It tells us where we hurt and what it feels like. The *motivational-affective component* influences the degree to which we desire to escape from the pain, either by withdrawing from its source, if possible, or by approaching and trying to attack or to eradicate its source. This component is responsible for the emotional reaction to the pain. The *cognitive-evaluative component* determines the meaning of the sensory experience. The pain from an injury on the battlefield may mean rest and relaxation from an aversive situation and may make it easier to cope with. The chronic pain associated with a terminal cancer in a young mother with three young children and an alcoholic husband has a different meaning. Her pain may signal impending death with associated feelings of anger and guilt. This appraisal may make the pain more difficult to tolerate. Figure 12-9 integrates the components of the gate control model as discussed.

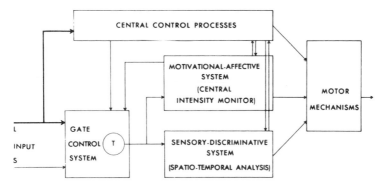

**FIGURE 12-9.** Integrated schematic of the sensory, motivational-affective, and central control mechanisms of pain. The output of the T cells of the gate control system projects to the sensory-discriminative system (via neospinothalamic fibers) and the motivational-affective system (via the paramedial ascending system). The central control trigger is represented by a line running from the large fiber system to central control processes; these, in turn, project back to the gate control system, and to the sensory-discriminative and motivational-affective systems. All three systems interact with one another and project to the motor system. From "Sensory, Motivational, and Central Control Determinants of Pain: A New Conceptual Model" by R. Melzack and K. L. Casey in *The Skin Senses* edited by D. Kenshalo. Copyright 1968 by Charles C Thomas, Publisher. Reprinted by permission.

## PSYCHOLOGICAL MODULATORS OF PAIN

Much research on the role of psychological factors in the modulation of pain has been conducted over the past decade. The early research emphasized the effects of psychological state (arousal level, anxiety level), personality style (introvert versus extrovert), and sociocultural background (ethnic affiliation) on measures of pain threshold and pain tolerance to laboratory or analogue pain stimuli (e.g., electric shock, thermal or radiant heat stimulation, cold pressor). Although the findings were somewhat complicated and, at times, conflicting, in general, these various psychological factors tended to influence the pain tolerance component of the pain response, but not the pain threshold or level at which pain was first experienced. Psychological factors were observed to influence the amount of pain (in terms of time) one was willing to endure (Weisenberg, 1977).

Later research focused on the use of various cognitive strategies to influence the pain experience. A great number of studies on the effects of attention diversion, sensory alteration, and mental imagery were conducted, and these indicated that such procedures can affect pain induced by laboratory methods. In conjunction with these findings, limited reports indicating that relaxation techniques and experimental manipulations that resulted in a sense of control or perceived self-control over the painful stimulus were also associated with increased pain tolerance and reduced reports of pain (Thompson, 1981).

Criticism over the use of analogue or laboratory pain stimulation as a means of understanding clinical pain, in general, and the psychological processes involved in clinical pain, in particular, was considerable. It was argued that the brief pain in the laboratory—a pain that was certain to cease—was quite different from the persistent pain observed in clinical pain states, such as chronic back pain or arthritis. This latter pain does not cease, and has a clearly different significance. One pain represents a brief annoyance, the other, a continuous aversive experience that may fluctuate in severity across a day or a week but is nevertheless persistent, and indicative of a degenerative condition or illness state. Even in the case where no clear pathology is apparent, as with certain chronic pain cases (see Chapter 9), the pain is a constant reminder that something is dysfunctional. In those cases with high disease conviction (see Chapter 9), the significance of the pain may be even more salient.

Partly in response to the criticisms regarding analogue pain and partly as a function of the increased interest in pain as a research problem with significant clinical implications, the study of clinical pain phenomena using various clinical groups has been emphasized. The research on psychological mechanisms of clinical pain can be divided into three major areas: (1) *environmental/behavioral*, (2) *cognitive/perceptual*, and (3) *psychophysiological/physiological*. Taken as a whole, these three areas represent a psychobiological approach to the study of chronic pain. It should be emphasized that this review is primarily directed at factors that may exacerbate and/or maintain chronic pain. There will be only minimal discussion of factors that may be responsible for the development of pain. Also, episodic or recurrent pain is not discussed in this section. A later section will discuss a conceptualization of the possible pathway for the development of one chronic pain disorder—chronic low back pain—proposed by Feuerstein, Papciak, and Hoon (1985). Recurrent pain is considered in the section on migraine headache. Let us review the three areas in order.

## Environmental/Behavioral Factors

One major hypothesis regarding the role of psychological factors in the exacerbation and maintenance of chronic pain is the concept that pain and pain behaviors can be influenced by the environment via learning processes. The three common learning mechanisms proposed to influence pain are *operant conditioning, respondent or classical conditioning,* and *modeling* or *observational learning*. Although these processes were briefly discussed in Chapter 9, under the category of social learning mechanisms as a means for explaining one form of chronic illness behavior (hypochondriasis), we will discuss the three types of learning processes and their specific relation to pain and pain behavior in greater detail in this section. The learning mechanisms hypothesis is a major approach to the understanding and management of chronic pain.

The classic behavioral approach to pain is based upon two concepts (Fordyce, 1978). The first is that behavior or the observable measurable overt actions of the organism are significant in their own right. That is, behavior does not need to be conceptualized as the final outcome of some underlying causative factor (e.g., conflict or anxiety). Behavior can stand on its own and not be necessarily tied to an inferred internal event. This concept represents the classical Skinnerian position and is argued by Fordyce. The second concept of the behavioral approach is an emphasis on operational measurement and observation. The phenomenon of interest is behavior, and as such, observational measurement of behavior is essential. Pain is a private event that must be brought into public observation. This can be achieved by measuring pain behavior (e.g., moaning, inactivity, medication use) and not inferred concepts. What factors influence this pain behavior?

When environmental circumstances increase or decrease the probability of a given behavior as a function of the rewarding or punishing consequences associated with the behavior, operant mechanisms are assumed to be present. That is, operant behavior is behavior that is effected by the environmental consequences of the behavior (reward/punishment). Once the behavior is modulated by such environmental consequences, other stimuli from the environment can facilitate the occurrence of the behaviors by serving as cues that the specific response will result in a certain consequence. These latter environmental cues are referred to as *discriminative stimuli* (SDs). An example of an operant process influencing pain is the case in which increased pain behavior on the part of a patient with chronic degenerative arthritis is associated with increased housework by spouse and family and increased attention and affection by a husband who is typically "too busy." In this case, the pain behaviors, defined as verbal complaints of pain and time in bed, are potentially influenced by the positive consequences associated with such behaviors (avoidance of housework, attention of spouse). The presence of such operant mechanisms is difficult to evaluate, however, and careful attention to the circumstances under which pain behavior occurs and the consequences of such behavior is required. Operant pain behavior does not require the occurrence of nociceptive (pain) input from a peripheral or central physiological process. The pain behavior can be totally independent of such nociceptive input, although typically there is some initial, continuous, or intermittent nociceptive input.

Family members often inadvertently serve to exacerbate or maintain the pain behavior in their efforts to provide solicitous assistance. Block (1980a,b) reported findings suggesting a possible basis for the role of spouse response in exacerbation of pain behavior. The spouses observed videotapes of painful and neutral facial expressions emitted by mates, hospitalized chronic pain patients, and performers. Spouses displayed greater increases in skin conductance to painful than neutral facial displays whether emitted by performers or patients. However, spouses reporting relatively high levels of marital satisfaction showed *greater* increases in skin conductance to painful displays of mates than unsatisfied spouses, although both groups provided similar ratings. Heightened autonomic reactivity to pain expression in satisfied spouses could play a role in influencing solicitous behavior in that heightened arousal *and* subjective distress may motivate spouse attempts at reducing pain (protection/care giving) in the patient. It would be of interest to test such a hypothesis by investigating the specific patterns of overt response to videotaped or live pain displays. Related to the role of the spouse in maintaining pain behavior is the finding that patients who reported their spouse as relatively nonsolicitous in response to pain behavior reported significantly lower pain levels in the spouse-observing condition than in the neutral-observer condition; the inverse was observed in patients with spouses perceived as solicitous, that is, high pain levels (Block, Kremer, & Gaylor, 1980b).

The role of reinforcers at a larger systems level has also been assumed to affect pain behavior. A frequently held assumption by health care providers and insurance carriers is that representation by attorneys and/or litigation in cases involving worker compensation claims is associated with increased pain behavior (i.e., higher utilization rates, increased medication use, greater number of work days lost). This hypothesis is based upon an operant-conditioning conceptualization of pain behavior in which such reinforcers as attention and excitement associated with the claims-processing procedures, in addition to the probable financial settlement, might influence the claimant's lawyer's nonverbal and verbal reinforcement of pain-related behavior, thus exacerbating and/or maintaining such behavior. Peck, Fordyce, and Black (1978) tested such a hypothesis, using worker compensation cases from the state of Washington. Although the data were not definitive, the results did *not* support the original hypothesis. Pending litigation against a third party with or without attorney representation was not associated with any consistent increase in pain behavior when compared with worker compensation cases in which there was no third party litigation (i.e., the standard worker compensation claim). The study was limited by the absence of a chronic pain group not involved in compensation settlement; however, the findings suggest that attorneys and related additional litigation procedures are not associated with concomitant increase in pain behavior. Peck *et al.* (1978) suggest that operantly influenced pain behavior may require more frequent exposure to reinforcement, as found in the family and work environment, in contrast to involvement with the legal system, and, therefore, contingencies within the legal system are not sufficient to reinforce pain behavior. Although there are several explanations for the absence of such an effect, a follow-up study to investigate the specific effects of compensation litigation as suspected reinforcers of pain behavior should be conducted.

In contrast, respondent pain is pain behavior that is controlled by a specific antecedent nociceptive stimulus (e.g., a burning sensation associated with nerve injury). In this learning mechanism, the burning sensation can be conditioned to a variety of environmental stimuli (places, people, thoughts). These environmental stimuli can then elicit the pain experience and/or associated pain behaviors. An example of the respondent conditioning process is the case in which a patient with chronic lumbar pain who reports consistent exacerbation of pain with muscle spasm in the evening, particularly around sleep onset, begins to associate the increased muscle spasm with sleep. The patient then begins to experience considerable anticipatory anxiety before retiring for the evening, which exacerbates the pain and the pain behavior. A similar phenomena may occur in relation to activity or movement in certain patients, when such movement produces excruciating increases in pain. Simply the thought of moving can then lead to increased fear or anxiety regarding pain, thus increasing the pain and pain behavior (e.g., increased time spent in bed-down time).

The role of avoidance has been hypothesized in the maintenance of pain behavior for years; however, little systematic study of this mechanism has been reported. Fordyce, Shelton, and Dundore (1982) presented a case investigating avoidance of aversive consequences as a mechanism for maintaining pain behavior. The conceptualization is as follows: during acute phase of injury, such avoidance behaviors as limping and decreased activity are effective in attenuating pain from nociception. Over time, with repeated learning trials, the avoidance behaviors become established. The patient learns to *anticipate* that certain behaviors will result in less or no pain and suffering. With chronic pain, the anticipation of suffering or the prevention of suffering may be sufficient for the long-term maintenance of the avoidance behaviors. Most discussions of the type of stimuli the chronic pain patient tends to avoid have been directed at such psychosocial factors as work or interpersonal interactions perceived as aversive. Fordyce *et al.* (1982) present a case in which certain pain behavior (limited activity, guarding, protective behaviors) appeared to be maintained by *anticipated internal nociceptive stimuli* and consequent pain. It is hypothesized that this avoidance behavior does not necessarily require intermittent nociception from the site of body damage, environmental reinforcement, or successful avoidance of aversive social activities to account for maintenance of guarding pain behavior because the avoidance behavior is assumed to be maintained by anticipation. Although a case study cannot provide confirmatory evidence for etiological mechanisms, the following case suggests the possible role of anticipatory avoidance behavior on chronic pain.

*The case was a 21-year-old male with a 15-year history of recurrent hospitalization for "abnormal abdominal pain" with no clear physiological basis. Following an accident, the patient became increasingly guarded because attempts to walk were associated with dizziness and pain. A markedly disturbed gait was observed and the patient was wheelchair-bound. Treatment goals were directed at free ambulation, achieved by reestablishing walking-related behaviors incompatible with guarding, using a flooding-like procedure during which the patient was guided through targeted activities with the goal of increasing speed. The patient became remobilized, ambulated freely, and returned to productive activity with gains maintained at 21 months posttreatment. Although reductions in pain/distress lagged behind the behavioral changes, as activities increased, the patient's pain report decreased.*

Prevalence data of the occurence of anticipatory avoidance behavior in chronic pain patients would be of considerable importance to determine the magnitude and clinical significance of this phenomenon. Clinical experience suggests that this type of behavior is quite common across a variety of environmental situations. Further research determining the cognitive attributions and physiological correlates associated with the presumed avoidance behaviors would appear to be important.

Research on the psychophysiology of fear, conducted in the 1960s and early 1970s, may provide a useful model for the study of the effects of fear, pain, and avoidance of activity. As Figure 12-10 illustrates, fear gradients (slope of curves) vary as a function of experience with the feared situation. Figure 12-10 presents self-ratings of fear, skin conductance, heart rate, and respiration rate responses recorded during a parachute jump sequence in novice (broken lines) and experienced (solid lines) parachutists. The figure illustrates a number of interesting observations, potentially applicable to activity avoidance in pain patients. The experienced parachutists reported increased fear in the initial stages of the jump sequence, which dropped considerably across the sequence and was lowest just before and during the jump, whereas the inexperienced parachutists displayed a gradual increase in fear from the night before the jump to reaching the airport, boarding the aircraft, receiving the "ready" signal (peak fear), etc. The physiological correlates of the jump sequence also indicated differences between experienced and novice parachutists. The greatest differences between the two groups occurred at the final altitude, before the jump; however, of greater interest to anticipatory fear and pain research was the finding of a steep slope (rise) in the skin conductance response from the time the novice parachutists became airborne, to 1,000 feet, midpoint altitude, and final altitude. This anticipatory fear and concomitant physiological arousal was *not* observed in the experienced parachutists.

A similar phenomenon may be operative in those chronic pain patients who report that it is simply "too painful to move or get out of bed." The anticipatory arousal inhibits activity and may also exacerbate pain in the absence of such movement, if increased arousal can exacerbate pain. A second possibility relates to the concept of *stress-induced analgesia* in which fear and arousal could actually *attenuate* the pain via endogenous opiate mechanisms, thus reinforcing the anticipatory fear response and low activity. In either case, the patient remains fearful and relatively immobile. Perhaps through gradual exposure, such fear can be extinguished. Unfortunately, unlike phobias, in which the fear has little or no basis in reality, the pain patient will experience exacerbations in pain. Therefore, efforts at teaching self-control strategies to attenuate pain would be necessary in conjunction with the gradual exposure to

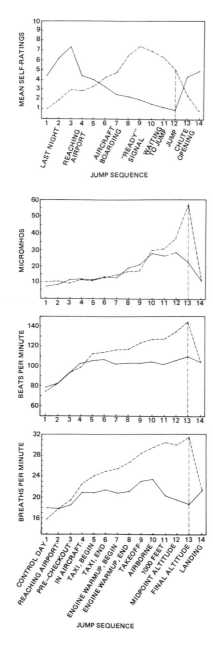

**FIGURE 12-10.** Anticipatory anxiety/fear gradients for self-report and physiological measures: The fear of skydiving. From "Gradients of Physiological Arousal in Parachutists as a Function of an Approaching Jump" by W. D. Fenz and S. Epstein, 1967, *Psychosomatic Medicine, 29,* 34–35. Copyright 1967 by Elsevier Science Co., Inc. Reprinted by permission.

pain-provoking situations. Direct empirical support for this approach to the understanding and modification of pain and pain behavior represents an important step in furthering our understanding of this mechanism and illustrates the integration of principles and techniques in psychophysiology, emotion, and behavior therapy.

The final learning mechanism proposed to explain the role of environmental factors on pain is vicarious or observational learning (Craig, 1978). Craig has demonstrated in an elaborate series of laboratory studies that observation of displays of pain and suffering and the consequences of such pain and suffering can influence the autonomic response of the observers (increased autonomic arousal) and the extent to which observers tolerate pain themselves. It is argued that this vicarious or observational learning forms the basis of acquiring new patterns of behavior in the absence of direct experience (Bandura, 1977). Moving from laboratory observations to the clinical situation, Craig (1978) hypothesized that modeling processes may form the basis for "inappropriate pain complaints and other sick role behaviors unrelated to verified organic pathology or for avoidance of treatment that is in the best interests of the individual" (p. 75). Although a potentially valid hypothesis, the majority of work on modeling mechanisms in pain has been in nonclinical subjects, with clinical support for the modeling concept obtained by indirect observation.

An example of indirect evidence is provided by Edwards, Zeichner, Kuczmierczyk, and Boczkowski (1985). These investigators indicated a significant positive relationship between the number of pain models in an individual's family and the frequency of current pain reports. Other correlational studies have indicated relationships between parental and offspring pain symptomatology for abdominal pain and low back pain (Craig, 1978) and headache (Turkat, Kuczmierczyk, & Adams, 1984). It has also been reported that individuals with a parental model who displayed work avoidance when ill reported greater avoidance of responsibility when ill than did individuals with no such parental model, which suggests a possible modeling process (Turkat, Guise, & Carter, 1983).

## Cognitive/Perceptual Processes

Recent models of pain emphasize the importance of cognitive/perceptual processes in the modulation of pain (Melzack & Wall, 1982). Such cognitive factors as perceived control over the painful event (Thompson, 1981), hypervigilance to somatic distress signals (Chapman, 1978), adaptation to high levels of nociceptive input (Naliboff, Cohen, Schandler, & Heinrich, 1981), variation and use of cognitive coping strategies (Rosensteil & Keefe, 1983), low self-esteem or poor self-concept (Thomas & Lyttle, 1980), cognitive distortion (Lefebvre, 1981), depression (Blumer & Heilbronn, 1982), and general perceptual defect or somatic amplification (Barsky & Klerman, 1983) have been proposed to explain certain clinical characteristics of chronic pain patients. These mechanisms have been typically invoked to account for the persistent preoccupation with somatic disturbance or the apparent constant monitoring and selective attention to pain sensations and other interoceptive stimuli. The perceptual defect hypothesis was discussed in detail in Chapter 9 and will not be reviewed here. The major difference between the concept applied to hypochondriasis and its possible application to chronic pain is that the chronic pain patient may or may not have a well-defined basis for the pain, whereas the "hypochondriacal" patient, according to the DSM-III, typically has no pathophysiological basis for the symptoms. It is the authors' belief that the presence of a physiological basis does not preclude the operation of several of the same psychobiological processes operable in the case in which such an organic basis is absent. Therefore, much of the discussion in Chapter 9 on cognitive and emotional factors is applicable to chronic pain. The factor that was not reviewed in Chapter 9, to any extent, was the role of coping strategies in chronic pain.

Rosensteil and Keefe (1983) have investigated the relationship between coping strategies and current adjustment in chronic pain. These investigators noted that praying, positive expectation, and coping self-statements (e.g., telling oneself that one can cope with the pain, regardless of how severe it becomes) were commonly used strategies. The use of reinterpreting pain sensation (e.g., imagine the pain sensation as numbness) was rarely reported. Patients reported their overall ability to control and decrease pain as quite low. The various coping strategies reported were subjected to a principal component analysis that revealed three factors (68% of the variance) described as *cognitive coping and suppression* (reinterpreting pain sensation, coping self-statement, ignoring pain sensation), *helplessness* (catastrophizing, increasing activity level, perceiving control over pain, believing in ability to decrease pain), and *diverting attention and praying.*

Results from the Rosensteil and Keefe (1983) research indicated that the type of coping strategy employed is not related to pain duration, disability status, or number of back surgeries, but rather that the three cognitive factors were predictive of average pain (22% of variance), depression (11%), state anxiety (14%), and functional capacity (12%). The coping factors did not predict down time. Patients scoring high on cognitive coping and suppression were more likely to report functional impairment than low scoring patients, whereas high scorers on helplessness were more depressed and anxious than low scorers; last, high scorers on attention diversion and praying experienced higher levels of pain and were more impaired functionally than low scorers. Interestingly, these results suggest that the use of certain previously hypothesized "coping" strategies are in fact related to *poorer* adjustment. These data reveal the complexities involved in assessing naturally occurring coping strategies in chronic low back pain patients. In general, the results indicate that increased helplessness (catastrophizing) is associated with increased distress, but not increased pain ratings. Given the frequently observed low correlation between pain report and pain behavior, further research on the relationship between helplessness and actual pain behavior may reveal an association more consistent with the hypothesis that negative cognitive appraisal is associated with increased pain. The Rosensteil and Keefe (1983) study also supported the role of pain history and somatization in adjustment to chronic low back pain. Disability status, number of previous surgeries, and duration of continuous pain were predictive of current down time, functional impairment, and pain level. These findings emphasize the need to identify and investigate factors contributing to duration of pain disorder on a prospective basis. Perhaps cognitive "coping strategies" may have a greater effect when pain first occurs. Such a hypothesis appears consistent with the observed effects of various cognitive strategies on acute experimental pain (e.g., Spanos, Horton, & Chaves, 1975).

## Psychophysiological Mechanisms

Research in the area of psychophysiological mechanisms of pain falls into two general categories: (1) identification of psychophysiological correlates of pain states and (2) research on hypothesized peripheral mechanisms of specific pain disorders. The research on correlates of pain states was conducted with healthy nonpatient volunteers and patient samples. This research is quite limited in terms of the number of studies available. An example of the type of investigation in this category is one that measures heart rate and skin conductance during baseline, anticipatory phase, pain stimulation, and recovery in healthy college student volunteers while also measuring pain tolerance to a cold pressor pain stimulus and McGill Pain Questionnaire (MPQ) responses of pain experience. Such a series of studies was conducted by Dowling (1982, 1983). The findings indicated a relationship between increased heart rate and pain reports on the MPQ only during anticipation of pain, and a negative relationship between skin conductance level and response on the evaluative scale of the MPQ. In regard to the skin conductance level, higher levels were associated with a report of less pain as reflected on the MPQ. This inverse relationship was noted during resting, anticipation, and pain periods, whereas the heart rate relationship was observed in anticipation of pain only. A later study investigating the relationship among heart rate, skin conductance, and pain tolerance (an indirect measure of pain behavior in the laboratory) revealed that skin conductance and heart rate during the anticipatory period were related to pain tolerance. Again, the direction of the relationship differed for the two measures. When the heart rate was lower, during anticipation of pain, pain tolerance was *greatest*. Higher levels of skin conductance during anticipation and immersion (pain), reflecting increased arousal, were associated with *greater* tolerance. The findings for heart rate suggest that increased autonomic arousal is associated with increased pain, while the skin conductance measure indicates the reverse. Why?

Dowling suggested that the findings may be confounded by differential levels of physical fitness (lower heart rates in the more physically fit), a factor not controlled for in these studies. Another possible explanation for the results may be the existence of preparatory cognitions, with an associated increased skin conductance during anticipation. During the anticipatory period, the subjects may have been psychologically preparing themselves for the pain. A third possibility is that stress can actually trigger an analgesic response. That is, animal research and limited human research has observed the existence of a stress-induced analgesia phenomenon. It may have been possible that the task produced such an increase in stress response that it was reflected by increased sympathetic discharge (increased skin conductance). The reason for the observation that heart rate did not follow a similar response may be associated with the bidirectional nature of heart rate, which has parasympathetic and sympathetic input.

A French physiologist has observed that humans display two types of responses to a painful electrical stimulus to the foot: (1) increased respiration, increased heart rate, and *inhibition* of nociceptive flexion reflexes and (2) increased respiration, decreased heart rate, and *facilitation* of nociceptive reflexes (Willer, 1975). No significant changes in physiology were observed for the experienced group (i.e., the group with previous exposures to painful stimuli). In a later study, using experienced subjects only, Willer and Albe-Fessard (1980) indicated that an *inescapable* noxious foot shock (experienced previously), delivered on a random schedule, induced cumulative anxiety, a progressive increase in respiration and heart rate, and *depression* of nociceptive reflexes (indicating reduction in pain) in all subjects. The stress-induced analgesia was modified using high doses of naloxone (a substance that competes for opiate receptor sites and serves as a narcotic antagonist). This finding suggests the role of CNS modulation via endorphin pathways for stress-induced analgesia in humans. (Refer to next section.)

Another approach to studying the physiological correlates of pain states is the research using brain-evoked potentials, a response of the CNS (cortical response) discussed in Chapter 4. Chen, Chapman, and Harkins (1979) reported that the amplitudes of the two earlier components of the human-evoked potential (cf. Figure 4-9) were related to the intensity of the stimulus (painful dental stimulation) when the effect of subjective painfulness was controlled for. The amplitudes of the two later components of the response, however, were associated with the subjective painfulness of the stimulus, *not* stimulus intensity. This study illustrates the use of a psychophysiological measure in pain research that appears to differentiate the cortical sensory transmission response from brain activity that involves *perception* of pain severity. Clinical research using this specific technique (dental pulp stimulation) is difficult to conduct for ethical reasons; however, continued research using the technique nonclinically may assist in identifying those variables influencing the brain's response to the perception of pain severity and perhaps permit a greater understanding of the specific role of attention, distraction, and anxiety/stress in the modulation of pain perception. Indeed, a recent clinical investigation has indicated significantly greater right hemisphere discharge during headache, in contrast to non-headache, consistently observed in the later components of evoked potential (Chen & Dworkin, 1982).

The second common approach to the psychophysiology of pain relates to determining whether the changes in the response of peripheral physiological indices assumed to relate to the pathophysiological process underlying the pain are indeed associated with the experience of pain. A corollary of this approach are studies directed at determining whether such measures are actually overreactive or hyperresponsive to stressors or movement or other stimuli assumed to trigger or to exacerbate the pain disorder. Muscular activity is a common physiological measure used in this type of research. In the study of low back pain, despite frequent assumption, it has not been found that the paraspinal lumbar muscles are (1) generally more active in patients than in controls, (2) more hyperreactive to stressors (psychological and physical) than controls, or (3) highly correlated with the pain experience. This work indicates the absence of a clear skeletal muscle difference between patients and controls. Recent research has also indicated that there are no differences in paraspinal muscle activity measured while patients engage in typical activities, over a 12-hour period, between back pain patients and matched controls (Feuerstein, Pistone, & Houle, 1985). This research typically suggests no or a minimal relationship between the hypothesized peripheral pain generator (skeletal muscle activity) and pain report or behavior, suggesting the possible role of central mechanisms in the pain experience. These findings, however, could be limited by the exclusive use of surface EMG recording techniques, which may not be sufficiently sensitive to monitor "hyperresponsivity" in the lumbar musculature. Other explanations include the possible role of a degenerative arthritic disorder in many patients with low back pain and the involvement of ligaments in pain. Clearly back pain, although highly common, is a complex disorder and little is known about its etiology (Turk & Flor, 1984).

## NATURAL PAIN SUPPRESSORS IN THE BRAIN AND SPINAL CORD

The psychological and psychophysiological findings discussed in earlier sections suggest the importance of central mechanisms of pain. The rapid growth in knowledge regarding the role of endogenous (internal) pain control systems in the brain over the past decade indicates the plausibility of such central control. These pain regulation mechanisms have been used to explain the role of various biobehavioral factors on pain, including hypotheses regarding the analgesic effects of such psychological treatment techniques as hypnosis. A brief review of endogenous pain control is essential when pain mechanisms are considered.

In the mid 1970s, physiological psychologists observed that electrical stimulation of certain brainstem sites in animals resulted in a profound analgesia *without* a general depression in behavior. This phenomenon is now called *stimulation-produced analgesia* (SPA). This SPA provided evidence for the existence of a system in the brain that produced analgesia, that is, an *endogenous analgesia system.* Several sites in the brain have been found to produce analgesia when stimulated; however, electrode placements in the *ventrolateral periaqueductal grey* area in or near the dorsal raphe nucleus are most consistently effective (Figure 12-2).

The stimulation of analgesia from selected brain sites was extended to clinical pain when Adams (1976) "successfully" employed electrical stimulation in the periventricular gray matter of a 54-year-old male patient with severe pain due to a diabetic neuropathy. Stimulation of a chronically implanted electrode resulted in complete relief of pain, with a latent period of from 10 to 15 minutes. Stimulation was typically maintained for anywhere between one and two hours, with the patient remaining pain-free for the next 22 to 23 hours. In addition to the clinical effect produced by this stimulation, the case highlights two interesting phenomena encountered in SPA: the *onset latency* and the *period of post-stimulation effectiveness.* Most research has indicated that stimulation does not produce immediate analgesia, but rather it develops gradually over a period of five minutes or longer (Melzack & Melinkoff, 1974). The period of post-stimulation effectiveness, the duration of such analgesia, varies in different species, with humans having the longest period. Stimulation-produced analgesia has been observed for both somatic and visceral pain.

Neuropharmacological studies have demonstrated the existence of receptors in the brain that are sensitive to opiate compounds. These *opiate receptors* are specific sites on cell surfaces that interact in a highly selective, stereospecific manner with opiate drugs. The concept of stereospecificity is somewhat similar to a lock and key, whereby a specific key (opiate drug) will only fit a specific lock (opiate receptor). The research on opiate receptors has shown that the affinity of an opiate binding to the receptor is correlated with its analgesic potency, which suggests that certain opiates have relatively specific receptor sites.

Since opiates do not occur naturally in animals, neurobiologists have reasoned that if opiate receptors exist in the brain, and these receptors have a physiological function, there must be a natural, opiate-like substance that binds to them. That is, some endogenous substance—a neurotransmitter or neuromodulator—that binds to the opiate receptor must exist. A search to isolate such an endogenous substance from the nervous system was thus begun (Goldstein, 1976; Snyder, 1977a). Two naturally occurring endogenous morphine-like substances (leucine-enkephalin and methionine-enkephalin) were subsequently discovered. The investigators coined the term *enkephalin* for the two peptides from the Greek "in the head." The term *endorphins* was coined for endogenous morphine-like substances. Other endorphins have also been identified. These substances have a powerful analgesic effect when administered intraventricularly (injected into the ventricles of the brain) or systemically (injected into the bloodstream). Opioid peptides of various structures have also been identified in the pituitary gland. These peptides are grouped together, based on their ability to mimic the effects of morphine on smooth muscle and to compete for binding to opiate receptors. The substance (a fragment of lipotropin) with the greatest opiate-like activity, in terms of binding to the opiate receptor, effect on smooth muscle, and analgesic ability, is β *endorphin*. Beta endorphin is assumed to account for most of the pituitary glands opioid activity, despite the existence of several other opiate-like peptides. The biological function of the *pituitary* opioid peptides, however, is unclear (Snyder, 1977b).

There is evidence that the enkephalins are neurotransmitters of specific neuronal systems in the brain involved in pain and emotional behavior. Variations in enkephalin levels tend to correlate with the distribution of opiate receptors, and the enkephalins appear to be localized in nerve endings (Synder, 1977a). Synder observed that the enkephalin nerve terminals are concentrated in the substantia gelatinosa of the spinal cord, the amygdala of the limbic system, and the thalamus. Each of these areas are believed to be intimately involved in the experience of pain. Interestingly, enkephalins have been detected in the gastrointestinal tract in many species, but not in other tissues.

Snyder (1977a) has proposed a model for the action of enkephalin on brain cells in an attempt to explain its effect on pain modulation. It is hypothesized that enkephalin has an *inhibitory* effect, that is, the cells fire at a generally lower rate. Opiates with specific opiate receptors also exert such an inhibitory effect. This inhibition could involve a number of mechanisms. Neurotransmitters are typically assumed to bind to receptors on the membrane of a receiving neuron to change some membrane property (e.g., ion permeability). The physiology of nerve transmission is reviewed here so that the reader can understand the proposed mechanism of action of enkephalin.

At rest, the nerve cell membrane is electrically polarized, so that the outside of the cell is electrically positive with respect to the inside. Excitatory neurotransmitters (e.g., acetylcholine) facilitate the firing of the receiving neuron by depolarizing the cell to produce an action potential or electrical signal. Inhibitory transmitters (e.g., glycine, gamma amino butyric acid) make the membrane more resistant to excitatory transmitter depolarization by increasing the permeability of the membrane to negatively charged chloride ions (hyperpolarization). Opiates and enkephalin, however, inhibit neuronal activity in some systems by blocking sodium influx by directly affecting the membrane of the receiving cell, rather than the excitatory neuron. An additional inhibitory mechanism for enkephalin has been proposed by Snyder (1977a). Snyder observed that receptors were localized on the nerve terminals as well as on the receiving cells, which suggests a second inhibitory mechanism. The mechanism is illustrated in Figure 12-11.

Essentially, rather than acting directly on the receiving cell, the enkephalin may *block* the release of excitatory neurotransmitters from the excitatory neuron. Snyder (1977a) describes the process as follows:

> Enkephalin released from a neuron binds to the opiate receptors on the terminal of an excitatory neuron, partially depolarizing the terminal membrane and reducing the net depolarization produced by the arrival of a nerve impulse. The amount of neurotransmitter released from the terminal is proportional to the net depolarization, so that less excitatory transmitter is released the receiving cell is then exposed to less excitatory stimulation and reduces its firing rate. (p. 54)

Snyder has hypothesized that a similar inhibitory system might modulate activity in ascending pain pathways in the spinal cord and

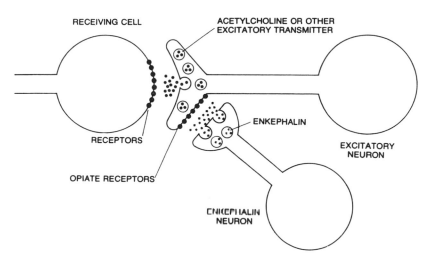

**FIGURE 12-11.** Neuronal mechanism of enkephalin inhibition. From "Opiate Receptors and Internal Opiates" by S. H. Snyder, 1977. *Scientific American, 236*, 54. Copyright 1977 by W. H. Freeman. Reprinted by permission.

brain and that opiate drugs might exert their effects by binding to free enkephalin receptors, thus potentiating the effects of the endogenous system.

The work on endogenous pain modulation is a major contribution to the understanding of the physiological substrate of pain. Although much controversy regarding the role of such mechanisms in clinical pain states exists, the discovery of the endorphins and the work on their mode of action is important to any psychobiological theory of pain. These endogenous mechanisms may also help further our basic understanding of treatment mechanisms.

## PSYCHOBIOLOGICAL FACTORS IN THE DEVELOPMENT OF PAIN: CHRONIC LOW BACK PAIN

To date, there have been no comprehensive prospective studies investigating the etiological role of psychobiological risk factors in chronic pain. Figure 12-12 is a model for such an investigation and highlights the possible variables and processes in which one type of chronic pain (chronic low back pain) may evolve (Feuerstein, Papciack, & Hoon, 1985). The figure identifies the accident or report of symptoms as the first stage. The majority of individuals experiencing back pain rest

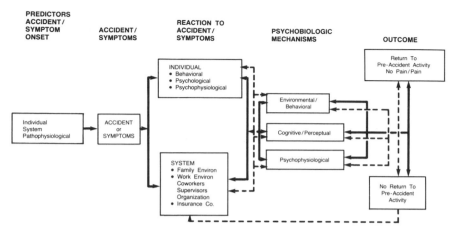

**FIGURE 12-12.** Psychobiological factors in the development of chronic low back pain.

and eventually improve. For those who do not, the reaction to the initial report of symptoms may play an important role in the development of long-term disability or chronicity. The reaction can occur at the individual level in terms of the patient's overt behavioral expression of pain and disability; at the psychological level in terms of subjective levels of anxiety, anger and frustration; and at the psychophysiological level, as a physiological stress response. The model also includes the responses of the family, co-workers, medical personnel, and insurance adjustors, all of whom can play a role. A set of complex interacting mechanisms at the environmental/behavioral, cognitive/perceptual, and psychological/physiological levels, as discussed in this chapter, are set into action to interact with the reaction variables of the individual. This model can be operationalized and tested. The schema provides an example of a psychobiological perspective.

## MEASUREMENT OF PAIN

As discussed earlier, pain is a multidimensional phenomenon. This is particularly the case with chronic pain. Therefore, a comprehensive psychological evaluation of pain often requires focusing on a number of target problems. Some of the major target areas for researcher and clinician include pain, activity level, medication use and/or abuse, mood state, psychological status, social climate or environment, and illness concept or attitude. These factors have been measured along several dimensions, including self-report, behavioral, and physiological, as appropriate. Table 12-1 lists some measures used to evaluate the several dimensions of pain. Pain itself can be divided into pain experience and pain behavior.

Reports of pain experience are obtained through patient self-monitoring, family monitoring, structured behavioral observation, and multidimensional self-report questionnaires. Self-monitoring by the patient is generally the most common and cost-efficient means of obtaining a general index of pain. Patients may monitor frequency, duration, degree of interference resulting from pain, medication use, location of pain, and severity of pain. Figures 12-3 and 12-4 illustrate the self-monitoring forms used by the authors in their research and clinical work. The problems associated with such monitoring is the validity of the self-reported data. Studies indicate that behavioral and self-report indices of pain often do not correlate. In addition, diurnal fluctuations have been reported with certain types of pain, and this may be problematic in certain cases. The type of scale used to monitor pain intensity is also a question for concern. Certain types of scaling produce skewed distributions of responses, whereas others (e.g., the Visual Analogue Scale) tend to be more reliable and sensitive and correlate with verbal pain intensity ratings. A visual analogue scale is presented in Figures 12-13 and 12-14.

Family monitoring or spouse monitoring of the patient's pain and well behavior also is a source of data important to a full understanding of the pain (Fordyce, 1976). Fordyce requests that family members complete a daily checklist of activities that the patient engages in.

Pain behavior is typically evaluated using behavioral observation in a structured environment. Keefe and Block (1982) report the development of a structured manipulation requiring a 1- and 2-minute sitting period, a 1- and 2-minute standing period, two 1-minute reclining periods, and two 1-minute walking periods. Patients were coded for bracing, rubbing, guarding, grimacing, and sighing (20 observations/patient; 20 seconds/observation). The investigators reported high reliability (.93–.99) and a significant correlation between pain rating with total frequency of pain behaviors ($r = .71$). The pain behaviors, however, were more apparent during movement.

Another device used as a behavioral observation measure is the *Pain Behavior Scale* (Richards, Nepomuceno, Riles, & Suer, 1982). This scale is a brief (five minutes/patient) measure of 10 target behaviors including vocal complaints—verbal, vocal complaints—nonverbal, down time, facial grimaces, standing posture, mobility, body language, use of visible supportive equipment, stationary movement, and medication. The patient is asked to (1) walk a short distance, (2) stand momentarily, (3)

**TABLE 12-1**
Measures Used to Evaluate Pain

| Measures | Characteristics |
|---|---|
| 1. *General Psychological Characteristics*<br>Minnesota Multiphasic Personality Inventory (MMPI) | |
| 2. *Pain*<br>Pain Questionnaire | History of pain problem, pain experience, sleep disturbance, activity level, medication use, prior medical intervention, impact on interpersonal relations, pain severity, location, and duration |
| Daily Pain/Mood Diary—3×/day | Pain frequency, severity, duration, interference, POMS mood-tension, depresion, anger, vigor, fatigue, confusion (provide index of pain–mood relationship) |
| McGill Pain Questionnaire | Sensory, affective, cognitive-evaluative components of pain experience |
| Pain Behavior Scale | Pain behavior—verbal complaints, nonverbal complaints, down time, facial grimaces, standing posture, mobility, body language, use of visable supports, stationary movements, medication |
| 3. *Illness Behavior/Attitude*<br>Illness Behavior Questionnaire | General hypochondriasis, disease conviction, psychological vs. somatic perception of illness, affective inhibition, affective disturbance, denial of problems, irritability |
| 4. *Environmental Strain*<br>Family Environment Scale (FES) | Cohesion, expressiveness, conflict, independence, achievement orientation, intellectual-cultural orientation, active- |

**TABLE 12-1** (*Continued*)

| Measures | Characteristics |
|---|---|
| Work Environment Scale (WES) | recreational orientation, moral-religious, organization, control Involvement, peer cohesion, supervisor support, autonomy, task orientation, work pressure, clarity, control, innovation, physical comfort |
| 5. *Substance Abuse Potential* McAndrew Scale | Possible index of substance abuse |
| 6. *Prognostic Indicators for Biobehav. TX* Self-Control Schedule (SCS) | Tendency to utilize self-control strategies in daily living |
| Schalling-Sifneos Personality Scale | Alexithymia—inability to readily access emotions, operative thinking |

move from sitting to standing, and (4) move from standing to sitting. The interrater reliability was .94 to .96, and the test–retest (50 patients, two consecutive days) was .89. In terms of preliminary validity data, a significant reduction in scores were observed following an operant pain program specifically designed to reduce pain behavior. In a random sample of chronic pain patients, daily measures of "well behaviors," including walking, sitting, and standing, were inversely correlated with pain behavior as measured on the Pain Behavior Scale. Interestingly, the Pain Behavior Scale did *not* correlate with a self-report measure of pain, the MPQ suggesting it may be measuring a different dimension of pain. The Pain Behavior Scale, as modified by the present authors for outpatient use, is presented in Figure 12-15.

The last types of pain index to be discussed are what may be termed multidimensional self-report measures of pain experience. An example of a widely used device is the *McGill Pain Questionnaire* (MPQ) (Melzack, 1983; Melzack & Torgerson, 1971). The MPQ is a series of adjective pain descriptors that classify pain into sensory, affective, and evaluative dimensions. Figure 12-16 illustrates the various components of the pain experience and the pain descriptors patients use, which form the specific pain components. Note the terms that fall under the various compo-

DATE: _____

| UPON AWAKENING | 4:00 P.M. | BEFORE BED |
|---|---|---|
| TIME:_____<br>(rate pain experienced during<br>sleep up to now) | (rate pain experienced since<br>morning) | TIME:_____<br>(rate pain experienced since<br>4:00 p.m.) |
| **PAIN PRESENT:** (circle)<br>YES            NO | **PAIN PRESENT:** (circle)<br>YES            NO | **PAIN PRESENT:** (circle)<br>YES            NO |
| **DURATION** in hours: (circle one)<br>1 2 3 4 5 6 7 8 9 10<br>Other: _____ | **DURATION** in hours: (circle one)<br>1 2 3 4 5 6 7 8 9 10<br>Other: _____ | **DURATION** in hours: (circle one)<br>1 2 3 4 5 6 7 8 9 10<br>Other: _____ |
| **SEVERITY:**<br>no pain            pain as bad as could be | **SEVERITY:**<br>no pain            pain as bad as could be | **SEVERITY:**<br>no pain            pain as bad as could be |
| **INTERFERENCE:**<br>no interference with daily activities            could not continue daily activity | **INTERFERENCE:**<br>no interference with daily activity            could not continue daily activity | **INTERFERENCE:**<br>no interference with daily activity            could not continue daily activity |
| **MEDICATION:**   # OF<br>TYPE       TABLETS<br>1. _____  _____<br>2. _____  _____<br>3. _____  _____ | **MEDICATION:**   # OF<br>TYPE       TABLETS<br>1. _____  _____<br>2. _____  _____<br>3. _____  _____ | **MEDICATION:**   # OF<br>TYPE       TABLETS<br>1. _____  _____<br>2. _____  _____<br>3. _____  _____ |
| **LOCATION:** (shade area where you currently experience pain) | **LOCATION:** (shade area where you currently experience pain) | **LOCATION:** (shade area where you currently experience pain) |

**FIGURE 12-13.** Self-monitoring form of daily pain.

nents. Examples of sensory-based terms include jumping, sharp, pinching, and hot; affective terms include sickening, suffocating, and fearful. The authors have found that the determination of the pattern of sensory and affective descriptors assists them in evaluating patients with chronic pain. Pattern analysis provides additional information as to the role of

How much pain did you experience when we asked you to stand, walk, and sit?

Indicate by pointing to area on the pain level scale below.

Pain Level

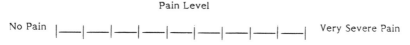

No Pain |—|—|—|—|—|—|—|—|—| Very Severe Pain

**FIGURE 12-14.** Example of a visual analogue scale.

psychological (i.e., affective) modulators of pain experience. As Table 12-1 indicates, other measures in addition to a clinical interview of patient and spouse are typically included in a clinical pain evaluation. The table illustrates such an evaluation.

## PSYCHOLOGICAL EVALUATION OF CLINICAL PAIN: CHRONIC PAIN SYNDROME

Clinical health psychologists are frequently requested to consult with various medical specialists on complicated cases of chronic pain. The health psychologist can integrate theory and technique to help understand the factors that might be contributing to, exacerbating, and maintaining the chronic pain. Their evaluation can also serve to document the impact the pain disorder has had in a number of psychological and social areas and assist in identifying specific intervention strategies for pain management. An example of a pain evaluation from the authors' case files is presented below.

*B.F. is a 53-year-old married white male referred by neurological surgery. B.F. reports a 19-month history of back, head, and leg pain which was reportedly caused by a job-related accident in May of 1982, in which he slipped and fell while carrying some plywood. In June 1982, the patient was hospitalized for reconstructive surgery, but he canceled because of anxiety over its outcome. Surgery was rescheduled and performed in September 1982, and the patient was placed in a body cast until December 8, 1982, at which time the cast was replaced with a lumbar–sacral corset. Spread of pain and weakness resulted in trials of physical therapy, including a TENS unit, and medication, including Darvon and Elavil (50 mg/day), during subsequent months. In April 1983, a decompressive laminectomy was performed, and the patient reported an immediate decrease in pain and weakness in his extremities post-surgery. Pain and weakness have reportedly increased gradually since this last surgery. During this time, he was treated with Tylenol, Percodan, Phenephen, Valium, and Tylox, all of which reduced his pain by approximately 10%. B.F. reports that a single trial of Demerol resulted in an increase in*

| | | DATE | M | T | W | T | F | S | S |
|---|---|---|---|---|---|---|---|---|---|
| *1. | Vocal Complaints: Verbal | None | 0 | 0 | 0 | 0 | 0 | 0 | 0 |
| | | Occasional | ½ | ½ | ½ | ½ | ½ | ½ | ½ |
| | | Frequent | 1 | 1 | 1 | 1 | 1 | 1 | 1 |
| *2. | Vocal Complaints: Non-Verbal | None | 0 | 0 | 0 | 0 | 0 | 0 | 0 |
| | (moans, groans, gasps, etc.) | Occasional | ½ | ½ | ½ | ½ | ½ | ½ | ½ |
| | | Frequent | 1 | 1 | 1 | 1 | 1 | 1 | 1 |
| 3. | Down-Time: | None | 0 | 0 | 0 | 0 | 0 | 0 | 0 |
| | (Time spent lying down | 0–60 min. | ½ | ½ | ½ | ½ | ½ | ½ | ½ |
| | per day because of pain.) | > 60 min. | 1 | 1 | 1 | 1 | 1 | 1 | 1 |
| *4. | Facial Grimaces | None | 0 | 0 | 0 | 0 | 0 | 0 | 0 |
| | | Mild and/or infrequent | ½ | ½ | ½ | ½ | ½ | ½ | ½ |
| | | Severe and/or frequent | 1 | 1 | 1 | 1 | 1 | 1 | 1 |
| *5. | Standing Posture | Normal | 0 | 0 | 0 | 0 | 0 | 0 | 0 |
| | | Mildly impaired | ½ | ½ | ½ | ½ | ½ | ½ | ½ |
| | | Distorted | 1 | 1 | 1 | 1 | 1 | 1 | 1 |
| *6. | Mobility | No visible impairment | 0 | 0 | 0 | 0 | 0 | 0 | 0 |
| | | Mild limp and/or mildly impaired walking | ½ | ½ | ½ | ½ | ½ | ½ | ½ |
| | | Marked limp and/or·labored walking | 1 | 1 | 1 | 1 | 1 | 1 | 1 |
| *7. | Body Language | None | 0 | 0 | 0 | 0 | 0 | 0 | 0 |
| | (clutching, rubbing | Occasional | ½ | ½ | ½ | ½ | ½ | ½ | ½ |
| | site of pain) | Frequent | 1 | 1 | 1 | 1 | 1 | 1 | 1 |
| *8. | Use of Visible, Supportive Equipment | None | 0 | 0 | 0 | 0 | 0 | 0 | 0 |
| | (braces, crutches, cane, leaning on furniture, TENS, etc.) | Occasional | ½ | ½ | ½ | ½ | ½ | ½ | ½ |
| | DO NOT score if equipment prescribed. | Dependent, constant use | 1 | 1 | 1 | 1 | 1 | 1 | 1 |
| *9. | Stationary Movement | Sits or stands still | 0 | 0 | 0 | 0 | 0 | 0 | 0 |
| | | Occasional shifts of position | ½ | ½ | ½ | ½ | ½ | ½ | ½ |
| | | Constant movement, position shifts | 1 | 1 | 1 | 1 | 1 | 1 | 1 |
| 10. | Medication | None | 0 | 0 | 0 | 0 | 0 | 0 | 0 |
| | | Non-narcotic analgesic and/or psychogenic medications as prescribed | ½ | ½ | ½ | ½ | ½ | ½ | ½ |
| | | Demands for increased dosage or frequency and/or narcotics, and/or medication abuse | 1 | 1 | 1 | 1 | 1 | 1 | 1 |
| | TOTAL BEHAVIOR (1, 2, 4, 5, 6, 7, 8, 9) | | | | | | | | | |
| | TOTAL DOWN-TIME AND MEDICATION | | | | | | | | | |

**FIGURE 12-15.** Pain behavior scale. From "Assessing Pain Behavior: The UAB Pain Behavior Scale" by J. S. Richards, C. Neponuceno, M. Riles, and Z. Suer, 1982, *Pain, 14,* 395. Copyright 1982 by Elsevier Biomedical Press. Reprinted by permission.

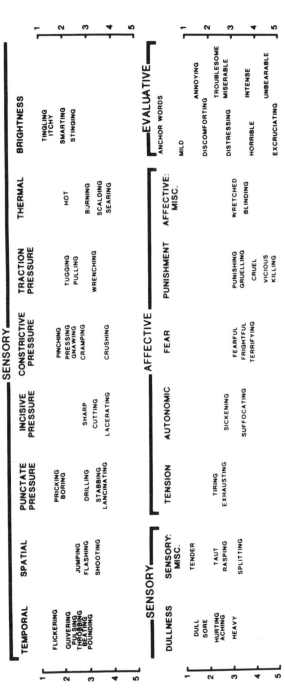

**FIGURE 12-16.** Pain descriptors used in the McGill Pain Questionnaire. Spatial display of pain descriptors based on intensity ratings by patients. The intensity scale values range from 1 (mild) to 5 (excruciating). From "On the Language of Pain" by R. Melzack and W. S. Torgerson, 1971, *Anesthesiology*, 23, 50. Copyright 1971 by J. B. Lippincott Co. Reprinted by permission.

pain, and that, in general, he avoids use of medication that "slow him down." B.F.'s medical history is significant for a lumbar laminectomy around 1962, which successfully eliminated his pain following a back injury similar to that which occurred in 1982. The patient reports that he was pain-free and able to engage in normal activities between 1964 and 1979, when he was involved in a motor vehicle accident, which resulted in severe headaches. The patient reports that successful surgery to remove bone spurs was conducted at that time. B.F. also reports that he was diagnosed as having a gastric ulcer during the summer of 1983, but that he currently avoids gastric discomfort by following a bland diet.

B.F. was evaluated by review of his medical record, interview of the patient, interview of Mrs. F., psychological testing (Pain and Stress Questionnaire, Minnesota Multiphasic Personality Inventory, Alexithymia Scale, Rosenbaum Self-Control Scale, Illness Behavior Scale, and Family Environmental Scale), and observation of his pain behavior on January 17, 1984.

B.F. describes his pain as a continuous stinging, burning, and throbbing sensation in his back, legs, feet, arms, shoulder, and hips. He reports numbness in his lower arms and hands and a tight, "bruised" sensation in his upper arm. Pain is increased with cold, dampness, massage, lifting, bending, vibration, sitting, and exercise. As a result of his pain, B.F. states that he has markedly decreased his participation in previously enjoyed activites, such as going out to dinner, playing cards, camping, hunting, fishing, dancing, and sexual intercourse. B.F. states that his pain is completely diminished by swimming, but that pain returns within 5 minutes after he leaves the pool. In addition to his back and extremity pain, B.F. reports that he experiences frequent headaches, which are broadly distributed over his forehead and scalp and may last 1 to 2 weeks. B.F. also describes episodes of weakness in both legs three to six times a day. In describing his pain, B.F. uses terms such as "vicious," "blinding," "sickening," and "exhausting," suggesting that he experiences a significant affective reaction to his pain. B.F. states that because of pain he experiences difficulty in falling asleep at night, and usually does not get to sleep until 5 or 6 A.M. However, he is typically awakened by pain, and by sleeping late and napping obtains approximately 8 hours of sleep a day. During the evaluation, B.F. was observed to show significant pain behavior: facial wincing and grimacing, a marked limp, and impaired standing posture.

B.F.'s responses on the MMPI and Illness Behavior Questionnaire suggest that he is currently experiencing marked anger, irritability, anxiety, depression, and worry, which are somatically focused. In addition, the MMPI responses suggest that he is socially withdrawn and may tend toward unconventional patterns of thinking. These results of testing were consistent with his interview report of helplessness, frustration over physical limitation, and loss of interest in previously enjoyed activities such as yardwork, hunting, and fishing. He reports that he now easily becomes angry at his wife, family, and friends and often feels guilty later over not being able to play with his five-year-old and 2-month-old sons. B.F. reports that he typically expresses anger by withdrawing from others and becoming uncommunicative, and this description was confirmed by his wife's reports. Both the patient and spouse report that B.F has crying spells every one to two weeks, and reports persistent suicidal thoughts, but denies suicidal intent because of concern about the effect on his children. Scores on the Rosenbaum and Alexithymia Ques-

*tionnaires were within normal limits, suggesting an average tendency to use cognitive self-control strategies to reduce the aversiveness of stressful situations, and an average ability to verbally describe his emotional feelings. B.F. reports episodes of dyspnea, tachycardia, and excessive sweating, approximately once per month. Results of the Family Environment Scale suggested that B.F. experiences little interpersonal conflict at home, but that a high degree of interpersonal dependence characterizes the family environment. Mrs. F. reports some resentment over the degree to which she has had to assume responsibility for managing the household, although she reports that over the last four months (i.e., since her return to work following the birth of their youngest son) he has been more helpful with housework and child-rearing. Mrs. F. reports that she often "ignores" his pain because she knows there is nothing she can do to decrease it. She also reports significant sexual frustration due to a decline in their frequency in sexual intercourse since his most recent accident.*

*B.F. indicated that he has been married three times previously and described himself as a recovered alcoholic who stopped drinking over the past two years for religious reasons. His work record suggests that he has had difficulty maintaining employment as a laborer for more than a few months at a time. He reports increasing use of pain medication, but not of alcohol, over the past six months, as his pain has increased, although he denies using medication at greater than prescribed dosages.*

## SUMMARY AND RECOMMENDATIONS:

*B.F. is a 53-year-old white male with a 19-month history of back pain subsequent to a work-related injury. Since his accident he has been operated on twice, with only transient relief. Medication decreases his pain only slightly, and physical therapy has been ineffective in reducing his pain. B.F.'s pain has spread and has been increasingly accompanied by weakness and numbness in his extremeties. Interview and test responses suggest that he is currently experiencing considerable anxiety and depression, which are somatically focused. These problems are confounded by marital and sexual difficulties. We recommend that B.F. become involved in an intensive pain management program, which would include the following components:*

1. *Relaxation training to decrease muscular tension, which may be contributing to his anxiety and pain, and sensory altering self-hypnosis techniques to modify his perception of pain.*
2. *A cognitive-behavioral approach to dealing with his depression.*
3. *Marital and sexual counseling to improve communication and help Mr. and Mrs. F. cope with difficulties presented by his pain.*
4. *Vocational counseling to help him find employment consistent with his physical limitations.*
5. *A trial of antidepressant medication to assist him in falling asleep, alter his mood, and possibly reduce pain. It is likely that his previous antidepressant medication was not prescribed at effective therapeutic levels.*
6. *Physical therapy to increase muscle flexibility and strength.*

*Given the magnitude of Mr. F.'s problems, and the distance he must travel for outpatient treatment, we believe that a program that involves daily involvement with our group appears to be a reasonable approach. Such a treatment program is likely to require four to six weeks of daily sessions, with follow-up sessions every three weeks for approximately 12 months. We have discussed these recommendations with B.F. and will be contacting him in the future regarding treatment.\**

## PSYCHOLOGICAL APPROACHES TO PAIN CONTROL

An increasingly greater number of psychological treatments are available for the management of chronic pain. In this section, the more frequently used approaches will be described. More detailed reviews of the outcome studies of the various approaches to be discussed can be found in Turner & Chapman (1981; 1982), Linton (1982), and Turk and Flor (1984). Different psychological treatment approaches are based on different theories and attempt to intervene according to those aspects emphasized by the theory. Interventions can be grouped in one of the four major areas: focus on pain behavior, modulation of the pain experience, modulation of mood, and cognitive-behavioral functioning.

### Operant Therapy

Operant therapy attempts to intervene at the level of pain behavior and applies learning principles to the treatment of chronic pain. Fordyce (1976) pioneered the operant treatment approach to chronic pain. The focus of this approach is on changing overt pain behaviors rather than on the patient's subjective experience of pain. Pain behaviors include avoidance of physical activity, medication use, verbal pain complaints, grimacing, and groaning. Thus, behaviors that can be *observed* and *measured* are the targets of intervention.

Pain behaviors are not assumed to solely reflect underlying pathophysiology, but rather are subject to the influence of a variety of factors, including systematic environmental consequences of the patient's actions. As discussed in the section on psychological factors con-

---

\* There are several approaches available for offering psychologically-oriented pain management therapy. Patients can be treated on an outpatient basis either weekly, twice weekly, or daily using a day treatment type of format (an out of town patient can live in a hotel rather than the hospital), or on an inpatient basis for two-six weeks, depending upon the extent of disability, narcotic analgesic abuse, and psychiatric complications. The format of treatment varies as a function of the type of facilities available, the set of presenting problems, the type of insurance coverage, and the current personal situation of the patient (e.g., childcare, travel distance).

tributing to pain, Fordyce and colleagues hypothesize the existence of two types of pain behavior—respondent and operant. Recall that respondent behavior is automatic whereby the pain behavior is controlled by a specific antecedent *nociceptive* stimulus; operant pain behavior, however, is under the control of the environment and other behavior-consequence relationships. The respondent and operant components of pain are differentiated by a behavioral analysis. The behavioral analysis attempts to identify the antecedent and consequences of pain *behavior* to provide a general sense of the extent to which conditioning factors may be present. This approach does not provide a differential diagnosis of operant/respondent versus "organic." It is assumed that components of pain with clear organic pathology and nociception can also be influenced by learning factors or environmental modulation. The behavioral analysis typically includes data from an interview of patient and spouse or significant other, along with an evaluation of activity diary data and direct behavioral observation of pain behavior. Table 12-2 illustrates the types of questions and specific areas that are typically covered in the interview. Treatment goals for an operant approach are specified in Table 12-3.

The goal of this form of treatment is to reduce pain behaviors, while simultaneously increasing well behaviors. Contingencies of pain behavior are modified. Behaviors incompatable with pain behavior, such as increased physical exercise, time spent on hobbies, and work are reinforced, and the patient's well behaviors are praised and attended to. In approaching chronic pain patients with this operant treatment procedure, it is recognized that the patient is experiencing subjective distress, but it is explained to the patient that this focus on the pain (defined by each individual's pain behavior observed and reported) will be reduced if physical and social activities are increased, despite the presence of pain. The use of selective reinforcement for non-pain behavior and extinction of pain behavior by staff, in the case of inpatients, or family, in the case of inpatient and outpatient cases, is a major component of this approach.

The operant approach is also helpful for the management of medication abuse whereby a patient is taking narcotic analgesics contingent upon exacerbations of pain. The approach assumes that such a contingent relationship (increased pain—increased medication) reinforces pain and pain behavior because of the positive consequence of the medication (pain relief or expected pain relief). The patient is therefore given medication at fixed intervals (e.g., every four hours), regardless of pain level. The analgesic is often mixed in cherry syrup, in what is referred to as a *pain cocktail*. Eventually, with the patient's approval, the amount of narcotic is gradually reduced and the patient is simply ingesting syrup.

TABLE 12-2
Behavioral Analyses of Chronic Pain: Interview Questions

| General topics and key phases | Relevant details and guidelines[a] |
|---|---|
| Time patterns<br>"Describe your pain experiences throughout a typical day." | Constant and unchanging = operant<br>Intermittent with fluctuating but existing pain-free intervals = respondent<br>Pain at night or during other environmental "shutdown" periods suggests respondent<br>Nocturnal pain ↑ corresponding to analgesic intake schedules suggests medication habituation rather than respondent pain. |
| Pain exacerbation<br>"Which activities or events bring on or increase your pain?"<br>Pain reduction<br>"List the activities or techniques which decrease your experience of pain." | Get specifics like lifting 15-kg parcels to waist level or higher rather than "lifting anything" or "any type of movement."<br>Specify rest intervals and time out from work in units of time required to consistently ↓ pain<br>List all medications (prescribed & "street" drugs) used for pain and the time delay before pain reduction occurs.<br>Immediate relief following medication or rest = conditioned or operant pain<br>Switching from one productive strategy to another for pain relief suggests respondent pain. |
| Pain related activity changes<br>"What physical, social, and work activities have been altered because of your pain problem?"<br>"Which of these would you like to resume?" | Identify discrepancies between avocational and vocational behavior change, given comparable physical demands. For example, in sitting tolerance at work with no change in sitting tolerance at the movies = operant pain.<br>Specify individual and couple activity changes in work and intercourse due to low back pain (where sexual activity has been enjoyable) suggests respondent pain. |
| Pain behavior<br>"If I were in the room and you were in pain, how would I know? What would you do or say?"<br>Environmental consequences of pain behaviors | Specify sounds, grimaces, and body movements used to indicate pain.<br>Medication usage or health care utilization = pain behavior.<br>List direct and indirect (via avoidance of stress or responsbility) reinforcement of pain behavior. |

**TABLE 12-2** (*Continued*)

| General topics and key phases | Relevant details and guidelines[a] |
|---|---|
| "How does your spouse react when you're in pain?" "What do you (spouse) do in response to his or her pain?" | No spouse and no job payoffs for pain suggest respondent pain. Angry or resentful spouse reactions can be reinforcing The more responsibilities or unpleasant activities assumed by the environment in response to pain, the higher the probability of operant pain. |

*Note.* From "Behavioral Health Care in the Management of Chronic Pain" by J. Steger and W. Fordyce in *Handbook of Clinical Health Psychology* (p. 477) edited by T. Millon, C. Green, and R. Meagher. Copyright 1982 by Plenum Press. Reprinted by permission.
[a]Many factors need to be considered in discriminating between operant and respondent pain; the examples listed should be treated as diagnostic signs, *not* proven indicators.

During this time, the patient is typically learning pain reduction and stress reduction techniques that can serve as substitute strategies to narcotic use, to assist the patient in pain control.

Most studies evaluating operant treatment programs for chronic pain have utilized single subject or uncontrolled, one group, pre/post

**TABLE 12-3**
Typical Treatment Goals of an Operant Approach to Pain Management

Increase activity level both generally and in regard to specific exercise or activity constraints

Reduction in pain behaviors associated with protective actions by others

Reduction in pain-related medication use

Restoration or establishment of effective well behaviors, including remediation of social skill and interpersonal problems previously limiting the ability to be well

Modification of the reinforcing contingencies to pain and well-behavior extent in the patient's milieu

Reduction in health care utilization related to pain problem including fruitless diagnostic and treatment procedures

*Note:* No mention of reduction in pain is included. Focus in on modification of pain behavior

*Note.* From "Learning Process in Pain" by W. E. Fordyce in *The Psychology of Pain* (p. 67) edited by R. A. Sternbach. Copyright 1978 by Raven Press. Reprinted by permission.

designs; only a few studies have used control conditions of some type (Linton, 1982). In general, operant programs have consistently shown clinically significant increases in activity levels and reduction of pain medications. However, the patient's self-report of the pain experience is only modestly reduced. On follow-up, good maintenance of treatment gains is seen.

The second type of psychological approach to the treatment of chronic pain emphasizes *modulation of the pain experience* itself. This can be accomplished by modifying psychophysiological aspects of the pain using biofeedback or relaxation techniques or modifying the patient's affective experience of the pain with the use of hypnosis for relaxation, sensory alteration, and attention diversion.

### Biofeedback Training

As discussed in Chapter 7, biofeedback training typically involves providing information about physiological functions that are normally not in the patient's awareness. A specified target response, such as cervical muscle tension, is electronically monitored and information about changes in the functioning of the targeted response is relayed to the patient via various feedback devices, such as a meter reading or an auditory signal. The goal is to use the feedback to teach the patient to control voluntarily physiological processes assumed to be related to the pain problem. Small, portable biofeedback devices can be used in the patient's natural environment. After the patient learns to control the response with feedback, he or she is then instructed to attempt to control the physiological response in the absence of feedback, both in the clinic and the natural environment; this is called *self-control*. For the treatment of chronic pain, EMG and skin temperature are the most frequently monitored physiological responses. More recently, studies suggest that EMG biofeedback may be useful in the treatment of such chronic pain as low back pain (Flor, Haag, Turk, & Kohler, 1983), although placebo-controlled studies (Bush, Ditto, & Feuerstein, 1985) suggest a strong nonspecific effect of such techniques.

### Relaxation Training

Another treatment that attempts to modulate the pain experience is relaxation training, which generally uses an adaptation of Jacobsen's progressive muscle relaxation procedure. As discussed in Chapter 7, most variations of muscle relaxation training involves progressively tensing and then relaxing major muscle groups in the body, particularly the muscles thought to be associated with the chronic pain problem. The patient continues practicing the relaxation procedure until he or she can relax all the muscles in the body through the recall of the relaxed state. The goal then is to teach the patient to discriminate between tensed and relaxed muscles, so that the patient can keep relaxed the muscles that are thought to cause muscular skeletal pain or contribute to pain associated with some other type of health problem when tense. The relaxation approach has been used with a variety of chronic pain problems, including temporal mandibular joint pain (TMJ), back pain, arthritis, muscle contraction headache, and migraine. It has been found that relaxation training can provide significant pain relief for both migraine and muscle-contraction headache sufferers (Feuerstein & Gainer, 1982). Electromyogram levels and the patient's self-report of pain seem to be significantly decreased for back, TMJ, and arthritic pain by relaxation training (Linton, 1982). There are experimental design problems with most of the studies reviewed, and better controlled investigations should be conducted. It should be noted that activity level is not typically assessed in studies of relaxation for chronic benign pain. A recent clinical investigation of relaxation training effects in the management of chronic pain was reported by Linton and Melin (1983). The investigators compared the combination of rehabilitation plus intensive training in relaxation skills, with one group receiving regular rehabilitation treatment only and a second control group of patients who were waiting for treatment. The patients were chronic pain patients in a physical rehabilitation unit at a major hospital. Treatment was conducted on an outpatient basis. The "regular rehabilitation" treatment included physical and occupational training and frequent consultations with social work and medical staff. Patients experienced a variety of chronic pain problems in addition to headache as the primary problem. Although the groups were relatively small, the results indicated that the rehabilitation plus relaxation group demonstrated a significantly greater change than either control group on subjective pain, medication intake, activity (distance cycled), and overall patient evaluation of treatment. The decrease in pain report was approximately 28%. Note that the treatment did not eliminate pain. This latter finding is important to emphasize. The various biobehavioral treatments are associated with the reductions in pain and an increase in activity, but typically do not totally eliminate the pain.

The Turner (1982) study comparing cognitive-behavioral group therapy with group progressive relaxation training for chronic low back pain discussed in Chapter 9 is a well-controlled investigation of the effects of relaxation therapy on chronic pain. Results indicated a general superiority of the cognitive-behavioral treatment. The cognitive treatment group maintained post-treatment improvement in pain intensity; the relaxation group had an *increase* in pain ratings. However, at one and one-half to two years following treatment, *both* groups had greatly de-creased health care use and pain intensity compared to pretreatment. These findings illustrate the need to consider multiple aspects or mea-sures of pain and disability and suggest that relaxation therapy may exert equivalent effects on certain measures on long-term follow-up. Yet, without the absence of a no-treatment control group, it is difficult to rule out alternative explanations for these results.

## Hypnosis

Hypnosis is also used to modulate the pain experience. The actual hypnotic procedure typically varies, depending on therapist or patient, but the goals are generally similar. Goals can include altering the pa-tient's negative perception of the pain, shifting it to a neutral or a positive one, enhancing positive self-statements, improving health-re-lated attitudes, and instilling feelings of deep relaxation potentially in-compatible with certain pain behaviors. The therapist will often instruct the patient in self-hypnosis. Clinical investigations, which are mostly case studies, have not provided a sufficient data base for meaningful evaluation. Since these group studies lack relevant controls and also fail to report independent evaluations of hypnotic susceptibility, such stud-ies can only suggest the use of hypnotic techniques for low back pain, migraine, cancer pain, burn patients, and childbirth pain (Barber, 1982).

In a review of the literature on hypnosuggestive procedures in the treatment of clinical pain, Barber (1982) highlights several of the more recent findings from laboratory research on hypnosis and pain relief that have implications for clinical work. These findings include the follow-ing: (1) subjects typically show as much pain reduction when provided with suggestions for reduced pain under waking conditions as under hypnosis; (2) many types of suggestions (without hypnotic procedures) are generally effective in reducing laboratory pain (e.g., reinterpret pain-ful sensations as numbness), (3) subjects highly responsive to a variety of general hypnosuggestions (e.g., arm becoming light and rising) are more responsive to pain reduction suggestions; and (4) when subjects are provided with pain reduction suggestions, either in a hypnosis or nonhypnosis condition, they typically attempt to distract themselves from the pain and attempt, when they do attend to the pain, to rein-terpret it as less bothersome, less painful, or less catastrophic. These findings have been incorporated into the clinical use of hypnosis in pain relief. It should be emphasized that hypnosis, as with all the techniques discussed, is rarely the exclusive treatment for pain management.

Another approach for modulating the pain experience is instructing the patient to focus his attention away from the pain through a variety of alternate responses. Hobbies, interesting activities, or nonpain-related thoughts can be used to help the patient redirect attention away from pain.

Approaches directed at pain refocusing are often associated with the cognitive approach to pain. This approach hypothesizes that the pain experience is mediated by cognition. Thus, if the pain is reinterpreted at the cognitive level, changes in pain experience, as well as in pain behavior, should be observed. At present, only a handful of poorly controlled studies have examined cognitive strategies for the reduction of *chronic* pain (Linton, 1982). However, the initial reports are promising. A comprehensive therapeutic framework that incorporates cognitive strategies, proposed by Turk and associates, will be discussed in greater detail in the next section.

A third approach to the treatment of chronic pain, and one that is not as well defined or studied as the other approaches, is modification of the patient's mood. Anger, anxiety, and depression are often reported by chronic pain patients. It is thought that these negative emotions interact with the patient's pain problem, resulting in an increased pain experience (cf. gate control theory). Therapies aimed at reducing anxiety, depression, or controlling anger are frequently used in clinical practice. Supportive therapy, as well as more direct approaches, are used. Some direct approaches to decreasing anxiety are systematic densensitization or stress management; a cognitive-behavioral approach that can be used to decrease depression; problem solving; and assertiveness training to help patients who have difficulty with anger and irritability (see Chapters 7 and 9 for a more detailed discussion of these treatment approaches). These treatment strategies are usually combined with a cognitive-behavioral or multimodal treatment program, such as those offered by Pain Centers (discussed in a subsequent section). It is difficult to make a statement regarding the relative efficacy of anxiety, depression, or anger management in the treatment of chronic pain, although these represent common goals in the management of chronic pain.

## Cognitive-Behavioral Approach: Pain Inoculation

A cognitive-behavioral approach conceptualizes chronic pain problems in terms of coping skill deficits in either the cognitive or behavioral domains. The goal is to help the patient develop more adaptive cognitive and behavioral responses to the physical problem. When discussing the cognitive approach, the patient is taught to identify negative, habitual thoughts related to pain; recognize the connection between thoughts and consequent feelings and pain; substitute more adaptive thoughts; and use coping strategies (such as relaxation, distraction, imagery) to reduce suffering. Often in conjunction with these cognitive strategies, the patient is introduced to operant conditioning principles, and a program is established to reinforce nonpain-related behavior, such as increased activity, and extinction of pain-related behaviors, such as medication use (Turk *et al.*, 1983).

We have discussed several psychological treatment approaches to chronic pain. The approaches appear to be more effective than no treatment in reducing a number of target goals (pain behavior, experience of pain). Although these procedures are recognized as useful, in many Pain Centers treatments from a number of disciplines are combined and several health care providers are consulted (e.g., physical therapists, vocational counselors) in an attempt to provide a more comprehensive and integrative treatment regime for the chronic pain patient. The next section will describe this integrative treatment approach.

## INTEGRATIVE TREATMENT APPROACH: THE PAIN CENTER

Pain Centers, which have developed rapidly over the last decade attempt to treat pain patients through a multidisciplinary team approach. It is increasingly recognized that chronic pain is a complex phenomenon involving neurophysiological, behavioral, and psychological factors; this has led clinicians to assume that chronic pain is perhaps best treated using a combination of treatment approaches. Multimodal asessment of chronic pain is one goal of the Pain Center. Pain Centers typically offer psychological intervention, physical therapy, occupational therapy, and vocational assessment and counseling; a physician is consulted on the patient's physical health, medication usage, and withdrawal of pain medication. Psychological intervention can include one or more of the approaches described in the previous section, for example, an operant program, cognitive-behavioral therapy, and techniques to modulate the pain experience, such as self-hypnosis or relaxation training. Physical therapy can include teaching patients specific exercises to strengthen muscles and using transcutaneous electrical stimulation and massage. Occupational therapy can provide experiences, skills, and hobbies to help broaden the patient's interest, increase activity level, and direct attention away from the pain. Ideally, the Pain Center can be thought of as an integrative approach to treating chronic pain since the individual patient is evaluated and treated by considering physiological, behavioral, and psychological factors. Professionals in a Pain Center typically include a multidisciplinary team of physicians (anesthesiologist, neurologist, psychiatrist, and internist), psychologist, physical therapist, occupational therapist, and vocational counselor. A job placement center representative and/or the patient's attorney are often consulted. The typical pain patient referred for pain treatment is one with a long history of unsuccessful medical and surgical treatment for a chronic pain problem. The patient is usually treated in an inpatient setting or in an all day outpatient program (day treatment) for several weeks. Unfortunately, many clinics that call themselves Pain Centers are not multidisciplinary treatment centers and commonly offer the patient an unidisciplinary approach to the pain problem (for example, a clinic that simply offers relaxation and biofeedback training). Although there are over 800 Pain Centers in the United States and Canada, there are only a few published reports of treatment results, and many of these studies are poorly designed and lack proper experimental control.

Guck, Skultety, Meilman, and Dowd (1985) have recently provided an example of a controlled study evaluating the efficacy of a multidisciplinary pain management center by comparing 20 treated pain patients with 20 no-treatment control patients who met the program's entrance criteria, wanted to participate, but could not because they did not have insurance coverage. The four-week, multicomponent, inpatient treatment program consisted of (1) a gradual reduction and eventual elimination of all non-narcotic, and psychotropic pain medication, (2) a progressively increasing program of daily exercise and physical activity, and (3) an attempt at identification and resolution of psychosocial issues related to or caused by the pain situation, including group discussions, individual and family therapy, relaxation and biofeedback, vocational counseling, and work simulation. Sixty per cent of the treated patients, compared to none of the untreated patients, reported less interference with activities, more "uptime," lower pain levels, less depression, and fewer hospitalizations at one to five years follow-up. A greater number of treated patients reported being employed, with fewer using either narcotic or psychotropic medication, at follow-up compared to untreated patients. The results of the controlled study by Guck *et al.*, therefore, indicate the potential long-term benefits to be derived from treatment at a multidisciplinary pain center.

Reports of clinics using an integrative approach tend, in general, to report positive results, particularly in terms of increasing physical activity and return to work, for *some* patients. An attempt is being made to identify patients early in the evaluation or treatment program who may become dissatisfied, drop-out, or not respond favorably, so that clinicians can make appropriate referrals or interventions at a different level with potential treatment failures. Ideally, a Pain Center will incorporate several disciplines and include multimodal assessment and treatment. Follow-up studies that report behavioral, psychological, and physiological outcome to the treatment program and compare those who succeed with those who do not over long periods of time are necessary. Now, let us shift our attention from chronic to recurrent pain, using headache as a model.

## RECURRENT HEADACHE: A BIOBEHAVIORAL APPROACH

The Ad Hoc Committee on Classification of Headache (1962) has differentiated 15 types of headache. As discussed in the first section on theories of pain, any type of persistent pain problem, including head pain, can be exacerbated or maintained by psychological factors. Psychological factors appear to play a considerable role in at least three major headache types: migraine headaches; muscle-contraction headaches; and mixed headaches, a combination of muscle and migraine symptoms (Adams, Feuerstein, & Fowler, 1980). This section will highlight the issues associated with recurrent pain and illustrate a psychobiological approach to such pain.

### Description

*Migraine headache,* as proposed by the Ad Hoc Committee of the Classification of Headache (1962), has two diagnostic categories, classic and common. In the classic form, the headache consists of two phases. During the first phase, prodromal symptoms are usually reported. Prodromal symptoms are symptoms that usually occur between 10 and 30 minutes before the onset of the headache. Common prodromes are scotoma (visual blind spots, flashing lights, or fortification spectra), abdominal pain, vertigo, and parathesias of the face or the hands (Waters & O'Connor, 1971).

During the second phase, the head aches. The headache phase is characterized by the onset of a throbbing or pulsating unilateral pain. The pain occurs most often in the temporal, orbital, or occipital cranial regions. Head pain is usually accompanied by nausea, photophobia, and constipation or diarrhea. Edema is often seen around the afflicted area of the head. This edema may exacerbate the pain and leave the area sensitive after the headache has ended.

Common migraine headache is similar to classic migraine in the type of pain experienced. The pain, described as pulsating or throbbing, is not well localized and is often bilateral. Nausea and vomiting may accompany the headache, but prodromal symptoms are not experienced.

Severe migraine can immobilize the patient, and most migraine patients report one to four headaches a month, which persist for less than 24 hours.

The *muscle-contraction* (or *tension*) headache, the most common type of headache, consists of a constant, nonpulsating, bilateral pain. The pain usually occurs in either the frontal or suboccipital areas of the head and then may radiate to the entire head. Head pain may vary from mild to severe and is often reported as a "bandlike pressure around the head." Headache frequency can vary from daily to once a year. *Mixed headaches* are characterized by a combination of symptoms from both the vascular and muscle-contraction headaches.

The remainder of this section on chronic headaches will discuss epidemiological, psychological, and psychophysiological aspects of migraine, muscle-contraction, and mixed headache. It will conclude with a psychological model of chronic headache, in an attempt to demonstrate an integrative approach to understanding this medical disorder.

## Epidemiological Research

Chronic headache is one of the most common chronic pain disorders and is reported by people of all races, ages, social class, and intellectual and educational levels: 10 to 30% of the population is thought to be affected. Studies of migraine headache in the general population reported varied results, ranging from less than 8 to more than 25% (Feuerstein & Gainer, 1982). Some factors that may account for these results are problems with diagnostic criteria and measurement; patient not contacting physician; poor response rate; and cross-cultural differences. In an attempt to overcome some of these difficulties, three epidemiological surveys involving 1,971 men and 2,237 women were conducted by Waters and O'Connor (1975). These studies indicate that the incidence of migraine is between 23 and 29% in women and 15 to 20% in men. A similar incidence of migraine, 23% in a sample of women age 15 to 44, was reported by Markush, Karp, Heyman, and O'Fallon (1975).

Based on descriptions of symptoms on a headache questionnaire, 170 males and 326 females were classified as having one of four types of headaches (classic migraine, common migraine, muscle contraction, and mixed) (Philips, 1977). Results revealed that, for the men, 1.6% had classic migraine, 12% migraine, 87% muscle contraction and 0.6% mixed. For the women, 3% had classic migraine, 18% common migraine, 77% muscle contraction, and 3% mixed. Philips reported no sex difference, yet other investigators have indicated that about 75% of subjects with tension headaches are female (Lance, 1978).

Chronic headache is one of the most common disorders seen in pediatric practice. The incidence of migraine is approximately 4% to 5% of children between the ages of 7 and 15 years (Feuerstein & Gainer,

1982). The prevalence of migraine increases with age and is rare under 2 years of age. Before puberty, the ratio changes, with more women than men reported as migraineurs (Waters & O'Connor, 1975; Thompson, 1980). The incidence of nonmigraine headache in children is approximately 13% to 15% for children between the ages of 7 and 15.

Epidemiological research is not only interested in determining the incidence of disease, but also in discovering factors that may predispose a person to, as well as those factors that may exacerbate, the disease.

Two factors have been studied as predispositional to migraine. One factor is a *genetic deficit,* manifested either as a peripheral cephalic vasomotor dysfunction in the temporal arteries (Dalessio, 1972) or a more central deficit in neurotransmission (Sicuteri, 1978). A migraineur's heightened physiological vulnerability, combined with such stressors as psychosocial problems, various foods, weather and hormonal changes, serves to activate the headache. Research strategies studying genetic predisposition have utilized family history or have taken a twin study approach, but the evidence in support of a genetic predisposition is minimal. Reports of a positive family history range from 10% to 71% across several studies involving large numbers of migraine patients and controls (Feuerstein & Gainer, 1982). Waters' (1971) approach was different, since he interviewed family members themselves rather than relying on the patient's report. Family incidence was 5.5% for a matched nonheadache control group and 10% for the migraine group.

Several twin studies again provide minimal positive data for a genetic predisposition. One of the larger studies reported data on 106 twin pairs (Ziegler, Hassenein, Harris, & Stewart, 1975). They used blood group, height, weight, and appearance to determine that 65 twin pairs were dizygotic and 51 were monozygotic. The combined data on family history and twin studies call into question the contribution of genetic factors in migraine headache.

The second predispositional factor associated with the development of headache is *psychosocial stress.* Most studies conceptualize psychosocial stress as important in exacerbating or triggering headache. Henryk-Gutt and Reese (1973) examined psychosocial stress as a potential predispositional factor in migraine and found that approximately 50% of their subjects reported that their migraines first began during a stressful period in their lives.

Factors that exacerbate or maintain chronic headache have been emphasized. Headache patients, and particularly migraine patients, will often report to clinicians that certain events seem to increase the frequency, duration, or intensity of their headaches. Although little systematic research has been done in this area, a few studies have looked at weather, hormonal changes, diet, sleep, and psychosocial stress in the exacerbation of chronic headache. Summaries of the findings of each of these factors are as follows.

*Weather.* An association has been thought to exist between certain weather conditions and muscle-contraction and migraine headaches. It was reported that 20% to 30% of a population exposed to the *Sharav* (sudden hot dry winds) in Israel experienced migraine attacks (Sulman, Levy, Lewy, Pfeifer, Superstine, & Tal, 1974). Wilkinson and Woodrow (1979) evaluated the relationship of a number of weather conditions (wind velocity and direction, barometric pressure, temperature, and humidity) to the onset of headaches. They studied this relationship with a heterogeneous group of 310 headache patients, including migraine and muscle-contraction headaches and migraine neuralgia. No significant relationships were observed between headache onset and the weather conditions. However, a consistent time of onset (6:00 A.M.–9:00 A.M.) was observed from these data. Further research in this area appears warranted, especially since recent psychophysiological findings suggest a relationship between physiological reactivity and weather conditions (relative humidity) in nonclinical subjects (Waters, Koresko, Rossie, & Hackley, 1979). This latter study also illustrates the use of psychophysiology to help explain an epidemiological finding.

*Sleep.* Many migraineurs report awaking in the morning with a headache, and this is consistent with the Wilkinson and Woodrow (1979) report of early morning headache onset. This clinical observation has been supported by evidence of a possible relationship between migraine onset, rapid eye movement (REM sleep), plasma serotonin levels (Dexter & Riley, 1975), and plasma catecholamine levels (Hsu, Crisp, Kalucy, Koval, Chen, Carruthers, & Zilkha, 1977). Basically, what occurs is that three hours before awakening with migraine, plasma norepinephrine levels rise, whereas with the onset of REM, plasma serotonin levels fall. Both studies reported that migraine onset was closely associated with REM. If this is so, then changes in norepinephrine and serotonin preceding or concomitant with REM may initiate the vasomotor pattern associated with migraine. Supporting the effect of REM on migraine onset is the finding that some drugs that are used to treat migraine (e.g., tricyclic antidepressants, barbiturates, caffeine, and amphetamines) decrease REM sleep, but do not increase stages III and IV slow-wave sleep.

*Hormonal Fluctuations.* Migraine in females frequently begins at menarche, improves during pregnancy, is aggravated by oral contraceptives, and disappears with menopause (Whitty, Hockoday, & Whitty, 1966). In males, migraine frequently improves during adolescence. Observations such as these imply sex hormone involvement, for example, estrogen, progesterone, and perhaps prolactin. Brown (1977) suggests that normal hormonal changes influence the occurrence of headaches in the genetically predisposed individual. Other investigators have reported that migraine frequency increases with decreasing serum estrogen levels. Graham (1981) hypothesizes that histamines, as well as antihistamines, increase during pregnancy. An alternative hypothesis to a direct effect is offered by Stein (1980), who suggests that hormones may act indirectly to influence the metabolism of such vasodilating substances as serotonin. In sum, several *theories* describe the role hormones may play in the exacerbation of migraine. No one theory has been adequately researched; thus, it is difficult to draw conclusions on the influence hormones have on the production of migraine headaches.

*Diet.* Approximately 25% of patients report the onset of migraine headache after the ingestion of various foods. The most commonly reported foods contain the vasoactive amines tyramine and phenylethylamine. Experimental studies in which migraine patients have been given either tyramine or phenylethylamine have produced conflicting findings. For example, Harrington, Horn, and Wilkinson (1970) reported a response to tyramine (125 mg) and virtually no placebo response. In contrast, Moffett, Swash, and Scott (1972), using a double blind design, found no differences between tyramine and lactose on headache incidence.

Medina and Diamond (1978) took an interesting approach by comparing three diets in a group of 24 patients. Diet A included items high in tyramine or other vasoactive substances and suggested avoiding tyramine-free foods. Diet B had no vasoactive items. Diet C had no restrictions. Twenty-four subjects were randomly assigned to their first diet. Once they completed the first diet, they were assigned the other two in sequence. Results suggested that foods containing tyramine and phenlethylamine were not related to an increase in headache attacks.

A number of other dietary factors have been implicated in vascular headaches; these include monosodium glutamate (the Chinese restaurant syndrome), transient and reactive hypoglycemia, sodium nitrate (contained in most cured meats to perserve them and to maintain red color), and alcohol (Feuerstein & Gainer, 1982). Although food appears to play some role in the etiology of migraine, recent research suggests the role is minimal.

*Stress.* Psychosocial stress is often thought to be associated with migraine and muscle-contraction headaches. However, there is little empirical evidence to support such an association. In the 1950s, Wolff and colleagues conducted observational studies with migraine patients in which they noted that headaches could be triggered by discussing personally relevant stressful material. Later studies relied on self-report by patients. In a study by Selby and Lance (1960), 67% of a group of 388 migraine patients reported "emotions" as initiating the onset of unilateral headaches. Henryk-Gutt and Reese (1973) took a more detailed approach, when they requested 100 migraine patients to monitor their headache activity, along with any triggering factors, for a 2-month period. There was no difference in the reported daily exposure to emotional stress between the migraine group and a matched nonheadache control group. Of significance, though, is that emotional stress was reported as a precipitating factor in 54% of headache attacks. In a third study, an epidemiological analysis of headache, subjects reported that the most common trigger for headache (type unspecified) was stress (Nikiforow & Hokkanen, 1978). Stress was indicated as responsible for the headache by 46% of the women and 35% of the men.

On face value, these studies point to stress as a likely trigger factor in headache. Caution must be taken, however, as no cause–effect relationship can be tested through self-report and large-scale epidemiological studies.

Factors that may predispose a person to headache or exacerbate headache have been reviewed and, given the state of empirical data available, one cannot draw firm conclusions. What about the factors that maintain chronic headaches? It is no surprise to find even less information available here. It has been suggested that *recurrent* exposure to a stressful environment, cyclic variations in hormonal levels, or a number of social learning factors can prolong the occurrence of chronic headache (Feuerstein & Gainer, 1982; Fordyce, 1976; Wooley, Blackwell, & Winget, 1978).

There is some preliminary data that social learning factors may be important in the maintenance of chronic headache. Specifically, certain pain behavior (e.g., verbal pain complaints, inactivity, frequent medication use) may be maintained through interaction of the patient and the environment. The reinforcing aspects of this interaction, such as attention for symptoms, the pleasant effects of some pain medication, and avoidance of unpleasant environmental demands; can increase the probability of later pain, and the problem is maintained. As reviewed in earlier sections of this chapter, preliminary support comes from two areas of research: (1) environmental factors have been reported in the context of more traditional chronic-pain problems, such as low back pain (Fordyce, 1976; Keefe & Block, 1982) and (2) patients report muscle-contraction headache in the absence of heightened skeletal muscle activity (Philips, 1978) and migraine headache in the absence of temporal artery vasodilation (Feuerstein, Bortolussi, Houle, & Labbe, 1983). These sources of information indirectly support the possible existence of such alternative social learning factors. A direct social learning analysis of pain behavior associated with either migraine or muscle-contraction headache could prove useful in enhancing our knowledge of behavioral factors maintaining headaches.

If we utilize the model of epidemiological research outlined in Chapter 3, the status of identifying risk factors for chronic headache is still in its initial phase. Systematic analyses employing matched-cohort studies or experimental studies should be conducted to identify relative risk ratios of these factors and the research on hypertension and coronary heart disease can be useful models for the epidemiology of chronic headache.

## Psychological Theories and Research

Historically, health care professionals have thought that psychological factors play a role in the development of headaches (Adams, Feuerstein, & Fowler, 1980; Dalessio, 1972). The migraine patient is described as rigid, sensitive, ambitious, unable to express anger, and overly cautious in interpersonal relationships. Muscle-contraction headaches are thought to result from tension and anxiety and are particularly prevalent in neurotic patients. Although clinical lore emphasizes personality and psychopathology, the empirical data reported to date on the role of psychological factors have been conflictual at best.

Studies of the psychological characteristics of muscle-contraction headache patients have employed standard psychological evaluation with few appropriate control groups. Investigations using the Minnesota Multiphasic Personality Inventory (MMPI) report elevations on hypochrondriasis (Hs) and hysteria (Hy) scales for muscle-contraction headache subjects. Elevated Hs and Hy scores are typical of individuals in pain, and, thus, this finding is not surprising (Sternbach, 1974). Philips (1976) compared groups of migraine, muscle-contraction and mixed headache patients in the general population on three personality dimensions (extraversion, neuroticism, psychoticism), as measured by the Eysenck Personality Questionnaire (EPQ). Philips reports that migraine patients are undistinguishable on EPQ scores. The data presented do not support the assumption that muscle-contraction headache patients are more emotionally labile than the general population.

Several investigations have searched for a typical "migraine personality," but no consistent or compelling findings have emerged. A variety of original, unstandardized questionnaires, as well as standardized measures (Wechsler Adult Intelligence Scale, MMPI, EPQ, Maudsley Personality Inventory, Cornell Medical Index, Buss-Durkee Scales of Hostile Attitude Behavior and Guilt, Rathus Assertiveness Schedule, and Beck Depression Inventory) have been used to study the migraine personality. An extensive review of the literature by Harrison (1975) indicates the absence of empirical data supporting a personality disorder or deficit for migraine patients. The only consistent findings, elevated Hs and Hy scores on the MMPI, are the same for migraine patients as for muscle-contraction headache patients. Thus, the hypothesis of inability to express anger, ridigity, and ambition as typical personality characteristics of migraine patients is not supported.

Researchers, disillusioned by the traditional trait approach, are now exploring other models, for example, a situation or trait-by-situation framework or one examining the relationship between stress, coping skills, and chronic headache.

### Hemodynamic and Biochemical Research

In the early 1950s, Wolff and colleagues specified that a complex change in the extracranial arteries preceded migraine headache. It was observed that 36 to 72 hours before a headache, the temporal artery undergoes a series of changes. The phases include an initial vasodilation, followed by increased lability (12 to 36 hours before the headache), and then by vasoconstriction 6 hours before the final phase of vasodilation and report of head pain. Figure 12-17 provides a schematic of the temporal artery changes proposed by the two- and four-stage models.

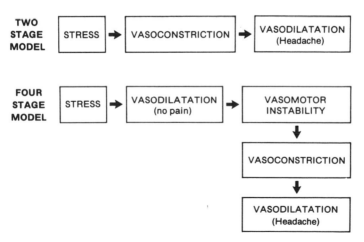

FIGURE 12-17. Schematic of two- and four-stage models of migraine. Stress is used as an example. The models hypothesize a variety of triggers.

The hemodynamic process involved in the *two-stage model* has been more widely recognized. This model includes an initial vasoconstriction followed by vasodilation and headache. Graham and Wolff (1938) first observed the vasodilation phase by recording pulsations of the extra-cranial temporal and/or occipital artery on the afflicted side during headache. Vasodilation was observed with the onset of head pain, and the injection of ergotamine tartrate, which is known to constrict smooth muscle, leads to a fairly abrupt termination of the migraine attack and also reduces by an average of 50% the amplitude of pulsations in the arteries. Intensity of headache has also been also associated with increased pulsation amplitude. Recent studies of cerebral blood flow in migraine, however, employ more sophisticated technology. In particular, a $^{133}$Xe-injection technique permits the quantification of regional cerebral blood flow (rCBF) and extracranial flow. Some investigators have found regional reduction of gray matter blood flow during the prodromal phase of migraine, with consistent increases in flow during the headache. Additional data on extracerebral flow in normal, migraine, and cluster headache subjects during different headache phases and under various experimental conditions have indicated that extra-cerebral blood volume and/or flow was significantly greater during the headache phase of both headache subjects, compared to normal subjects at rest.

In general, most of the CBF studies support the hemodynamic changes associated with the two-stage model of migraine. However, methodological limitations of these studies, such as sampling biases and small number of subjects, must not be overlooked, as well as occasional reports of contrary evidence. For example, 16 cases were reported in which intramuscular injection of ergotamine tartrate had no effect on rCBF (Hachinski, Norris, Edmeads, & Cooper, 1978). Also, the rCBF for the three migraine patients did not change during the prodromal or headache phase. Hachinski *et al.* suggest that there may be considerable variation within and between individuals in the cerebral hemodynamics of headache.

Although the evidence for hemodynamic changes before and during headache is substantial extracranial vasodilation is not sufficient to explain the headache experience. Two sources of data suggest that extra-cranial vasodilation may be necessary, but not sufficient to produce head pain. First, bilateral hyperpulsation of the temporal arteries can be observed during *unilateral* migraine headaches (Graham & Wolff, 1938), and second, extracranial distension equal to or greater than that recorded during headache attacks has been observed during headache-free periods (Dalessio, 1972). Chemical substances have been implicated in both arterial distention and a lowering of the pain threshold. Among these, the serotonin and norepinephrine hypotheses have been more widely studied and supported.

The *serotonin hypothesis,* in which released serotonin affects both the extracranial vessels and the pain threshold, is outlined by Fanchamps (1974). It is postulated that the blood platelets release serotonin at the beginning of an attack, as histamine proteolytic enzymes are released from cells. An increase in capillary permeability promotes the transudation of a plasmakinin into the vascular wall, and both plasmakinin and serotonin reduce the pain threshold of the arterial wall receptors. Also, as the plasma serotonin level falls, the tonus of extracranial vessels is reduced, and capillary constriction induces a passive extracranial dilation. Serotonin has a vasoconstrictive effect on extracranial arteries and a vasodilative effect on capillaries. Thus, the two necessary physiological changes thought to be involved in the headache experience are present: extracranial arterial distension and a lowered pain threshold.

A second biochemical theory implicates norepinephrine in migraine headache production. It is suggested that the increased release of norepinephrine from nerve endings to the affected vessels causes the vasoconstriction of the prodromal phase. Following this vasoconstriction, a rebound vasodilation, and concomitant pain, occurs. Research findings in support of the norepinephrine hypothesis comes from several areas (Johnson, 1978). These include (1) adrenegic vasoconstriction innervation of the larger cerebral vessels, (2) decreased CBF in humans or induced scotomata following an intravenous infusion of norepinephrine, (3) apparent changes in the diameter of cerebral vessels following electrical stimulation of their innervation in man and baboons, (4) increased concentration of plasma norepinephrine and dopamine β-hydroxylase during the prodromal phase, and (5) reversal of norepinephrine-induced cerebral vasoconstriction by adrenoceptor blockade (e.g., ergotamine).

The physiological basis of muscle-contraction headaches is not well known. It is often thought that environmental or psychological stressors induce sustained contraction of the muscles in the head, neck, and shoulders, as well as a relative ischemia in the involved muscles. Some additional, possibly inherited factor is thought by Lance (1978) to be involved, rather than just an inability to relax these muscles. Lance suggests that potential factors contributing to this disorder include a vascular reactivity in the muscles of the scalp and neck, along with an accumulation of pain-provoking substances or a central deficit of inhibitory neurotransmittor substances.

The muscles seem to be tense in muscle-contraction headache, although it is unclear whether such tension is secondary or primary to the pain (Dalessio, 1972). Vasoconstriction of scalp vessels in tension headache subjects suggests a relative ischemia in the involved muscles. The vasoconstriction could be directly associated with the pain, particularly because such substances as the dilator alcohol or constrictor ergotamine can relieve or exacerbate, respectively, the headache. Other workers have suggested that a central deficiency of monoamine transmitters might be involved, which would disrupt the antinociceptive system (Sicuteri, 1977).

### Psychophysiological Research

A psychophysiological approach to headache attempts to address a number of questions including (1) whether headache sufferers have different physiological responses to nonaversive and aversive stimuli, compared to nonheadache controls; (2) whether different headache types differ in terms of psychophysiological responsivity; and (3) how the physiological and psychological activity preceding and during a headache can be described. The primary focus of psychophysiological research has been the identification of possible mechanisms linking exposure to stressors to headache onset and exacerbation. For migraine patients, research has focused on temporal artery lability and/or the phasic temporal artery vasomotor response (i.e., dilation or constriction). With muscle-contraction headache, the focus has been on the skeletal muscle system.

Differences in certain psychophysiological measures between headache patients and no-headache controls and between headache types have been reported in many studies. However, a critical examination of the methodology used in these studies do not allow definitive conclusions to be drawn regarding psychophysiological mechanisms of headache. For instance, before reliable measures can be taken during a nonaversive or aversive situation, a stable baseline of the physiological responses must be obtained, and this often requires that the subject sit quietly for about 15 minutes before baseline and stressor conditions are measured; this has rarely been done. Other methodological problems include small sample size, lack of information on inclusion and exclusion criteria, no or poor matching for key demographic variables, the use of inappropriate measurement and analyses procedures, a limited use of control groups, and usually the measurement of just one physiological response system or one stimulus condition (Andrasik, Blanchard, Arena, Saunders, & Barron, 1982). Andrasik *et al.*'s (1982) review of investigations since 1970 indicate that only six studies are sufficiently rigorous, methodologically. Three of the psychophysiological studies found that migraine patients have *higher* levels of forehead muscle tension during rest *and* stress, two of these studies found that migraine patients have higher muscle tension than muscle-contraction patients, and that muscle-contraction patients have higher muscle tension than controls. The other three studies reported no muscle tension differences among controls and headache groups. Of the three studies that measured cephalic blood flow, one reported no difference between headache groups, one indicated that migraine patients were slower to return to prestress vasomotor levels than controls, and one found that the headache groups respond with similar vasomotor activity, with controls revealing an opposite pattern. Three studies that employed other measures, including hand surface temperature, finger blood volume, heart rate, blood pressure, and electrodermal activity, reported no differences among headache groups and controls during stress and rest. In sum, conflictual findings occur in even those studies with reasonably acceptable methodology.

In response to these findings, Andrasik *et al.* (1981) attempted to control for previous methodological difficulties in a study of 138 individuals with recurrent headache (migraine, 39; muscle contraction, 62; mixed, 37) and 58 individuals with no chronic headache problems. All groups were studied under a variety of experimental conditions (rest, self-control, and stressor). Physiological recordings were obtained for forehead and forearm EMG, temporal artery blood flow, hand surface temperature, heart rate, and skin resistance level. The findings indicated no group differences or consistent group by condition interactions. In support of these results, Feuerstein, Bush, and Corbisiero (1982) observed no difference for migraine, muscle-contraction, mixed headache, and nonheadache control subjects in temporal artery activity when aversive pain stimuli were applied to the index finger. Although there were no differences between the groups, all the groups generated a pattern of digital blood volume pulse, frontal EMG, and spontaneous resistence responses indicative of a general arousal response. Temporal artery dilation also occurred to the aversive stimuli. In another recent, well-controlled study, different and positive results were obtained for headache groups and nonheadache controls (Cohen, Williamson, Monguillat, Hutchinson, & Gottlieb, 1983). Using discriminant analysis, the headache groups were differentiated from the nonheadache control groups on two conditions after a period of relaxation and as a function of psychophysiological responsiveness to a stressor (26 questions of increasing difficulty). The stress condition also differentiated the various headache groups. The headache groups demonstrated a higher level of arousal and were more responsive to stress than the controls. However, the response pattern of the headache groups differed in the stress condition, with muscle-contraction subjects demonstrating higher frontal EMG and classic and mixed headache groups responding with greater cardiovascular responses (heart rate).

Another approach to studying headache from a psychophysiological standpoint is to measure stressors or one possible outcome of a stressor (i.e., subjective distress and physiological activity before and during a headache). In an attempt to determine the relationship among temporal artery activity, pain, and anxiety/stress in migraine, the present authors monitored daily temporal artery, frontal EMG, systemic blood pressure, peripheral temperature, heart rate, and anxiety levels for four days preceding a typical migraine attack and then during the headache (Feuerstein, Bortolussi, Houle, & Labbe, 1983). The subjects were 12 female migraineurs. The results indicated the presence of an increased variability in the right temporal artery *three* days preceding the migraine, but no change in general autonomic and skeletal muscle measures. Considerable individual differences in temporal artery amplitude were observed, necessitating an analysis of individual patients; this revealed a general pattern of dilation three days before the attack and constriction the day before the attack. Stress, as measured by the State-Trait Anxiety Inventory—state form, increased on the day of headache. Elevations in anxiety level four days before the attack were associated with the increased temporal artery variability observed three days before the attack. However, anxiety experienced on the headache day was not related to changes in temporal artery amplitude variability or pain. Finally, report of pain site (i.e., left or right temporal area) was not consistently associated with temporal artery dilation. In summary, this study provides preliminary evidence for a relationship between temporal artery variability and stress, with stress possibly occurring several days before the headache. The findings also suggest the possible involvement of central mechanisms in the experience of the headache itself. This study provides a model for future studies on chronic recurrent headache and stress. Physiological responses were sampled over time and attempts were made to assess the impact of stressors in the natural environment, as well as recording data during the headache itself. It would be interesting to conduct similar studies with larger samples and other stress measures and include muscle-contraction headache, mixed headache, and nonheadache controls, perhaps using the ambulatory monitoring equipment discussed in Chapter 4.

Before the traditional psychophysiological approach to the study of headache (i.e., single recording in laboratory) can be considered fruitless, several additional problems should be considered. Although the more recent laboratory studies are better controlled, the generalization of findings to the natural environment is questionable, since the stressors presented may not be representative of the stressors experienced by the subjects and are usually measured only once. It has been increasingly recognized that a stressor for one person may not be a stressor for another person, for such reasons as coping style and type of social environment (see Chapter 5). Also, the physiological responses in these studies were not sampled over time or when the subject was moving freely and interacting with his environment. At the methodological level, studies can be improved with greater use of personally relevant stressors and coordinated laboratory and ambulatory monitoring of physiological reactivity in the natural environment.

We have examined epidemiological, biochemical, hemodynamic, and psychophysiological research areas and theories. Each area has provided some insight into understanding chronic headache, but no one area can account for all the phenomena seen in chronic headache patients. An integrative approach that combines these areas in a more comprehensive way may provide a useful model for the investigation of chronic headache.

## An Integrative Perspective

In proposing an alternative model of chronic headache, we need to consider several factors to integrate our approach. First, the approach must account for a dynamic situational rather than a static or trait-like framework of the headache process and the individual involved. Second, in considering the individual patient, we need to evaluate several levels of functioning and explain each level's contribution to the production of headache. This includes cognitions, behaviors, mood, and physiology. These aspects of the individual should be thought of not only as stimuli related to the onset of headache, but as responses as well. The responses can be either adaptive or contribute further to the disorder. Third, we must consider the influence of the environment, both in terms of operant factors and exposure to stressors. Pain behavior can be influenced by both subtle and obvious environmental conditioning. The possible influence of stress has been noted, and an understanding of how major life changes and daily "hassles and uplifts" contribute to chronic headache is needed.

For migraine headache, any explanation of the role of behavioral, cognitive, and emotional factors in triggering the onset of or maintaining the headache must take into account current pathophysiological models of migraine. Although several factors are assumed to be involved in the pathophysiology of migraine, the classic model hypothesizes that migraine is associated with a two-stage neurovascular process whereby extracranial and intracranial arteries proceed from a stable state to vas-

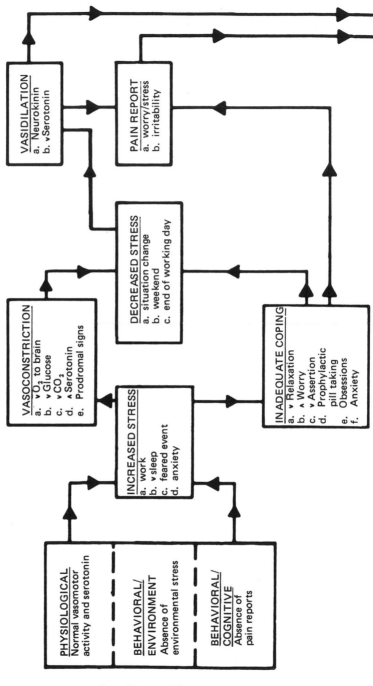

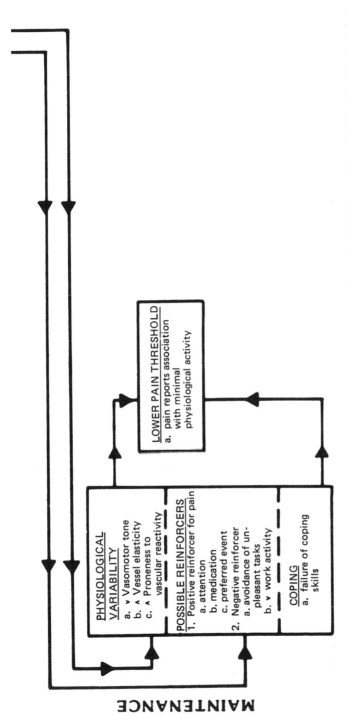

**FIGURE 12-18.** Psychobiological model of the development and maintenance of migraine headache. This theoretical model identifies the physiological factors in the top portion of the figure and the behavioral/environmental and behavioral/cognitive variables in the center and lower portions, respectively. From "Behavioral Treatment of Migraine Headaches" by P. M. Cinciripini, D. A. Williamson, and L. H. Epstein in the *Comprehensive Handbook of Behavioral Medicine* (Vol. 2, p. 210), edited by J. M. Ferguson and C. Barr Taylor. Copyright 1981 by Spectrum Publications, Inc. Reprinted by permission.

oconstriction, followed by vasodilation and pain. Environmental, cognitive, and behavioral events are thought to contribute to the development and maintenance of these neurovascular changes. Cinciripini, Williamson, and Epstein (1981) proposed a model based on Wolff's headache studies and Dalessio's (1980) unified theory of migraine. Cinciripini *et al.* note that, although earlier researchers assumed that psychological factors were important, they did not elaborate on the possible mechanisms involved. Figure 12-18 shows a theoretical model that attempts to specify how psychological and environmental factors interact with pathophysiology. The figure indicates that prolonged vasoconstriction and the absence of adequate coping skills may make it difficult for the headache sufferer to lower environmental stressors or alter physiological activity. Some event then occurs that lowers the stress level; this is associated with relaxation, a rebound vasodilation, and headache. Pain behavior and decreased coping ability are examples of two responses that may act to promote or maintain the headache. For example, on a physiological level, repeated migraine attacks may produce structural changes in the vessel wall or the pain threshold may be lowered biochemically. The model proposed by Cinciripini *et al.* integrates several levels of an individual's functioning, the environment, and the process whereby a response can serve to facilitate or inhibit the migraine process.

A similar model that also offers a more explicit account of the possible "dynamic" nature of this recurrent pain phenomenon is the four-stage model proposed by Tunis and Wolff (1953) and elaborated by Feuerstein and Gainer (1982); this was also discussed in Chapter 6. In a recent psychobiological model of health and illness, it is argued that temporal "windows," in which an individual's psychobiological responsivity to psychosocial factors may be greater, may exist, but that at other points in time the responsivity is equivalent to that of individuals not experiencing the disorder (Schwartz, 1983). This type of dynamic model is particularly appealing for an investigation of the role of stress on such recurrent pain phenomena as migraine, in which the pain period may vary considerably.

As discussed earlier, Tunis and Wolff (1953) proposed such a time-dependent or window model whereby temporal artery activity and mood followed a specific sequence of changes preceding the onset of the migraine headache. In their initial studies, they observed that the temporal artery undergoes a four-stage series of changes 36 to 72 hours before onset of the headache. These vascular modifications were accompanied by changes in the emotional state of the subjects, and it was suggested that these modifications were the "sequel of adaptive reactions to life stress" (p. 268). The sequence of psychophysiological change proposed by Tunis and Wolff was an early attempt at conceptualizing the effects of stress on migraine as a *dynamic* process, rather than as the consequence of a static deficit. Whichever pathophysiological model (the four-stage or two-stage) of headache proves to be more accurate, recent elaborations on these models help specify more clearly the role of environmental, cognitive, behavioral, and emotional factors. This psychobiological approach provides a more integrated framework for evaluation.

A psychobiological approach to muscle-contraction headache would have to consider issues similar to those raised in the discussion of migraine. In considering environmental influences on muscle-contraction headache, several operant conditioning theories have been proposed (Epstein & Cinciripini, 1981). This approach suggests that such psychological events as increased muscle tension can be regarded as antecedent stimuli that set the occasion for reporting pain. Pain behavior may then be reinforced by such environmental occurrences as attention, sympathy, and relief from responsibility. The patient may then be more likely to report pain at lower levels of physiological activity (i.e., less muscle tension). Although this model is plausible, and helps explain the frequent observation of a lack of correlation between muscle hyperactivity and pain in muscle-contraction headaches, other factors must be considered; these include the role of stress, coping abilities, depression, and the pathophysiology of muscle-contraction headaches, such as a possible CNS modulation of pain.

## SUMMARY

This final chapter reviewed various theories of pain with emphasis on the gate control theory, which is a major psychobiological model of pain. Specific psychological factors that have been demonstrated to influence the pain experience were also presented. Environmental/behavioral, cognitive/perceptual, and psychological/physiological mechanisms were reviewed. The findings related to endogenous pain modulation, a system that may help explain a number of findings related to psychological influences on pain, and pain treatment were also presented— the emphasis was on specific physiological regulatory processes within this so-called endorphin system. Our discussion of mechanisms concluded with the presentation of a potentially useful framework for future efforts at identifying psychobiological risk factors of chronic pain, using low back pain as a model problem.

Procedures used to measure clinical pain were discussed and specific approaches designed to measure pain severity, pain behavior, and pain experience were illustrated. A clinical evaluation from the authors' cases was presented. Common psychological approaches to chronic pain management were reviewed and Pain Centers were discussed.

The final section of the chapter reviewed the mechanisms of headache in detail, to illustrate a biobehavioral approach to these common pain disorders. This last section illustrates the several variants of headache, reviews suspected causal agents, discusses the pathophysiology, and provides examples of attempts within health psychology to explain how various psychological factors contribute to the pathophysiology of recurrent pain.

## REFERENCES

Ad Hoc Committee on Classification of Headache. (1962). Classification of headache. *Journal of the American Medical Association, 179,* 717–718.

Adams, H. E., Feuerstein, M., & Fowler, J. L. (1980). Migraine headache: Review of parameters, etiology, and intervention. *Psychological Bulletin, 87*(2), 217–237.

Adams, J. E. (1976). Naloxone reversal of analgesia produced by brain stimulation in the human. *Pain, 2,* 161–166.

Andrasik, F., Blanchard, E. B., Arena, J. G., Saunders, N. L., & Barron, K. D. (1982). Psychophysiology of recurrent headache: Methodological issues and new empirical findings. *Behavior Therapy, 13,* 407–429.

Bandura, A. (1977). *Social learning theory.* Englewood Cliffs, NJ: Prentice-Hall.

Barber, T. X. (1982). Hypnosuggestive procedures in the treatment of clinical pain. In T. Millon, C. Green, & R. Meagher (Eds.), *Handbook of clinical health psychology.* New York: Plenum Press.

Barsky, A. J., & Klerman, G. L. (1982). Overview: Hypochondriasis, bodily complaints and somatic styles. *American Journal of Psychiatry, 140*(3), 273–283.

Beecher, H. K. (1956). The subjective response and reaction to sensation: The reaction phase as the effective site for drug action. *American Journal of Medicine, 20,* 107–113.

Block, A. R., Kremer, E., F., & Gaylor, M. (1980a). Behavioral treatment of chronic pain: Variables affecting treatment efficacy. *Pain, 8*(3), 367–375.

Block, A. R., Kremer, E. F., & Gaylor, M. (1980b). Behavioral treatment of chronic pain: The spouse as a discriminative cue for pain behavior. *Pain, 9,* 243–252.

Blumer, D., & Heilbronn, M. (1982). Chronic pain as a variant of depressive disease: The pain-prone disorder. *The Journal of Nervous and Mental Disease, 170*(7), 381–406.

Bonica, J. J. (1979). Importance of the problem. In J. J. Bonica & V. Ventafridda (Eds.), *Advances in pain research and therapy* (Vol. 2). New York: Raven Press.

Brown, J. K. (1977). Migraine and migraine equivalents in children. *Developmental Medicine and Child Neurology, 19,* 683–692.

Bush, C., Ditto, B., & Feuerstein, M. (1985). A controlled evaluation of paraspinal EMG biofeedback in the treatment of chronic low back pain. *Health Psychology, 4,* 307–321.

Chapman, R. (1978). Pain: The perception of noxious events. In R. A. Sternbach (Ed.), *The psychology of pain.* New York: Raven Press.

Chen, A. C. N., & Dworkin, S. F. (1982). Human pain and evoked potentials. In J. Courjon, F. Mauguiere, & M. Revol (Eds.), *Clinical applications of evoked potentials in neurology.* New York: Raven Press.

Chen, A. C. N., Chapman, C. R., & Harkins, S. W. (1979). Brain evoked potentials are functional correlates of induced pain in man. *Pain, 6*(3), 365–374.

Cinciripini, P. M., Williamson, D. A., & Epstein, L. H. (1981). Behavioral treatment of migraine headaches. In J. M. Ferguson & C. Barr Taylor (Eds.), *The comprehensive handbook of behavioral medicine* (Vol. 2). New York: Spectrum Medical.

Cohen, R. A., Williamson, D. A., Monguillot, J. E., Hutchinson, P. C., Gottlieb, J., & Waters, W. F. (1983). Psychophysiological response patterns in vascular and muscle contraction headaches. *Journal of Behavioral Medicine, 6*(1), 93–107.

Craig, K. D. (1978). Social modeling influences on pain. In R. A. Sternbach (Ed.), *The psychology of pain*. New York: Raven Press.

Dalessio, D. J. (ed.). (1980). *Wolff's headache and other head pain*. New York: Oxford University Press.

Dexter, J. D., & Riley, T. L. (1975). Studies in nocturnal migraine. *Headache, 15*(1), 51–62.

Dowling, J. (1982). Autonomic indices and reactive pain reports on the McGill Pain Questionnaire. *Pain, 14,* 387–392.

Dowling, J. (1983). Autonomic measures and behavioral indices of pain sensitivity. *Pain, 16*(2), 193–200.

Edwards, P. W., Zeichner, A., Kuczmierczyk, A. R., & Boczkowski, J. (1985). Familial pain models: The relationship between family history of pain and current pain experience. *Pain, 21,* 379–384.

Epstein, L. H., & Cinciripini, P. M. (1981). Behavioral control of tension headaches. In J. M. Ferguson, & C. Barr Taylor (Eds.), *The comprehensive handbook of behavioral medicine* (Vol. 2). New York: Spectrum Medical.

Fanchamps, A. (1974). The role of humoral mediators in migraine headache. *Canadian Journal of Neurological Sciences, 1,* 189–195.

Feuerstein, M., & Gainer, J. (1982). Chronic headache: Etiology and management. In D. M. Doleys, R. L. Meredith, & A. R. Ciminero (Eds.), *Behavioral medicine: Assessment and treatment strategies*. New York: Plenum Press.

Feuerstein, M., Bush, C., & Corbisiero, T. (1982). Stress and chronic headache: A psychophysiological analysis of mechanisms. *Journal of Psychosomatic Research, 26,* 167–182.

Feuerstein, M., Bortolussi, L., Houle, M., & Labbe, E. (1983). Stress, temporal artery activity, and pain in migraine headache: A prospective analysis. *Headache, 23,* 296 304.

Feuerstein, M., Papciak, A. S. & Hoon, P. E. (1985). *Biobehavioral mechanisms of chronic low back pain*. Manuscript submitted for publication.

Feuerstein, M., Pistone, L., & Houle, M. (1985). *Ambulatory monitoring of paraspinal skeletal muscle, autonomic and mood-pain interaction in chronic low back pain*. Manuscript submitted for publication.

Flor, H., Haag, G., Turk, D. C., & Kohler, H. (1983). Efficacy of EMG biofeedback, pseudotherapy, and medical treatment for chronic rheumatic back pain. *Pain, 17,* 21–31.

Fordyce, W. E. (1976). *Behavioral methods for chronic pain and illness*. St. Louis: Mosby.

Fordyce, W. E. (1978). Learning processes in pain. In R. A. Sternbach (Ed.), *The psychology of pain*. New York: Raven Press.

Fordyce, W., Shelton, J., & Dundore, D. (1982). The modification of avoidance learning pain behaviors. *Journal of Behavioral Medicine, 4,* 405–414.

Goldstein, A. (1976). Opioid peptides endorphins in pituitary and brain. *Science, 193*(4258), 1081–1086.

Graham, J. (1981). The migraine connection. *Headache, 21,* 246.

Graham, J. R., & Wolff, H. G. (1938). Mechanism of migraine headache and action of ergotamine tartrate. *Archives of Neurology and Psychiatry, 39,* 737–763.

Guck, T. P., Skultety, F. M., Meilman, P. W., & Dowd, E. T. (1985). Multidisciplinary pain center follow-up study: Evaluation with a no-treatment control group. *Pain, 21,* 295–306.

Hachinski, V., Norris, J. W., Edmeads, J., & Cooper, P. W. (1978). Ergotamine and cerebral blood flow. *Stroke, 9,* 594–596.

Harrington, E., Horn, M., & Wilkinson, M. (1970). Further observations on the effects of tyramine. In *Background to Migraine: Third British Migraine Symposium.* London: Heineman.

Henryk-Gutt, R., & Reese, W. L. (1973). Psychological aspects of migraine. *Journal of Psychosomatic Research, 17,* 141–153.

Hsu, L. K. G., Crisp, A. H., Kalucy, R. S., Koval, J., Chen, C. N., Carruthers, M., & Zilkha, K. (1977). Early morning migraine. Nocturnal plasma levels of catecholamines, tryptophan, glucose, and free fatty acids and sleep encephalographs. *Lancet, 1*(8009), 447–451.

Johnson, E. S. (1978). A basis for migraine therapy—the autonomic theory reappraised. *Post-Graduate Medical Journal, 54,* 231–243.

Keefe, F. J., & Block, A. R. (1982). Development of an observation method for assessing pain behavior in chronic low back pain patients. *Behavior Therapy, 13,* 363–375.

Lance, J. W. (1978). *Mechanisms and management of headache* (3rd ed.). London: Butterworth.

Lefebvre, M. F. (1981). Cognitive distortion and cognitive errors in depressed psychiatric and low back pain patients. *Journal of Consulting and Clinical Psychology, 49*(4), 517–525.

Linton, S. J. (1982). A critical review of behavioural treatments for chronic benign pain other than headache. *British Journal of Clinical Psychology, 21*(Pt. 4), 321–337.

Linton, S. J., & Melin, L. (1983). Applied relaxation in the management of chronic pain. *Behavioral Psychotherapy, 11,* 337–350.

Markush, R. E., Karp, H. R., Heyman, A., & O'Fallon, W. M. (1975). Epidemiologic study of migraine symptoms in young women. *Neurology, 25*(5), 430–435.

Medina, J. L., & Diamond, S. (1978). The role of diet in migraine. *Headache, 18*(1), 31–34.

Melzack, R. (1983). The McGill Pain Questionnaire. In R. Melzack (Ed.), *Pain measurement and assessment.* New York: Raven Press.

Melzack, R., & Melinkoff, D. F. (1974). Analgesia produced by brain stimulation: Evidence of a prolonged onset period. *Experimental Neurology, 43,* 369–374.

Melzack, R., & Torgerson, W. S. (1971). On the language of pain. *Anesthesiology, 34,* 50–59.

Melzack, R., & Wall, P. D. (1965). Pain mechanisms: A new theory. *Science, 150,* 971–979.

Melzack, R., & Wall, P. D. (1982). *The challenge of pain.* New York: Basic Books.

Moffett, A., Swash, M., & Scott, D. F. (1972). Effect of tyramine in migraine: A double-blind study. *Journal of Neurology, Neurosurgery and Psychiatry, 35,* 496–499.

Naliboff, B. D., Cohen, M. J., Schandler, S. L., & Henrich, R. L. (1981). Signal detection and threshold measures for chronic back pain patients, chronic illness patients, and cohort controls to radiant heat stimuli. *Journal of Abnormal Psychology, 90,* 271–274.

Nikiforow, R., & Hokkanen, E. (1978). An epidemiological study of headache in an urban and a rural population in Northern Finland. *Headache, 18*(3), 137–145.

Peck, C. J., Fordyce, W. E., & Black, R. G. (1978). The effect of the pendency of claims for compensation upon behavior indicative of pain. *Washington Law Review, 53,* 251–278.

Philips, C. (1976). Headache and personality. *Journal of Psychosomatic Research, 20*(6), 535–542.

Philips, C. (1977). Headache in general practice. *Headache, 16*(6), 322–329.

Philips, C. (1978). Tension headache: Theoretical problems. *Behavior Research and Therapy, 16,* 249–261.

Richards, J. S., Nepomuceno, C., Riles, M., & Suer, Z. (1982). Assessing pain behavior: The UAB pain behavior scale. *Pain, 14,* 393–398.

Rosensteil, A., & Keefe, F. (1983). The use of coping strategies in chronic low back pain patients: Relationships to patient characteristics and current adjustment. *Pain, 17*, 33–44.

Schwartz, G. E. (1983). Disregulation theory and disease: Applications to the repression/cerebral disconnection/cardiovascular disorder hypothesis. *International Review of Applied Psychology, 32*(2), 95–118.

Selby, G., & Lance, J. W. (1960). Observations on 500 cases of migraine and allied vascular headache. *Journal of Neurology, Neurosurgery and Psychiatry, 23*, 23–32.

Sicuteri, F. (1977). Monoamine supersensitivity in non-organic pain (idiopathic headache). *Excerpta Medica, 427*, 194–199.

Sicuteri, F. (1978). Endorphins, opiate receptors and migraine headache. *Headache, 17*(6), 253–257.

Snyder, S. H. (1977a). Opiate receptors and internal opiates. *Scientific American, 236*(3), 44–56.

Snyder, S. H. (1977b). Opiate receptors in the brain. *The New England Journal of Medicine, 296*(5), 266–271.

Spanos, N. P., Horton, C., & Chaves, J. F. (1975). The effects of two cognitive strategies on pain thresholds. *Journal of Abnormal Psychology, 84*, 677–681.

Steger, J., & Fordyce, W. (1982). Behavioral health care in the management of chronic pain. In T. Millon, C. Green, & R. Meagher (Eds.), *Handbook of clinical health psychology*. New York: Plenum Press.

Stein, G. S. (1980). Headaches in the first post-partum week and their relationship to migraine. *Headache, 21*, 201–205.

Sternbach, R. A. (1974). *Pain patients: Traits and treatments*. New York: Academic Press.

Sulman, F. G., Levy, D., Lewy, A., Pfeifer, Y., Superstine, E., & Tal, E. (1974). Air-ionometry of hot, dry desert winds (sharav) and treatment with air ions of weather-sensitive subjects. *Journal of International Biometerology, 18*, 313–318.

Thomas, M. R., & Lyttle, D. (1980). Patient expectations about success of treatment and reported relief from low back pain. *Journal of Psychosomatic Research, 24*, 297–301.

Thompson, J. A. (1980). Diagnosis and treatment of headache in the pediatric patient. *Current Problems in Pediatrics, 10*, 1–52.

Thompson, S. C. (1981). Will it hurt less if I can control it? A complex answer to a simple question. *Psychological Bulletin, 90*(1), 89–101.

Tunis, M. M., & Wolff, H. G. (1953). Studies on headache: Long-term observations of the reactivity of the cranial arteries in subjects with vascular headache of the migraine type. *Archives of Neurology and Psychiatry, 70*, 551–558.

Turk, D. C., & Flor, H. (1984). Etiological theories and treatments for chronic back pain. II. Psychological models and interventions. *Pain, 19*, 209–234.

Turk, D. C., Meichenbaum, D., & Genest, M. (1983). *Pain and behavioral medicine: A cognitive behavioral perspective*. New York: Guilford Press.

Turkat, I. D., Guise, B. J., & Carter, K. M. (1983). The effects of vicarious experience on pain termination and work avoidance: A replication. *Behavior Research and Therapy, 21*, 491–493.

Turkat, I. D., Kuczmierczyk, A. R., & Adams, H. E. (1984). An investigation of the etiology of chronic headache: The role of headache models. *British Journal of Psychiatry, 145*, 665–666.

Turner, J. A. (1982). Comparison of group progressive-relaxation training and cognitive-behavioral group therapy for chronic low back pain. *Journal of Consulting and Clinical Psychology, 50*, 757–765.

Turner, J. A., & Chapman, C. R. (1981). Psychological interventions for chronic pain: A critical review. I. Relaxation training and biofeedback. *Pain, 12*(1), 1–21.

Turner, J. A., & Chapman, C. R. (1982). Psychological interventions for chronic pain. A critical review. II. Operant conditioning, hypnosis, and cognitive-behavioral therapy. *Pain, 12*(1), 23–46.

Waters, W. E. (1971). Epidemiological aspects of migraine. In J. N. Cummings (Ed.), *Background to migraine.* London: Heinemann.

Waters, W. E., & O'Connor, P. J. (1971). Epidemiology of headache and migraine in women. *Journal of Neurology, Neurosurgery, and Psychiatry, 34,* 148–153.

Waters, W. E., & O'Connor, P. J. (1975). Prevalence of migraine. *Journal of Neurology, Neurosurgery, and Psychiatry, 38*(6), 613–616.

Waters, W. F., Koresko, R. L., Rossie, G. V., & Hackley, S. A. (1979). Short-, medium-, and long-term relationships among meterological and electrodermal variables. *Psychophysiology, 16,* 445–451.

Weisenberg, M. (1977). Pain and pain control. *Psychological Bulletin, 84,* 1008–1044.

Whitty, C. W. M., Hockaday, J. M., & Whitty, M. M. (1966). The effects of oral contraceptives on migraine. *Lancet, 1,* 856.

Wilkinson, M., & Woodrow, J. (1979). Migraine and weather. *Headache, 19,* 375–378.

Willer, J. C. (1975). Influence de l'anticipation de la douleur sur les fréquences cardiaque et respiratoire et sur le réflexe nociceptif chez l'homme. *Physiology and Behavior, 15,* 411–415.

Willer, J. C., & Albe-Fessard, D. (1980). Electrophysiological evidence for a release of endogenous opiates in stress-induced analgesia in man. *Brain Research, 198,* 419–426.

Wooley, S. C., Blackwell, B., & Winget, C. (1978). A learning theory model of chronic illness behavior: Theory, treatment and research. *Psychosomatic Medicine, 40,* 379–401.

Ziegler, D. K., Hassanein, R. S., Harris, D., & Stewart, R. (1975). Headache in a non-clinic twin population. *Headache, 14*(4), 213–218.

# INDEX